EVIDENCE-BASED NURSING

The Research-Practice Connection

FOURTH EDITION

Sarah Jo Brown, PhD, RN

Consultant Emeritus
Evidence-Based Practice
Norwich, Vermont

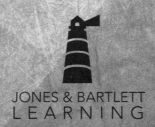

JONES & BARTLETT
LEARNING

World Headquarters
Jones & Bartlett Learning
5 Wall Street
Burlington, MA 01803
978-443-5000
info@jblearning.com
www.jblearning.com

Jones & Bartlett Learning books and products are available through most bookstores and online booksellers. To contact Jones & Bartlett Learning directly, call 800-832-0034, fax 978-443-8000, or visit our website, www .jblearning.com.

Substantial discounts on bulk quantities of Jones & Bartlett Learning publications are available to corporations, professional associations, and other qualified organizations. For details and specific discount information, contact the special sales department at Jones & Bartlett Learning via the above contact information or send an email to specialsales@jblearning.com.

The content, statements, views, and opinions herein are the sole expression of the respective authors and not that of Jones & Bartlett Learning, LLC. Reference herein to any specific commercial product, process, or service by trade name, trademark, manufacturer, or otherwise does not constitute or imply its endorsement or recommendation by Jones & Bartlett Learning, LLC and such reference shall not be used for advertising or product endorsement purposes. All trademarks displayed are the trademarks of the parties noted herein. *Evidence-Based Nursing: The Research–Practice Connection, Fourth Edition* is an independent publication and has not been authorized, sponsored, or otherwise approved by the owners of the trademarks or service marks referenced in this product.

There may be images in this book that feature models; these models do not necessarily endorse, represent, or participate in the activities represented in the images. Any screenshots in this product are for educational and instructive purposes only. Any individuals and scenarios featured in the case studies throughout this product may be real or fictitious, but are used for instructional purposes only.

The authors, editor, and publisher have made every effort to provide accurate information. However, they are not responsible for errors, omissions, or for any outcomes related to the use of the contents of this book and take no responsibility for the use of the products and procedures described. Treatments and side effects described in this book may not be applicable to all people; likewise, some people may require a dose or experience a side effect that is not described herein. Drugs and medical devices are discussed that may have limited availability controlled by the Food and Drug Administration (FDA) for use only in a research study or clinical trial. Research, clinical practice, and government regulations often change the accepted standard in this field. When consideration is being given to use of any drug in the clinical setting, the health care provider or reader is responsible for determining FDA status of the drug, reading the package insert, and reviewing prescribing information for the most up-to-date recommendations on dose, precautions, and contraindications, and determining the appropriate usage for the product. This is especially important in the case of drugs that are new or seldom used.

10075-4

Production Credits
VP, Executive Publisher: David D. Cella
Executive Editor: Amanda Martin
Associate Acquisitions Editor: Rebecca Stephenson
Editorial Assistant: Danielle Bessette
Editorial Assistant: Emma Huggard
Editorial Assistant: Christina Freitas
Associate Production Editor: Rebekah Linga
Senior Marketing Manager: Jennifer Scherzay
Product Fulfillment Manager: Wendy Kilborn
Composition: S4Carlisle Publishing Services
Rights & Media Specialist: Wes DeShano
Media Development Editor: Troy Liston
Cover Image: © LeksusTuss/Shutterstock
Printing and Binding: Edwards Brothers Malloy
Cover Printing: Edwards Brothers Malloy

Library of Congress Cataloging-in-Publication Data
Names: Brown, Sarah Jo, author.
Title: Evidence-based nursing : the research-practice connection / Sarah Jo
  Brown.
Description: Fourth edition. | Burlington, Massachusetts : Jones & Bartlett
  Learning, [2017] | Includes bibliographical references and index.
Identifiers: LCCN 2016030106 | ISBN 9781284099430 (pbk.)
Subjects: | MESH: Evidence-Based Nursing | Nursing Research
Classification: LCC RT81.5 | NLM WY 100.7 | DDC 610.73--dc23
LC record available at https://lccn.loc.gov/2016030106

6048

Printed in the United States of America
19 18 17 16   10 9 8 7 6 5 4 3 2 1

Contents

Lead-In

"Evidence is stronger than argument."
—*from* The Celebrity
by Winston Churchill, 1897

Healthcare professionals apply specialized knowledge and skills in the interest of patients. This text is about the production and use of new knowledge produced by research. As a professional nurse, you should know something about how knowledge for practice is produced and how to use that knowledge in what you do every day.

Aims

In the first part of the text, the focus is on how clinical knowledge is produced—from original studies, to research summaries, to the translation of research evidence into practice guidelines. Just enough of the basics of conducting research are explained so you can understand research reports, research reviews, and evidence-based guidelines published in clinical journals. Then in the second part of the book, the use of research in practice settings is examined. This includes locating, appraising, and translating research evidence into clinical protocols and standards of care.

Features of Note

- *Emphasis on Using Research Evidence* Systematic research reviews and evidence-based clinical practice guidelines receive considerable attention as the most ready-to-go forms of research evidence. Basing care on one or even several individual studies is viewed as the fallback position—for reasons that are explained early on. In the second part of the text there is a strong emphasis on developing skills in appraising the quality and applicability of the various forms of research evidence.

▪ *Easy to Read* An online reviewer of the third edition said it was easy to understand because it was written almost like a blog. Although some persons may view these descriptions as an indication that the book is not "academic," I feel good about them because I have made considerable effort to write so that complex information is conveyed in a clear and de-jargonized way. I hope you find it readable and clear—even interesting.

▪ *Format* In Part I, a profile and discussion is provided for each exemplar research report you read; this material is presented in a consistent WHY-HOW-WHAT format to assist you in breaking a research article down into its key parts.

▪ *Exemplars* As in previous editions, actual research reports are used to illustrate the different types of research evidence. Careful reading of these exemplars is essential to acquiring understanding of how nursing research is conducted and reported. Four exemplars are printed in full, whereas the citation and abstract are provided for the other three. We are unable to print these three in full here due to copyright restrictions. The full reports should be easily obtained through college, university, and medical center libraries.

▪ *Statistics* You will note that there is not a chapter about statistics; instead specific statistical tests and their interpretations are incorporated into the explanations of results of the exemplar reports. Students have told me that learning about a statistical test in the context of an actual study is quite helpful. The index indicates the page(s) on which each statistic is explained.

▪ *Gender References* As with all texts that include examples with unknown persons, there is the *she-her/he-him* conundrum. There are various ways to deal with it, but I have chosen to sometimes refer to the nurse as *she* and other times as *he*—the same with references to an individual patient.

Sarah Jo Brown, PhD, RN

PART I

Nursing Research

The level of knowledge required to understand research reports published in clinical journals is somewhat akin to being a savvy computer user. To be a competent computer user, you do not have to understand binary arithmetic, circuitry, program architecture, or how central processing units work. You just need to know some basic computer language and be familiar with the features of the hardware and software programs you use. Similarly, as a professional nurse in clinical care, you do not need to know all the different ways of obtaining samples, how to choose an appropriate research design, or how to decide on the best statistical test. But you do need to be able to read study reports with basic understanding of the methods used and what the results mean.

The goal of the first part of the text is to introduce you to research methods and different kinds of research evidence. To accomplish this, seven research articles have been chosen as exemplars of each major research method. The use of exemplar articles allows me to explain research methods and results by pointing them out in the context of an actual study. For reasons explained in the Lead-In, an abstract and citation is provided for the first three exemplars; the next four are reprinted in full.

I strongly recommend that you read all the articles in full, whether they are reprinted in full herein or not. Getting to the full articles for the first three articles using your college or university library access should not be difficult. Admittedly, you might *get by* reading just the abstract. But *if* you really want to acquire the knowledge and skills needed to become a nurse who is able to read and put into practice professional health literature, you will have to read the exemplar articles in full. Doing so will help you acquire: (1) understanding of research methods and results, (2) the ability to extract key information from research reports; and (3) skill in evaluating whether the research evidence is trustworthy and applicable to your practice. The abstract is just a sketch and lacks the details needed to acquire the needed knowledge and skills.

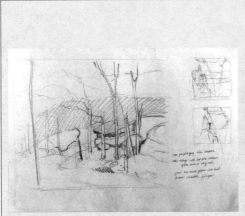 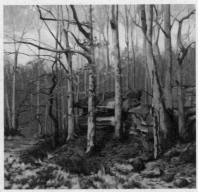

Courtesy of Abby Laux, Landscape Artist of Indiana, U.S.A.

One other advisory: Research and evidence-based practice knowledge is built piece by piece from the simple to the more complex across the text. If you don't master early information, you will struggle when more complex information is presented later in the text.

For readers who like to know where their learning will take them, an overview of the text's learning progression is graphically displayed in **Figure PI-1**. The main learning goals are in the chevrons on the left side. More specific learning issues associated with each goal are shown to the right.

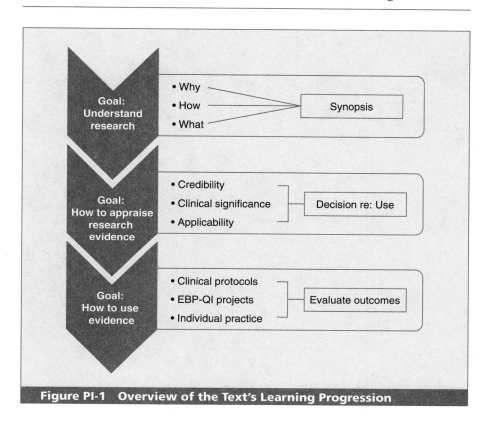

Figure PI-1 Overview of the Text's Learning Progression

CHAPTER ONE

The Research–Practice Connection

Effective nursing practice requires the application of knowledge, information, judgment, skills, caring, and art to take care of patients in an effective and considerate way. An important part of the knowledge used in making decisions about care is produced by research findings. Ideally, all key decisions about how patients are cared for should be based on research evidence (Institute of Medicine, 2001). Although this is not a completely attainable goal, large bodies of healthcare research provide considerable guidance for care. This text introduces you to the basics of how knowledge is produced by conducting research studies and to the application of that knowledge to nursing practice.

Research to Practice

In the healthcare professions, research is conducted to develop, refine, and expand clinical knowledge about how to promote wellness and care for persons with illness. The development of clinical knowledge about a clinical issue plays out over time proceeding from a single study about the issue, to several similar and related studies, to a systematic summary of the finding of the several studies, to a translation of the summary conclusions into a clinical action or decision recommendation. Thus, research evidence develops as a progression from knowledge that has limited certainty to greater certainty and from limited usefulness to greater usefulness. Actually, clinical nursing knowledge is quite variable with some issues having been examined by only one or two studies and other issues having been studied and summarized sufficiently that research-based recommendations have been issued by respected organizations and associations.

The end users of research evidence are healthcare delivery organizations and individual care providers. The healthcare delivery organization could be nurses on a particular unit or ward of a hospital, a nursing department, a multidisciplinary clinical service line, a home care agency, a long-term care facility, or a rehabilitation team; in short: a group of providers or an organization with a commitment to basing the care they deliver on research evidence.

Use of research evidence by provider groups and organizations often takes the form of clinical protocols that are developed using the research evidence available. In contrast, individuals use research evidence in a softer, less prescribed way—meaning that they incorporate it into their own practice as a refinement or slight change in how they do something. After reading a research summary about patient education methods for children learning to give themselves insulin, a nurse might alter her teaching approach; or after reading a study about sleep deprivation in hospitalized adults, a nurse working the night shift might pay more attention to how often patients are being awakened and try to cluster care activities to reduce interruptions of sleep.

Clinical Care Protocols

Clinical protocols are standards of care for a specified population that are set forth by caregiving organizations with the expectation that providers will deliver care accordingly. A population is a group of patients who have the same health condition, problem, or treatment. A population can be defined broadly, for example, as persons having surgery; or narrowly, as elderly persons having hip replacement surgery. Some clinical protocols set forth a comprehensive plan of care for the specified population; for example, perioperative and postoperative care of elderly persons having hip surgery, whereas others address just one aspect of care such as body temperature maintenance in the elderly having hip surgery. Still others are even narrower and could be called a clinical procedure, for example, blood salvage and transfusion during hip surgery. Generally, multidisciplinary groups produce protocols that address many aspects of care, whereas nursing staff members produce protocols that address clinical issues that nurses manage, such as preventing delirium in ICU patients.

Clinical protocols are set forth in various formats: standardized plans of care, standard order sets, clinical pathways, care algorithms, decision trees—all are guides for clinicians regarding specific actions that should be taken on behalf of patients in the specified population.

> **PROTOCOLS**
>
> - **Standardized plans of care**
> - **Standard order sets**
> - **Clinical pathways**
> - **Care algorithms**
> - **Decision trees**
> - **Care bundles**

Evidence

To produce effective and useful clinical protocols, project teams combine research evidence with other forms of evidence, including:

- Internal quality monitoring data
- Data from national databases
- Expert opinion
- Scientific principles
- Patient/family preferences

There is wide agreement among healthcare providers that research findings are the most trustworthy sources of evidence and that clinical protocols should be based on research evidence to the extent possible. However, when research evidence is not available or does not address all aspects of a clinical issue, the other forms of evidence come into play. In recognition of the fact that multiple sources of knowledge and information are used to develop clinical protocols, they are commonly called *evidence-based protocols*. Research evidence is an essential ingredient, although, as you will learn, the strength of the research evidence will vary. From here forward I will use the descriptor *evidence-based,* often abbreviated *e-b,* to describe protocols and care actions that are based to a major degree, but maybe not entirely, on research findings.

Evidence-Based Practice

When research findings are used to develop a protocol and the protocol is followed in daily practice, everyone involved (patients, healthcare professionals, the caregiving organization, third-party payers, and accrediting agencies) can have confidence that patients are receiving high-quality care. This is the case because the recommended actions have been scientifically studied, and people with expertise in the field have considered their application. In addition, the consistency of care achieved with standardized e-b protocols reduces variability and omissions in care, which enhance even further the likelihood of good patient outcomes.

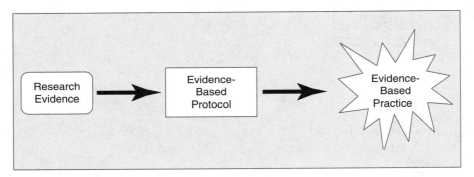

Using Clinical Protocols

In any care setting, care protocols do not exist for every patient population and every care situation. Healthcare organizations develop protocols to promote effective clinical management and to reduce variability in the care of their high-volume and high-risk patient groups. If a protocol exists, it should be followed unless there is good reason for not doing so. Protocols should be adhered to but with attentiveness to how they are affecting individual patients. Nurses are patient advocates and as such look out for patients' welfare; this requires that nurses be constantly aware of patients' responses to protocols. If a nurse observes that a protocol is not producing effective results with a patient, a clinical leader should be consulted to help determine whether a different approach to care should be used. A protocol may be evidence-based and may work well for most patients; however, it may not be right for every patient.

Scenario   Suppose you are providing care to a patient 2 days after he had a lumbar spinal fusion and you observe that he does not seem as comfortable as he should be even though the postoperative protocol is being followed; he has no neurological deficit and the surgeon's notes indicate that there are no signs of complications. You should then ask yourself questions such as, "Why isn't he getting good pain relief? Should we get a different pain medication approach? Would applying ice packs to his lower back reduce muscle spasm that could cause his pain? Is he turning in bed and getting up using proper technique? Should he be sitting less? Should he use his brace more?" The advisable course of action would be to talk with the patient and then with your nurse manager or a clinical leader about how to supplement or change some aspect of his care.

> **Protocols ≠ Recipes**

So, now you know a bit about how research evidence contributes to good patient care. In the rest of Part I of this text, I will walk you through the methods used to develop clinical practice knowledge. In later chapters of Part II, I will turn your thinking once again to e-b protocols and to how you as an individual can locate research evidence when there is no protocol for a clinical condition or situation.

As a Staff Nurse

After you have been in the staff nurse role for a while, you may be asked to participate in a project to develop or update a care protocol or procedure. Often, your organization will be adapting an evidence-based guideline that was issued by a professional association, leading healthcare system, or government organization. Other times, an evidence-based guideline will not be available, but a research summary relative to the clinical issue will have been published, and its conclusions will be used in developing the protocol. To contribute to a protocol project, you will need to know how to read and understand research articles published in professional nursing journals and on trustworthy healthcare Internet sites.

Scenario You are working in a pediatric, urgent care clinic and are asked to be a member of a work group revising the protocol for evaluating and treating children with fever who are suspected of a having a urinary tract infection. You may be asked to read, appraise, and report to the group about an evidence-based clinical guideline produced by a leading pediatric hospital. To fulfill this assignment, you should be able to formulate a reasonably informed opinion as to the extent to which the guideline recommendations are evidence based (e-b) and were produced in a sound manner. If the recommendations are deemed credible, then the protocol work group will rely heavily on them while developing their protocol.

In this anecdote, do note that the protocol project team was building on the works of others who had produced an e-b guideline on the issue. E-b guidelines and protocols may sound similar but they are different in an important way. E-b guidelines (1) draw directly on the research evidence, (2) are produced by experts from a variety of work settings, and (3) consist of a set of e-b recommendations that are not intended for a particular setting. In contrast, clinical protocols are produced by providers in a healthcare setting for that setting; often they are translations of an e-b guideline that keep the essential nature of the guideline recommendations but tweak them to fit into the routines and resources of the particular setting.

> **GUIDELINE:** A set of recommendations for the care of a patient population that is issued by a professional association, leading healthcare center, or government organization. Guidelines are not setting specific.
>
> **PROTOCOL:** A set of care actions for a patient population that has been endorsed by the hospital, agency, clinic, or healthcare facility. Protocols are setting specific.

Short History of Evidence-Based Nursing Practice

The nursing profession has been conducting scientific research since the 1920s, when case studies were first published, and calls for research about nursing practice were first issued in the *American Journal of Nursing*. Now, nursing research is being conducted in countries around the world, and reports of clinical research studies are published in research journals and clinical journals in many languages. In many countries, nursing research is funded by the government, and over 50 countries have doctoral programs in nursing. The growing cadre of nurses with doctoral degrees has propelled both the quantity and quality of clinical nursing research being conducted. In the United States, the National Institute of Nursing Research (www.ninr.nih.gov), a component of the National Institutes of Health, is a major source of funding for nursing research. Many other countries have similar organizations.

In the mid-1970s, visionary nurse leaders realized that even though clinical research was producing new knowledge indicating which nursing methods were effective and which were not, practicing nurses were not aware of the research. As a result, several projects were started to increase the utilization of research-supported actions by practicing nurses. These projects gathered together the research that had been conducted on issues such as preoperative teaching, constipation in nursing home residents, management of urinary drainage systems, and preventing decubitus ulcers. Studies were critiqued, evidence-based guidelines were developed, and considerable attention was paid to how the guidelines were introduced into nursing departments (Horsley, Crane, & Bingle, 1978; Krueger, Nelson, & Wolanin, 1978). These projects stimulated interest in the use of nursing research in practice throughout the United States; at the same time, nurses in other countries were also coming to the same recognition. By the 1980s and 1990s, many research utilization projects using diverse approaches to making nurses aware of research findings were under way.

During this time, interest in using research findings in practice was also proceeding in medicine. In the United Kingdom, the Cochrane Collaboration at Oxford University was formed in 1992 to produce rigorous research summaries with the goal of making it easier for clinicians to learn what various studies found regarding the effectiveness of particular healthcare interventions. At the McMaster Medical School in Montreal, Canada, a faculty group started the evidence-based practice movement. This movement brought to the forefront the responsibility of the individual clinicians to seek out the best evidence available when making clinical decisions in everyday practice. The evidence-based practice (EBP) movement in medicine flowed over into nursing and reenergized the use of research by nurses.

Three other things were happening in the late 1990s and early 2000s:

- Considerably more clinical nursing research was being conducted.
- The EBP movement was proceeding in a somewhat multidisciplinary way.
- National governments in the United States, the United Kingdom, Canada, and many other countries funded efforts to promote the translation of research into practice.

Today, high-quality evidence-based clinical practice guidelines and research summaries are being produced by healthcare organizations around the world, and nursing staffs are increasingly developing clinical protocols based on those guidelines and summaries. Also, individual clinicians are increasingly seeking out the best available evidence to use as a guide for the care they provide to patients. The most recent development is an area of research called *implementation research* or translational research. These studies examine how to implement evidence-based innovations in various practice settings so the changes are taken up by direct care providers and become part of routine care.

Your Path to Evidence-Based Practice

I want to emphasize that the point of this text and of the course you are taking is not to prepare you to become a nurse researcher, but rather to help you be an informed consumer of nursing research, i.e., a true professional clinician. The exemplar research articles you will be reading were published in clinical journals, not research journals. They were written for clinicians; thus they do not go into the fine points of research methodology. In Part I you will start by learning about individual studies, then about research summaries, and last about clinical practice guidelines—the three major forms of research evidence. Your goal in reading about them will be to grasp *why* the study/summary/guideline was done, *how* it was done, and *what* was found.

Because this text is a primer, only the most widely used and important types of research are presented. Also, the information provided is selective, which means that it is not a comprehensive reference source regarding research methodology. It does not delve deeply into methodological issues; it does not explain all research designs, methods, and statistics. However, it does provide an introduction to research methods and results that serves as a foundation for making a judgment about the credibility of a study/summary/guideline.

In Part II you will learn about using research evidence in nursing practice. You will revisit the studies/summaries/guidelines you read in Part I, to learn how to critically appraise their soundness, and consider their applicability to a particular setting. You will also learn about how organizations use research evidence to develop clinical protocols and how to use research evidence in your own individual clinical practice.

You, the Learner

The exploration of evidence-based nursing in this text assumes that you (1) have had an introduction to statistics course; (2) have some experience in clinical settings; and (3) are committed to excellence in your professional practice.

Other Learning Resources

In reading this text, and indeed in your reading of research articles once you have graduated, you may want to have a statistics book handy to look up statistical terms and tests you have forgotten or never learned. Your statistics text need not be new. Earlier editions are often available very inexpensively—and statistics do not change much from edition to edition. Do make sure you use a basic book, not an advanced one written for researchers. If in doubt, ask your instructor for a suggestion.

For a full suite of learning activities and resources, use the access code located in the front of your text to visit this exclusive website: http://go.jblearning.com/brown4e. If you do not have an access code, you can obtain one at the site.

REFERENCES

Horsley, J. A., Crane, J., & Bingle, J. (1978). Research utilization as an organizational process. *Journal of Nursing Administration, 8,* 4–6.

Institute of Medicine. (2001). *Crossing the quality chasm: A new health system for the 21st century.* Washington, DC: National Academy of Sciences. Retrieved from http://www.nap.edu/html/quality_chasm/reportbrief.pdf

Krueger, J. C., Nelson, A. H., & Wolanin, M. O. (1978). *Nursing research: Development, collaboration, and utilization.* Germantown, MD: Aspen.

CHAPTER TWO

Research Evidence

The term *research evidence* needs to be defined. First, perhaps obvious, scientific research is the methodical study of phenomena that are part of the reality that humans can observe, detect, or infer; it is conducted to understand what exists and to acquire knowledge about how things work. More particularly, nursing research is the study of phenomena in and relevant to the world of nursing practice; nursing phenomena can be grouped into five categories (adapted from Kim, 2000). The categories and examples of phenomena within each are:

- The Client as a Person (motivation, anxiety, hope, exercise level, and adherence to treatments)
- The Client's Environment (social support, financial resources, and peer group values)
- Nursing Interventions (risk assessment for skin breakdown, patient teaching, and wound care)
- Nurse–patient Relationship and Communication (person-centered talk, collaborative decision making)
- The Healthcare System (access to health care, quality of care, cost)

In brief, nursing phenomena are personal, social, physical, and system realities that exist or occur within the realm with which nursing is concerned.

As a student new to the science of nursing, when mention is made of research evidence, you will naturally think of the findings of a scientific study. However, as you proceed through this course, you will come to see that research evidence can take several forms, namely:

- Findings from a single, original study
- Conclusions from a summary of several (or many) original studies
- Research-based recommendations of a clinical practice guideline

Building Knowledge for Practice

A finding of a single original study is the most basic form of research evidence. Most studies produce several findings, but each finding should be considered as a separate piece of evidence because one finding may be well supported by the study whereas another finding may be on shaky ground. Although a finding from an original study is the basic building block of scientific knowledge, clinical knowledge is really more like a structure made up of many different kinds of blocks.

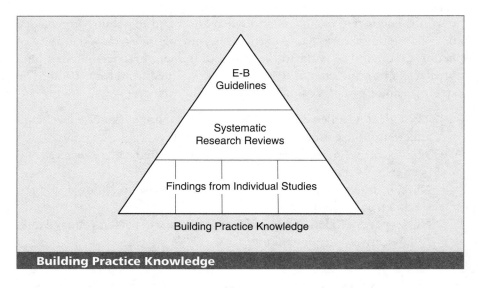

Building Practice Knowledge

Findings from several/many soundly conducted studies are necessary to build reliable knowledge regarding a clinical issue. Insistence on confirmation of a finding from more than one study ensures that a knowledge claim (or assertion) is not just a fluke unique to the patients, setting, or research methods of one study. If a finding is confirmed in several different studies, clinicians have confidence in that knowledge because it held up across diverse settings, research methods, patient participants, and clinician participants.

There are several recognized ways of summarizing findings from two or more studies; as a group these methods are called *systematic research reviews*, most often shortened to *systematic reviews*. Conclusions from systematic reviews may then be translated into evidence-based recommendations by expert panels. A group of e-b recommendations is called an evidence-based clinical practice guideline. Although one could make a case that evidence-based recommendations are technically derivations of research evidence, when they are true to the underlying research results they are considered research evidence for practical purposes. In this chapter, each of these forms of research evidence is introduced briefly in turn. Later in the text, each is considered in depth.

Findings from an Original Study

Most people think of a research study as involving (1) a large number of subjects who are (2) randomly assigned to be in one of several intervention groups; (3) research environments that are tightly controlled; and (4) data that are meticulously obtained and then analyzed using statistics to produce results. In fact, research using these methods is common and valuable; however, it is only one type of scientific study—there are many other kinds. The most common way of thinking about research methods is to categorize them as qualitative and quantitative.

Qualitative Research

Qualitative research can be used to study what it is like to have a certain health problem or healthcare experience. Qualitative research methods are also used to study care settings and patient–provider interaction. The following are examples of phenomena a nurse researcher might study using qualitative methods:

1. The experience of being a physically disabled parent or the experience of recovery from a disability.
2. The interpersonal support dynamics at a social center for persons with chronic mental illness.
3. How intensive care unit (ICU) staff members interact with family members of unconscious patients.
4. How a family who has entered a family weight loss program makes changes in eating and physical activity over time.

These kinds of social experiences and situations are typically tangles of issues, forces, perceptions, values, expectations, and aims. They can be understood and sorted out best by methods of inquiry that will get at participants' perceptions, feelings, daily thoughts, beliefs, expectations, and behavior patterns.

Qualitative researchers have an overall plan for how they will approach potential informants and position themselves in situations of interest. However, they are also committed to going where the data leads them and following up leads suggested by prior informants. Data collection methods such as in-depth interviewing, extended observation, diary keeping, and focus groups are used to acquire insights regarding subjective and social realities. Qualitative data consists of what people say, observational notes, and written material. The data are analyzed in ways that preserve the meanings of the stories, opinions, and comments participants offer. The goal of qualitative research is understanding—not counting, measuring, averaging, or quantifying in any way. Qualitative research is described in more depth in Chapter 4.

Quantitative Research

Quantitative research methods provide a different perspective on how the world works. Quantitative researchers assume a basic understanding of phenomena that allows numerical measurement of them. They then use numerical measurements to confirm the level at which phenomena are present and explore the nature of relationships among them under various conditions. For instance, the quantitative measurement of body temperature using a degree scale on a thermometer is a precise way of determining body temperature at a point in time and tracking it over time. It is also makes possible the study of the relationship between body temperature and blood alcohol level by 2-axis graphing and by statistical analysis. Measurement is also used to test how well a nursing intervention works compared to another intervention by measuring the outcomes achieved by both intervention groups to determine if there is a difference.

Quantitative researchers have specific study questions they want to examine; most often the questions involve several phenomena. For example, a researcher whose main interest is preoperative anxiety may ask a research question pertaining to how patients' levels of perceived risk for a bad outcome affect anxiety. Perceived risk and preoperative anxiety are the phenomena that make up the research question. In research lingo, however, the phenomena of interest are called *variables* because they are not constants—they exist at more than one level and vary in time, place, person, and context.

> ### Variables are phenomenon that exist
> ### at more than one level

The following are examples of study purposes that could be studied using quantitative research methods:

- The strength of relationship between health-related phenomena (e.g., between mothers' hours worked outside the home and mothers' level of fatigue).
- Test a hypothesis about the effectiveness of an intervention (e.g., A smoking cessation program delivered to small groups of sixth graders by a school nurse will result in a lower level of smoking in 3 years than will an interactive computer program delivered and evaluated in the same time frame. The intervention in this study is one variable (it is a variable because it has two forms); level of smoking at 3 years is the other variable.
- Predict good or bad health outcomes (e.g., Determine predictors of re-hospitalization within 30 days for persons discharged on newly prescribed anticoagulants. Several predictor variables could be tested, such as: type of anticoagulant, frequency of blood level monitoring, age, or lives alone. Re-hospitalization (yes/no) is the outcome variable).

Researchers then choose a research design that will produce answers to their questions. A research design is a framework or general guide regarding how to structure studies conducted to answer a certain type of research question. The four quantitative research designs used most often in nursing research are:

1. Descriptive designs
2. Correlation designs
3. Experimental designs
4. Quasi-experimental designs (Burns & Grove, 2009)

After choosing a design that will answer their research questions and is feasible given their resources, they develop a detailed study plan that spells out specifically how their study will be conducted—sample size, how participants will be recruited, data to be collected, statistical analysis that will be done, etc.

Mixed Methods Research

Researchers sometimes use qualitative and quantitative methods in combination with one another. Using mixed methods may produce a more complete portrayal of an issue than can one method alone. For instance, researchers used mixed methods to identify health concerns in an African American community; they conducted focus groups and analyzed the results of a community health survey. They concluded that "Although quantitative approaches yield concrete evidence of community needs, qualitative approaches provide a context for how these issues can be addressed" (Weathers et al., 2011, p. 2087).

Conclusions of a Systematic Review

Systematic reviews are an important and useful form of research evidence. A systematic review is a research summary that produces conclusions by bringing together and integrating the findings from all available original studies. The process is often referred to as *synthesis* because it involves making a new whole out of the parts. The integration of findings from several or many studies can be done using tables and logical reasoning and/or with statistics. To reduce bias resulting from the process used to produce the conclusions, the methods used for conducting a systematic review are rigorous and widely agreed upon.

Systematic reviews, when well done, bring to light trends and nuances regarding the clinical issue that are not evident in the findings of individual studies. I suggest that now you take a look at an abstract of a systematic review, because reading and using the conclusions of systematic reviews is one of the destinations on your learning path, and looking at one will give you a sense of this important learning destination.

1. Go to the CINAHL database in your library's website or go online to PubMed (http://www.ncbi.nlm.nih.gov/pubmed). PubMed is a free, online database of healthcare articles.
2. Type the following text in the search box: "facilitated tucking Obeidat" and click on the *Search* button. (Facilitated tucking involves holding or swaddling an infant so his arms and legs are slightly flexed and close to his body.)

3. That should bring up the citation and abstract for a systematic review of five studies about facilitated tucking of preterm infants during invasive procedure to modulate their responses to pain; the review was conducted by Obeidat, Kahalaf, Callister, & Froelicher and published in 2009.

4. Note that the abstract provides information about how many articles were included in the review, the outcomes that were examined, and the main conclusion of the review. Remember: You are reading a very short synopsis of the review, not the entire report.

From this quick look at the abstract of a systematic review, you should get a sense of the groundwork that has been done by the persons who did this review. In the process of doing the review, they did the following:

- Searched for articles
- Sifted through them for relevant studies
- Extracted information from each study report
- Brought the findings together in a coherent way

Clearly, this saves clinical nurses a great deal of time when they are looking for the research evidence about an issue in care. You will delve more deeply into systematic reviews in later chapters.

Recommendations of an Evidence-Based Clinical Practice Guideline

The third form of research evidence is the recommendations of an evidence-based clinical practice guideline. A clinical practice guideline consists of a set of recommendations, and when the recommendations are based on research evidence, the whole guideline is referred to as an evidence-based clinical practice guideline. These guidelines are most often developed by organizations with the resources (money, expertise, time) required to produce them. I think it will be informative for you to now briefly look at a guideline to get a feel for how the recommendations and supporting research evidence are linked. (You will be examining a guideline in more depth in Chapter 10.)

1. Go to the website of the Registered Nurses' Association of Ontario (RNAO; http://www.rnao.org).

2. Click the *Best Practice Guidelines* tab; scroll down to the search box, enter "dyspnea," and click *Search*. The search result will bring up the

guideline *Nursing Care of Dyspnea: The 6th Vital Sign in Individuals with Chronic Obstructive Pulmonary Disease.*

3. Double click to open the page for the guideline.
4. Low on the page under Related File(s), you will see *COPD Summary*. Open that by double clicking and you will see a list of recommendations.

The developers of this guideline looked at the research evidence regarding nursing assessment and management of stable, unstable, and acute dyspnea associated with COPD. Based on the evidence, they derived the recommendations listed. (I suggest that you look at the Practice Recommendations [1–5] and ignore the Education Recommendation and Organization & Policy Recommendations that follow.)

The strength of the evidence supporting each recommendation is indicated in the right column, and definitions of those levels are provided at the end of the table; do not get caught up in that right now, although you should know that level Ia is very strong research evidence whereas level IV evidence was obtained from expert opinion evidence (i.e., no research exists, so consensus of an expert panel was the best available evidence). The evidence levels that support the recommendations are mostly either Ia or IV, indicating that considerable research evidence is available for some issues but none for quite a few others.

Remember that you are looking at part of a much larger report. The other document, the complete 166-page guideline (viewable by clicking on *Free Download* tab), presents more specific guidance and detailed review of the evidence that led to each recommendation. It also informs the reader how the search for evidence was conducted and how the 2010 update of the original 2005 guideline was done.

As you can see, evidence-based clinical practice guidelines are even more ready to go for use in practice than systematic reviews and definitely more ready to go than tracking down the original research articles and trying to get an overall sense of them. For time-pressed protocol development teams, evidence-based clinical practice guidelines and systematic reviews are the short roads to evidence-based protocols, as portrayed in **Figure 2-1**. If starting the development of a care protocol by retrieving individual research articles is like baking a cake from scratch, and systematic reviews are like using a cake mix, then starting with an evidence-based clinical practice

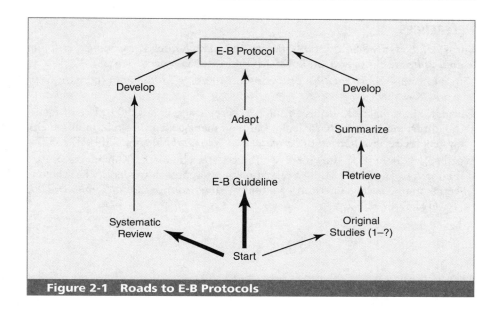

Figure 2-1   Roads to E-B Protocols

guideline is like buying a cake at the bakery and adding a personalized top-ping or presentation.

Going Forward

In Chapter 3, you will begin to learn how to read research reports of indi-vidual studies. Then in Chapters 4 through 8, you will be guided through reading of exemplary articles reporting five different types of research (one qualitative study and four types of quantitative studies). After that, you will read a systematic review and learn how one type of systematic review is conducted, and then you will read an evidence-based clinical practice guideline and learn how they are produced.

Note that this order is the reverse of the order in which care design proj-ect teams search for research evidence—they first look for evidence-based guidelines and systematic reviews. If they exist and are well done, the team can build on them rather than reinventing the wheel. The order of presen-tation in this book is reversed because proceeding from original studies to systematic reviews to evidence-based clinical practice guidelines is a more natural learning order.

REFERENCES

Burns, N., & Grove, S. K. (2009). *Practice of nursing research: Conduct, critique, and utilization* (6th ed.). St. Louis, MO: Elsevier Saunders.

Kim, H. S. (2000). *The nature of theoretical thinking in nursing* (2nd ed.). New York, NY: Springer.

Obeidat, H., Kahalaf, I., Callister, L. C., & Froelicher, E. S. (2009). Use of facilitated tucking for nonpharmacological pain management in preterm infants: A systematic review. *Journal of Perinatal and Neonatal Nursing, 23*(4), 372–377.

Weathers, B., Barg, F. K., Bowman, M., Briggs, V., Delmoor, E., Kumanyika, S., . . . Halbert, C. H. (2011). Using a mixed-methods approach to identify health concerns in an African American community. *American Journal of Public Health, 101*(11), 2087–2092.

CHAPTER THREE

Reading Research Articles

To get the most out of a research article one has to be intellectually engaged. One way to be intellectually engaged is to annotate or mark your copy of the article: underline, circle phrases, highlight, or jot comments in the margin—whatever helps you keep track of important information and connect the various parts of the study. When reading a pdf file in Acrobat Reader, you can click "Comment" on the tool bar and use the Comment and Annotation tools. Also, some people prefer to make notes in a file on their computer—fine, whatever works for you.

I tend to annotate right on my paper copy of articles. I write something like "n = 54" in the margin so I can quickly locate the sample size, underline important definitions, outcomes or findings, circle abbreviations that will be used in the report and the parts of a table that are most important or unexpected. I put question marks where a statement does not fit with what was said earlier or does not make sense. When reading a pdf file electronically, I use the sticky note feature and/or the highlight and underline tools. Of course, it is possible to over-annotate and in so doing produce clutter. However, if you annotate selectively, you will be able to find important information easily when you return to the article at a later time.

In this chapter, I make suggestions about how to read reports of individual studies. At this point in your learning, the goals in reading a research article about a study are to identify (1) why the study was done, (2) how it was conducted, and (3) what was found. After you are have mastered extracting these aspects of a study, you will add the goals of (4) determining whether the study was soundly conducted, and (5) relevant to the care of patients to whom your agency or unit provides care.

The emphasis in this chapter and in all of Part I of the book is on understanding the why, how, and what of a study (goals 1–3). As you read you may wonder whether the data really showed what the researcher claimed it did or think about the patients to whom the results would and would not apply. That's fine—just put your thinking about credibility and applicability (goals 4 and 5) on the back burner for now and we'll take them up in Part II when we revisit the studies with the aim of appraising them. Also, in reading this chapter, you may see a few terms that are unfamiliar to you. For now, just look them up in the glossary to get a sense of what they mean; they are explained in full as you proceed through the first part of the text.

Starting Point

Is this a report of an original research study? This seems like it should be an easy question to answer, but at times it is not. Some articles read like research articles, but they are in fact other kinds of reports. An article with tables and percentages may lead you to think you are reading a research study, but the article may just be providing numerical data to describe a clinical program. Such data is anecdotal and naturally occurring with no control over its quality or the conditions under which it was collected. As you will learn, it takes more than numerical data to call an evaluation report *research*.

Most often, the author of a research report, which is often referred to as a research article, will refer to "the study" early in the report, but sometimes you have to read quite far into an article to determine that it has the essential elements of a study. The essential elements of a research study include the following:

- A specified research question, hypothesis, or purpose
- Specified, systematic methods of data collection
- Data analysis and results

■ Findings (interpreted results)
■ Conclusions

If all these elements are present, then the likelihood that you are reading a research study report is very high. Remember, however, that there are many types of research methods and designs, and the essential elements of each type look quite different. Most quantitative studies address specific research questions or hypotheses, whereas qualitative studies may have a broad aim or purpose. Quantitative studies report results with tables, graphs, and statistics, whereas the data of qualitative studies consist of extended quotes and narrative descriptions. Qualitative studies often have small sample sizes (e.g., $N = 6$); most quantitative nursing studies use moderate sample sizes (e.g., $N = 40–200$). In short, research articles are diverse but should include at a minimum a clear purpose statement, a description of methods used to collect and analyze data, results and/or findings, and conclusions.

Format of Study Reports

Research reports of original studies are organized in a very logical way, and the formats used are similar from one journal to another. This standardization of format helps you as a reader because you will learn where to expect, and later locate, various kinds of information about the study. The following is a brief orientation to the format of research reports.

Title and Abstract

The title tells the reader what the study examined and often the patient group of interest. These are your first clues as to whether the report is likely to be of interest to you. However, titles can be misleading because a phrase or term used in the title may be different from the one used in your practice setting.

Abstracts almost always precede the main body of the article. An abstract provides a brief summary of the study—typically 300 words or less. The section headings used in the abstract are similar but not identical to those used in the full report. The abstract distills the main points of the study, and after reading it you should know whether the study is of interest.

Let us assume that you have decided to read the whole study. Rather than read straight through the first time, you might want to read the introduction and then jump to the discussion section. The discussion summarizes the important findings and places them in the context of findings from earlier studies. Having read the introduction and the discussion, you should have a sense for the context of the study—and be ready to read the article from start to finish in its entirety.

Introduction

In the introduction of a research study report, the researcher presents a view of the current state of knowledge regarding the issue or problem being investigated; this includes what is known and what are the gaps in knowledge. Study purposes are often set forth in the introduction section. Mark them in some way because they are important and you will want to refer to them.

Theoretical Framework   In the introduction section of a research study report, a theory that has been used to organize thinking about the issue and that serves as a conceptual context for the study may be specified. A theory is made up of assumptions, concepts, definitions, and/or propositions that provide a cohesive, although often tentative, explanation of how a phenomenon in the physical, psychological, or social world works. Propositions are suggested linkages among the concepts of the theory that have not yet been proven.

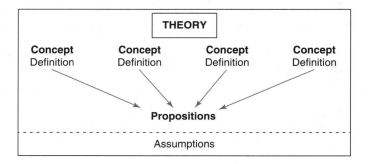

To make the preceding paragraph a bit more rooted in the real world, consider the following illustration. The *theory of community empowerment* was developed to provide direction for improving health in communities (Persily & Hildebrandt, 2008). Consider two propositions from this theory:

1. Involving lay workers in a community health promotion program extends access to health promotion opportunities.
2. Access to health promotion information leads to adoption of healthy behaviors.

Lay workers, access, health promotion opportunities, and *adoption of healthy behaviors* are concepts of the theory.

A researcher conducting a study about improving the health of elders living in their own homes might use the *theory of community empowerment* as a source of ideas for the study. By translating the two theoretical propositions into more concrete terms, the following two study hypotheses are formed:

1. Trained volunteers who collect healthy living questions from elders once a month at the weekly senior lunch and deliver answers the following week will increase access to health promotion information.
2. Health promotion information of personal interest will produce changes in health-related behaviors.

The questions submitted are given to a nurse practitioner who answers them via video recording shown at the next week's lunch. Adoption of new health behavior outcomes will then be measured at 3-month intervals for 1 year. Thus, the theory has served the research by bringing into a trial program a component that otherwise might not have been included and by providing a knowledge context for the findings. At the same time, the study acts as a test of the theory because the study has translated the abstract concepts of the theory into concrete realities that can be examined. If the study hypotheses are supported, the theory is supported because the hypotheses represent the theory.

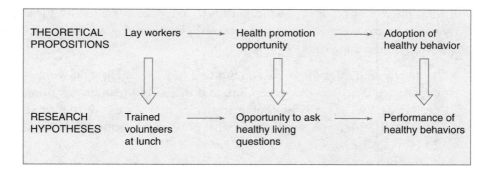

Not all study reports stipulate a theoretical framework; many researchers, particularly those testing physiological hypotheses, do not locate their studies within a theoretical framework; instead, they locate their study in a review of what is known from previously conducted research and what is still not known with certainty. Clearly, much more could be said about the relationship between theory and research; however, doing so would be a diversion from the topic of this chapter, which is how research articles are formatted.

Study Purposes

A reason for doing a study may be stated as a purpose statement, aims, objectives, research questions, or as hypotheses that will be tested by the study. Purpose words and phrases you will encounter in nursing study reports include:

- Acquire insights about . . .
- Understand
- Explore
- Examine
- Describe
- Compare
- Examine the relationship/association between . . .
- Predict
- Test the hypothesis that . . .

In the early stages of studying an issue, research is directed at acquiring understanding of the various aspects of the issue—the problems people with the condition are experiencing, social or psychological forces at work, and what the condition or experience means to individuals. Generally, these early studies use qualitative research methods. The following are study purposes from qualitative studies:

- "The research question in this qualitative study was: How do women experience miscarriage, conception, and the early pregnancy waiting period, and what types of coping strategies do they use during these periods" (Ockhuijsen, van den Hoogen, Boivins, Macklon, & de Boes, 2014, p. 267)?
- "The objective of this study was to examine how skilled nursing facility nurses transition the care of individuals admitted from hospitals, the barriers they experience, and the outcomes associated with variation in the quality of transitions" (King et al., 2013, p. 1095).

Note how both purposes set forth issues that will be examined, but they do not get highly specific about what they are looking for because they want the study participants to highlight the important aspects of their situation and experiences.

After the condition or situation is well understood at the experiential or social process level, subsequent studies may determine the frequency with which it occurs in different populations or measure the degree to which aspects of the condition or situation are present. Later, when several studies have been done and the situation is fairly well mapped, researchers will propose and quantitatively test associations between aspects of the situation or effectiveness of interventions directed at it.

The following examples illustrate several ways of stating quantitative research purposes:

- "The specific research question was 'What patient characteristics, clinical conditions, nursing unit characteristics, medical pharmacy, and nursing interventions are associated with falls during hospitalization of older adults'" (Titler, Shever, Kanak, Picone, & Qin, 2011, p. 129)?
- "The purpose of this study was to compare the time needed to reach a specified temperature and the efficiency of two warming methods— warm cotton blankets and a radiant warmer—for hypothermia patients in a postanesthesia care unit after spinal surgery" (Yang et al., 2012, p. 2).
- "The hypothesis is that the outcomes from nurse-led clinics will not be inferior to those obtained by the rheumatologist-led clinics, but at a lower cost and greater patient satisfaction" (Ndosi et al., 2011, p. 996).
- In a study of the association between depression and health-risk behaviors in high school students, two competing explanations became the hypotheses that were tested in the study: (1) Early depressive symptoms predict increases in risk behaviors over time; and (2) Early participation in health-risk behaviors predicts increases in depressive symptoms over time (Hooshmand, Willoughby, & Good, 2012).

Methods

In the methods section, the author describes how the study was conducted, including information about the following:

1. The overall arrangements and logistics of the study
2. The setting or settings in which the study was conducted
3. The institutional review board (IRB) that gave ethical approval to the study

4. How the sample was obtained
5. How data were collected
6. Any measurement instruments that were used (i.e., scales, question-naires, physiologic measurements)
7. How the data were analyzed

Each of these steps will be discussed in detail specific to different research designs later. Briefly here, I will just say that the information about the sample should be sufficient to inform the reader about the likelihood that the sample is a good representation of the target population or provide enough profile information about the sample to let readers decide to whom the results would likely apply.

The information about how the data were obtained includes a statement about the organization that gave ethical approval to the study, procedures used to collect data, and descriptions of the measurement instruments used. For now, you should come away from reading the methods section of the reports with an understanding of the characteristics of the people who were included in the study, the sequence of steps in the study, and the data collected.

Results/Findings

In the results/findings section, a profile of the sample and the results of the data analysis are reported. The profile of the sample lists characteristics of the sample as its composition determines the population to whom the results can be generalized. Results are the outcomes of the analyses. In quantitative studies, results are shown in tables, graphs, percentages, frequencies, and statistics. There should be results related to each of the research questions, hypotheses, or aims. To illustrate, consider the following hypothetical statement that might be found in the results section of a quantitative study: "The t-test comparing the functional status scores of those in intervention group A and intervention group B indicated a significant difference (mean A = 8.4; mean B = 6.1; $p = .038$)." This is a result statement; it reports the results of the statistical analysis.

The interpretation of a result is called a finding. A finding for the result statement just given would be stated something like, "The group who received nursing intervention A had a significantly higher functional level than did the group who received intervention B." Note how the findings statement interprets the statistical result but does not claim anything more than the statistical result indicated. Findings statements are usually found in the conclusions or discussion section of quantitative study reports.

To illustrate further, consider the results and findings of a hypothetical quantitative study comparing the effects of a new method for osteoporosis prevention education to standard education among high school students. A t-test was used to compare the scores of the two groups on an osteoporosis prevention questionnaire; the result of that test was $t = 1.99, p = .025$. This result indicates that the statistical calculation comparing the scores of the two groups resulted in a t-value of 1.99, which is statistically significant at the $p = .025$ level. The finding was this: The new educational method on average produced higher osteoporosis knowledge levels than standard education did, and there is a very low chance that this claim would not hold up in other similar situations. The concept of p-values will be explained in detail in Chapters 6 and 7.

Results → Findings → Conclusions

In qualitative research reports, data (observations, quotes) and findings (e.g., themes) are often intermingled. Generally, qualitative study reports do not have a results section; rather, they have a findings section in which themes, narrative descriptions, or theoretical statements are presented along with examples of data that led to them. Chapter 4 provides more explanation of the analytical processes used by qualitative researchers.

When you first begin reading research articles, you may have a tendency to skip over the tables and figures. However, you really should pay attention to them because that is where you will find the real meat of the results. Most authors highlight or summarize in the text what is in the tables, but others assume the reader will get the information from the tables, thus they do not restate that information. In examining tables and figures, it is important to carefully read their titles so you know exactly what you are looking at. Also, within tables, the column and row labels are critical to understanding the data provided. Reading tables is a bit like dancing with a new partner—with a bit of practice, you will quickly get good at it.

Discussion and Conclusions

In the discussion section, the researcher ties together several aspects of the study and offers possible applications of the findings. The researcher will usually open this section by stating the most important findings and placing them in the context of what other studies on the topic or question have found. In discussing the findings, many researchers describe what they think are the clinical implications of the findings. Here, they are allowed some latitude in saying what they think the findings mean. In the osteoporosis education for high school students example just given, the researcher might say, "The findings indicate that a short educational session is effective in increasing high school students' knowledge regarding osteoporosis prevention." This conclusion statement is close to the findings. On the other hand, if the researcher said, "Short educational sessions are an effective way of increasing osteoporosis prevention behaviors in high school students," the findings statement would be beyond the results. Because the study only measured the outcome of knowledge, not behaviors, the author is adding an assumption to the results, namely, that knowledge produces behavior change—and that is a big assumption.

Authors are also expected to consider alternative explanations for their findings. This would include noting how research methods may have influenced the results, such as "The sample size may have been too small to detect a difference in the treatment groups" or "The fact that a high proportion of patients in the intervention group didn't return for follow-up may have made the outcomes of the intervention group look better than they would have been if post-data had been available from everyone in that group." At the end of this section, the authors usually comment on what they view as the limitations of the study and the implications of the findings for future research.

References

The references list should include complete information for all citations made in the text. You might find it useful to mark in the text and in the reference list any articles that you want to obtain and read for greater understanding or because they studied a population of interest to you, for example, elderly persons living independently in the inner city. Perusal of the reference list also reveals other current work on the issue, who has done research on the issue, and which journals have published research articles about the issue.

> **WHERE TO LOOK FOR THE WHY? HOW? WHAT?**
>
> - **Why was the study done—to what purpose?**
>   Found in *INTRODUCTION and its subsections; includes Background,*
>   *Literature Review, Theoretical Framework, Purpose, Hypotheses*
> - **How was the study done?**
>   Found in *METHODS and its subsections; includes Design, Setting,*
>   *Sample, Data Collection, Measuring Instruments, Data Analysis*
> - **What was found?**
>   Found in *RESULTS, DISCUSSION, CONCLUSIONS*

Reading Approach

When you first read research reports, they may seem difficult to read. It is really like any new undertaking—at first it is confusing. However, the fog lifts rather quickly: you get the hang of the lingo, the whole picture comes into focus, and the relationships between the parts become clear. Importantly, even seasoned readers of research reports find it necessary to read a research report at least twice. The first time you may only get a general sense of why the study was done, how it was done, and what was found. A second reading usually results in greatly improved identification of the essential elements of the study.

Wading In

Having considered how research reports are organized and having noted some difference between the formats of qualitative and quantitative study reports, it is now time to delve into reading one of them. Your instructor may have you choose one or assign one for everyone in the class to read. Alternatively, several studies are listed on the text's website.

The studies in subsequent chapters are considered *exemplars* in that they are typical or representative of a particular type of healthcare research. Most of the exemplar studies were also very well conducted, but they were not chosen because they are perfect models—all studies have warts. Rather, they were chosen because they used a research design that is widely used in healthcare research. I hope you will spend enough time with these studies to acquire a fairly detailed understanding of them.

REFERENCES

Hooshmand, S., Willoughby, T., & Good, M. (2012). Does the direction of effects in the association between depressive symptoms and health-risk behaviors differ by behavior? A longitudinal study across the high school years. *Journal of Adolescent Health, 50*(2), 140–147.

King, B. J., Gilmore-Bykovskyi, A. L., Roiland, R. A., Polnaszek, B. E., Bowers, B. J., & Kind, A. J. H. (2013). The consequences of poor communication during transitions from hospital to skilled nursing facility: A qualitative study. *Journal of the American Geriatrics Society, 61*(7), 1095–1102.

Ndosi, M., Lewis, M., Hale, C., Quinn, H., Ryan, S., Emery, P., . . . Hill, J. (2011). A randomized controlled study of outcome and cost effectiveness for RA patients attending nurse-led rheumatology clinics: Study protocol of an ongoing nationwide multi-centre study. *International Journal of Nursing Studies, 48*(8), 995–1011.

Ockhuijsen, H. D. L., van den Hoogen, A., Boivins, J., Macklon, N. S., & de Boes, F. (2014). Pregnancy after miscarriage: Balancing between loss of control and searching for control. *Research in Nursing & Health, 37*(4), 267–275. doi:10.1002/nur.21610

Persily, C. A., & Hildebrandt, E. (2008). The theory of community empowerment. In M. J. Smith & P. R. Liehr (Eds.), *Middle range theory for nursing* (2nd ed., pp. 131–144). New York, NY: Springer.

Titler, M. G., Shever, L. L., Kanak, M. F., Picone, D. M., & Qin, R. (2011). Factors associated with falls during hospitalization in an older adult population. *Research and Theory for Nursing Practice: An International Journal, 25*(2), 127–134.

Yang, H-L., Lee, H-F., Chu, T-L., Su, Y-Y., Ho, L-H., & Fan, J-Y. (2012). The comparison of two recovery room warming methods for hypothermia patients who had undergone spinal surgery. *Journal of Nursing Scholarship, 44*(1), 2–10.some quantitative studies use a very large number of participants (e.g., $N = 3,200$).

CHAPTER FOUR

Qualitative Research

Research methods that seek to understand human experiences, perceptions, social processes, and subcultures are referred to as qualitative research. As a group, qualitative research methods:

- Recognize that every individual is situated in an unfolding life context—that is, a set of circumstances, experiences, values
- Respect the meanings each individual assigns to what happens to and around him or her
- Recognize that cultures and subcultures are diverse and have considerable effect on individuals

Qualitative researchers are of the opinion that a person's experiences, preferences, decisions, and social interactions are not reducible to numbers and categories—they are much too complex for that. They believe that the researcher attempting to understand subjective and social experiences must let the participant's words and accounts lead the researcher to understandings that would remain hidden without open-minded and probing exploration (Munhall, 2007). Thus, qualitative researchers go into their exploration with as few assumptions as possible so as to let participants describe their situation and what they think is happening.

Data in qualitative research may take the form of observations with field notes, recording and transcripts of interviews, diaries, or other documents. The researcher spends considerable time going back and forth through data and field notes to identify important connections. As the researcher gains greater insight into the issue, the questions asked of subsequent study participants may change, or new, potentially informative sources of data may be identified (Swanson, 2001). The researcher works inductively—that is, moving from the details of what was said or observed to a slightly more encompassing phrase or concept, back to the data, and finally to a set of categories, themes, or even to a theory that portrays important aspects of the subjective experience, social process, or culture.

Research Traditions

The term *qualitative research* actually refers to an array of methodologies with diverse aims, data collection methods, and analysis techniques. Several methodological traditions, developed in sociology, anthropology, and psychology, have been adopted by nursing. The three traditional methods that have been used the most in nursing are: (1) grounded theory research; (2) ethnographic research; and (3) phenomenological inquiry (see Table 4-1). Nursing researchers use grounded theory methodology to understand the fundamental social processes involved in healthcare situations, such as the communication processes involved in emergency care transports or how families make the decision for a child to have an organ transplant. A study using grounded theory methodology examined how adults with inadequately controlled pain moved through the healthcare system and interacted with providers to achieve pain control (McDonald, 2014). Interaction at 23 ambulatory medical visits were recorded and transcribed, and 4 patients and 4 providers were interviewed in depth.

The ethnographic research tradition as used in nursing creates detailed descriptions of healthcare subcultures, such as chronic renal dialysis units or Alzheimer's disease support groups—from the insider perspective. A recent ethnographic study examined how nurses think and talk about patients in a critical care unit in the United Kingdom. Data were collected over 8 months through 92 hours of observation and 13 interviews (McLean, Coombs, & Gobbi, 2015).

The phenomenological research tradition is useful in gaining insight into human experiences, such as living with a severe facial deformity. A study using phenomenological methodology explored how patients who had a stroke think and feel about the whole experience from the perspective of 3 months after being discharged home (Simeone, Savini, Cohen, Alvaro, & Vellone, 2015).

These methods aim to produce deep, complex, and comprehensive portrayals of their subject matter. Each of these traditions specifies a research process and set of methods and techniques for collecting and analyzing

TABLE 4-1 Qualitative Research Traditions

Tradition	Common Aim in Nursing Studies	Data Collection Techniques	Data Analysis Techniques
Phenomenologic research	Understanding and description of the lived experience of persons with a particular health condition or situation	1. Select persons who are living or have lived the experience. 2. Set aside preconceived ideas. 3. Engage in dialogue with each participant. 4. Explore the person's lifeworld. 5. Assist person to be reflective about his or her experiences and what they mean to him or her. 6. Stay in the setting until no new insights are emerging and all issues are understood.	1. Transcribe interviews. 2. Look for segments in the account. 3. Identify significant phrases. 4. Group phrases with common thoughts into themes. 5. Confirm themes with the participants.
Ethnographic research	A rich portrayal of the norms, values, language, roles, and social rules of a health or healthcare culture or subculture	1. Immerse self in the culture/setting, typically for long periods of time. 2. Observe social interactions. 3. Seek out and informally question good informants. 4. Analyze documents. 5. Take detailed notes.	1. Identification of social rules and understandings. 2. Analysis of social networks. 3. Confirmation of interpretations. 4. Produce a coherent account of the culture. 5. Check out description with key informants.

(continued)

TABLE 4-1 Qualitative Research Traditions (continued)

Tradition	Common Aim in Nursing Studies	Data Collection Techniques	Data Analysis Techniques
Grounded theory research	A theory (i.e., a tentative, coherent explanation) about how a social process works, particularly social interaction	1. Gain access to the social setting. 2. Observe social interactions. 3. Identify key informants. 4. Conduct informal interviews. 5. Keep field notes. 6. Identify useful written materials. 7. Interweave data collection and analysis. 8. Stay in the setting until no new insights are emerging and all issues are well understood.	1. Intermix data collection and analysis. 2. Name what is happening in the data with codes. 3. Analyze the use of language. 4. Proceed from concrete codes to theoretical ones. 5. Constantly compare new data with previously acquired data. 6. Generate core concepts and hypotheses and check them out with participants.

data appropriate to its purposes. These methodologies were developed for building scholarly knowledge about various issues rather than for acquiring useful knowledge for clinical practice—although the knowledge produced can be quite informative for clinicians. As you can tell from the studies just described and from Table 4-1, conducting studies using these methodologies requires considerable planning, time spent in collecting data, and skill in interviewing, observing, and data analysis. However, data analysis and management of coding is greatly aided by software designed specifically for the purpose.

Three other qualitative research traditions are discourse analysis, historical analysis, and case study analysis. Discourse analysis is used to analyze the dynamics and structure of conversations, such as patient–provider dialogue. Historical research examines past events and trends, usually through records, documents, articles, and personal diaries from the past. Case studies are used to achieve a holistic understanding of a single case in its real-world context. The case may be an individual in a particular situation, an event, or an organization. Case studies are useful in gaining knowledge about experiences or happenings that play out over considerable time or occur rarely.

Qualitative Description

In the clinical fields, knowledge that is more focused and straightforward than that produced by the traditional methodologies is often quite useful. For instance, clinicians could interact more sensitively with teenagers who have been told that they are going to have to have hemodialysis while they wait for a kidney transplant if they knew what these young people think about during the interval after learning of the necessity of the dialysis and up to actually starting it. A study could be designed that focuses on just that issue by interviewing them shortly after they start on dialysis. They would be asked what thoughts were going through their heads, what worried them the most, how they handled their worries, and what helped them during the time prior to starting dialysis. No attempt would be made to understand how the bigger picture of their lives, their philosophical approach to life, social support, or medical history shaped different responses during that time. Typically, no observations of them would be made during that time and no attempt to interview parents or care providers would be made. The knowledge produced would not be complex, but it could provide useful insights for clinicians who give care to these young people.

Goals

Qualitative description   Methodology produces straightforward descriptions of the perceptions, thinking, worries, attitudes, and coping methods of a group of people (Neergaard, Olesen, Andersen, & Sondegaard, 2009; Sandelowski, 2010). The goal of qualitative description is to capture the important elements of an experience or situation and to produce a descriptive summary of them. The researchers "stay close to their data and to the surface of words and events" (Sandelowski, 2000, p. 334); in so doing they preserve the everyday language of what participants said and impose a minimum of conjecture about what the participant meant.

Methods

Commonly used methods of qualitative description include, but are not limited to the following:

1. Sampling of sources for depth and breadth of information
2. Data collection by informal or semistructured interviews of individuals or focus groups
3. Data analysis by qualitative content analysis
4. Findings rendered in the form of categories, themes, or patterns that capture what the study participants said (Sandelowski, 2000)

Purposive sampling can have one of several objectives, most commonly a sample of: (1) typical persons in the predefined group; (2) a diverse representation of the predefined group; or (3) persons with the demographic characteristics of the predefined group proportionally represented (Trochim, 2006).

If you think about it, you will realize that interviews and focus groups produce an abundance of data—pages and pages of transcripts of interviews or focus group discussion. To extract meaning from all this raw data, researchers use a technique called *content analysis*. Actually, there are quite a few types of content analysis and they are quite diverse in purpose and methods. However, conventional content analysis, which aims to produce a descriptive summary of an experience or situation of interest, is the most common type used in nursing studies—so only it is described here.

Most commonly, researchers first identify small sections of data that convey an idea and assign it a word or phrase code that captures its essence. The code should be data derived, i.e., it should closely represent what was said (Sandelowski, 2010). In assigning a code to a section of transcribed narrative or a section of a diary, the researcher is always aware that an interpretation is being made, and therefore must be careful that the code does not change the original meaning of what was said.

Content analysis is not a linear, constantly forward-moving process. Rather, it is dynamic and reflexive. If none of the previously used codes captures the meaning of a section of text, the researcher will create a new code. The new code may or may not lead the researcher to revise the coding of already coded text. At some point, several closely related codes may be combined into one. Thus, there is quite a bit of back-and-forth in the data and an emerging feel for what participants were saying across all interviews or observations. Fortunately, software programs are available to search through the data, identify and track words and codes, and apply new codes, thereby assisting the researcher to move around in the data and evolve categories, patterns, and themes.

A list of codes can be informative, but it may be more useful if coding is taken a step further. By identifying similarities in the codes, it may be possible to group similar codes without losing the meaning of the first round of codes. This broader or more abstract grouping may be a category, a chronological order, or a theme. Again, the researcher is on guard to not lose the meaning of the original data and codes. To illustrate, a study was conducted to explore and clarify the lived experience of older people who are delirious post-orthopaedic surgery (Pollard, Fitzgerald, & Ford, 2015). Eleven interviews were audio-recorded and transcribed. Sections of what patients said were coded as: *the feeling, suspicion and mistrust, being trapped, abandonment,* and *disconnection.* Those codes were then combined to the slightly more abstract categories of *The Suffering* and *The Predicament,* which capture the experience a bit more broadly. These two categories were then identified as relating to *Living the Delirium,* which was different from *Living After the Delirium,* which included categories related to how patients later felt and thought about having been delirious.

Original quote → Code
Several similar quotes → Code modification
Several similar codes → Category or Theme

In summary, qualitative description is a very pragmatic approach to doing qualitative research. It is characterized by using a combination of techniques that produces a useful description of the experience, perceptions, or events of interest. Any interpretation produced should not be far removed in meaning from the data provided by the study participants. Lastly, I would note that qualitative description is perhaps the most frequently used qualitative method used in published nursing studies.

Uniqueness of Qualitative Studies

Findings from qualitative research often are useful in their own right and others produce questions and hypotheses that require further study using more in-depth qualitative methods or quantitative methods. Certainly, many study descriptions of patients' experiences of illness and health care provide insights that are directly useful to nurses in understanding what their patients are experiencing and in communicating sensitively with them. They may also be useful in developing nursing assessment guides and teaching plans. When a qualitative study uncovers or alludes to an issue but doesn't fully explore it, a more in-depth qualitative study or a quantitative study may be valuable. A qualitative study could produce a deeper understanding of the dynamics of the situation, whereas a quantitative study could test hypotheses pertaining to possible causal relationships or quantify prevalence of perceptions and attitudes in a population.

At first, qualitative research methods may seem unscientific to you. Although it is true that they are very different from what most people view as scientific, the reality is that these methods have been developed to acquire insights into subjective experiences and social processes—complex human realities that cannot be broken apart, manipulated, and examined the way physical realities can be. The rich and nuanced understandings of human experiences and social interaction produced by qualitative methods cannot be achieved using methods that reduce human characteristics to numbers and the context of human lives to the status of variables.

Qualitative studies are sometimes criticized for having small sample sizes or for not being objective. These criticisms are based on a lack of understanding of what qualitative studies aim to produce and how their methods produce unique and valuable forms of knowledge for clinical practice. Both qualitative and quantitative research methods have a place in the scientific toolbox of the clinical professions. Just as a house cannot be built with only one type of tool, e.g., hammers, so it is that producing the full range of knowledge required for clinical practice requires the use of both qualitative and quantitative research methods.

Exemplar

Reading Tips

Before reading the exemplar, it will be helpful for you to note the structure of this chapter because the same structure will be used in the rest of the chapters in Part I of this text.

Each chapter is made up of three sections:

1. Introductory information about the featured research method in an opening section such as what you have just read about qualitative methods.
2. A reprinted abstract and reference information for the exemplar article in which the featured method was used; some exemplars will be reprinted in full in the text itself.
3. A profile and commentary on the exemplar article.

Again, I would stress (nag, nag, nag) that reading just the abstract will not help deepen your knowledge about qualitative research methods and the meaning of the findings. For this study in particular the conclusions in the abstract do not come close to the very interesting, more fine-grained insights described in the results section of the article. Similarly, the Profile & Commentary section will only make sense if you have the exemplar article in front of you and refer to it.

O'Lynn, C., & Krautscheld, L. (2011). How should I touch you? A qualitative study of attitudes on intimate touch in nursing care. *American Journal of Nursing, 111*(3), 24–31.

Abstract

Objective: Although touch is essential to nursing practice, few studies have investigated patients' preferences for how nurses should perform tasks involving touch, especially intimate touch involving private and sometimes anxiety-provoking areas of patients' bodies. Some studies suggest that patients have more concerns about intimate touch from male than female nurses. This study sought to elicit the attitudes of laypersons on intimate touch provided by nurses in general and male nurses in particular.

Methods: A maximum-variation sample of 24 adults was selected and semistructured interviews were conducted in four focus groups. Interviews were recorded and transcribed; thematic analysis was performed.

Results: Four themes emerged from the interviews: "Communicate with me," "Give me choices," "Ask me about gender," and "Touch me professionally, not too fast and not too slow." Participants said they want to contribute to decisions about whether intimate touch is necessary, and when it is they want information from and rapport with their nurses. Participants varied in their responses to questions on the nurse's gender. They said they want a firm but not rough touch and for nurses to ensure their privacy.

Conclusions: These findings suggest that nurses and other clinicians who provide intimate care should be more aware of patients' attitudes on touch. Further research on the patient's perspective is warranted.

Profile & Commentary

STUDY PURPOSE

Strange as it may seem, even though touch is an integral part of nursing, it has received very little research attention. The fact that the authors found no prior study asking patients or the general public about how nurses should touch them when intimate touch is necessary is astounding. However, a similar study has since been conducted in China (Lu, Gao, & Zhang, 2014).

The clearest statement of the exemplar study's purpose is in the abstract where it says, "This study sought to elicit the attitudes of laypersons on intimate touch provided by nurses in general and male nurses in particular" (p. 24). They expanded on this in the text: "Our study aimed to gain information from the public that could help nurses, both male and female, in providing care in a way that communicates professionalism and respect" (p. 25). Intimate touch is defined as task-oriented touch to areas of patients' bodies—genitalia, buttocks, perineum, inner thighs, lower abdomen, and breasts—that may produce feelings of social discomfort, anxiety, or fear in patients or caregivers.

The delineation of different types of touch is informative, and they acknowledge that even the term *intimate touch* is controversial among nurses. Also, note that the study did not explore expressive touch, which is patting or resting a hand on the hand, arm, shoulder, or knee to convey reassurance or sincerity or to comfort. I would commend the authors for their clear definitions because definitions are essential to the precision of an investigation and eventually to the application of its findings. Finally, the inclusion of gender as an issue in the study yielded valuable insights about how people view intimate touch by male nurses.

METHODS
HOW

Design Although the study is described as "an exploratory, qualitative investigation," it has all the characteristics of qualitative description as I have defined it:

- A fairly narrow purpose
- Data collection in focus groups using questions that elicited laypersons' perceptions, preferences, and suggestions
- Analysis of transcript data using a technique that went back and forth between data and assigned categories, i.e., codes
- Offered themes that are close to what patients said
- Produced knowledge that is useful for clinical practice

Sample A purposive sample aimed at achieving diversity by recruiting college students through on-campus ROTC and middle-aged and older persons from a Catholic and a Protestant church.

Data Collection The way the focus groups were conducted is well described. The focus group interview questions start broad then pose "pretend questions." The pretend questions may seem leading, however, the results indicate that the situations posed in them helped participants who had not experienced intimate touch by nurses think concretely about how they would react in the future. They also seem to have helped persons who had experienced intimate touch remember their reactions. It is doubtful that questions asking about intimate touch more generally would have brought forth such vivid responses. The reason for stopping data collection at four groups is explicitly stated, and a profile of participants is provided.

Data Analysis   The table of demographic characteristics informs the reader of the extent to which diversity was achieved. At first, I thought that the fact that only 42% of the participants had actually received intimate touch by a nurse was a limitation of the study but on further reading I realized that the mix of those who had experienced it and those who had not brought out how actually experiencing intimate touch by nurses changed attitudes toward it, particularly as it pertains to care by male nurses.

The data analysis method was described as "thematic analysis." From the description provided, it can be determined that this technique is similar, if not identical, to what I have described as content analysis. In fact, *thematic content analysis* is a form of content analysis, and you need not be concerned about its fine points since the authors described quite well how they analyzed the data. The important issue is that both authors spent considerable time muddling around in the data and refining themes so as to richly capture the data.

Ethics Review   It is unusual that this report makes no explicit mention of the study having undergone ethics review and been approved by an institutional review board (IRB). However, it does say, "Each participant reviewed and signed a consent form approved by our university's institutional review board" (p. 26). This implies, but does not actually say, that the study as a whole was reviewed and approved by the IRB. So, I wrote the lead author for clarification and he responded by saying that the study was approved by the IRB of the University of Portland, but that the sentence conveying that information was inadvertently dropped in the editing and revision of the article. A full discussion of IRB review may be found in Chapter 5.

 RESULTS

The four themes that were derived from analysis of the interview transcripts are useful and practical. Sufficient participant quotes are provided to reassure the reader that the themes emerged from what the participants said. In fact, many of the participants' quotes are quite powerful in and of themselves. The themes are valuable reminders for experienced nurses and worth passing on to nursing students. Specific nurse communication that annoyed patients and that which they preferred are worth keeping in mind;

they resonate with experienced nurses as representing what patients prefer but rarely ever say. So, the results at the direct quote level, at the category level, and at the theme level are clinically informative.

The discussion and recommendations are an excellent summary of how people view being intimately touched by nurses and locates the findings in the context of the few prior studies on the topic. The limitations discussion reminds the reader of whom these views about intimate touch may and may not represent.

REFERENCES

Lu, N., Gao, X., & Zhang, S. (2014). Attitudes on intimate touch during nursing care in China. *International Journal of Nursing Practice, 20*(2), 221–225.

McDonald, D. D. (2014). Trialing to pain control: A grounded theory. *Research in Nursing & Health, 37*(2), 107–116.

McLean, C., Coombs, M., & Gobbi, M. (2015, Feb. 25). Talking about persons—thinking about patients: An ethnographic study in critical care. *International Journal of Nursing Studies*, pp. 122–131. doi: 10.1016/j.ijnurstu.2015.02.011

Munhall, P. (2007). The landscape of qualitative research. In P. Munhall (Ed.), *Nursing research: A qualitative perspective* (4th ed., pp. 3–36). Sudbury, MA: Jones and Bartlett.

Neergaard, M. A., Olesen, F., Andersen, R. S., & Sondergaard, J. (2009). Qualitative description—the poor cousin of health research? *BMC Medical Research Methodology, 9*, 52–57. Advance online publication. Retrieved from http://www.biomedcentral.com/1471-2288/9/52/prepub

O'Lynn, C., & Krautscheld, L. (2011). How should I touch you? A qualitative study of attitudes on intimate touch in nursing care. *American Journal of Nursing, 111*(3), 24–31.

Pollard, C., Fitzgerald, M., & Ford, K. (2015). Delirium: The lived experience of older people who are delirious post-orthopaedic surgery. *International Journal of Mental Health Nursing, 24*, 213–221.

Sandelowski, M. (2000). Focus on research methods: Whatever happened to qualitative description? *Research in Nursing & Health, 23*, 334–340.

Sandelowski, M. (2010). What's in a name? Qualitative description revisited. *Research in Nursing & Health, 33*, 77–84.

Simeone, S., Savini, S., Cohen, M. Z., Alvaro, R., & Vellone, E. (2015). The experience of stroke survivors three months after being discharged home: A phenomenological investigation. *European Journal of Cardiovascular Nursing, 14*(2), 162–169.

Swanson, J. M. (2001). Questions in use. In J. M. Morse, J. M. Swanson, & A. J. Kuzel (Eds.), *The nature of qualitative evidence* (pp. 75–110). Thousand Oaks, CA: Sage.

Trochim, W. M. K. (2006). *Research methods knowledge base*. Retrieved from http://www.socialresearchmethods.net/kb/sampnon.php

CHAPTER FIVE

Quantitative Descriptive Research

Quantitative researchers approach scientific inquiry very differently from qualitative researchers. While qualitative researchers seek to understand the meaning of human experiences and social interaction, quantitative researchers aim to determine the characteristics, variability, and connections of the world. Quantitative researchers measure and count phenomena, then analyze the numbers to portray the phenomena and determine its relationship with other phenomena. Quantitative research is not a research method; rather it is a collection of quite a few methods that have in common collection and analysis of numerical data of some sort. In this and Chapters 6, 7, and 8, the quantitative research methods most widely used in nursing research will be explained.

Methods

A useful early step when building knowledge about patients' wellness behaviors, illnesses, or caregiving situations, is to learn about the frequency of occurrence of the phenomena of interest as well as the elements and features that comprise them. In quantitative descriptive research (from now on just called *descriptive research*), data are obtained under natural conditions, with no attempt to manipulate the situation in any way—no treatment or intervention is given. For this reason, descriptive studies are classified as nonexperimental or observational designs. The aim is to capture naturally occurring features of the phenomenon being studied.

To create detailed descriptions of phenomena, researchers with descriptive aims collect numerical or categorical data, which could consist of any of the following:

- Measurements of physiologic states that produce a number value, e.g., heart beats/minute
- Questionnaires with choice answers that can be scored, e.g., always (2), sometimes (1), never (0)
- Observations that are categorized and/or counted, e.g., Readmitted within 30 days/readmitted between 31 and 60 days/not readmitted; distance walked in 6 minutes

Some quantitative data are obtained directly in numerical form (e.g., white blood cell count), whereas other quantitative data are produced by converting occurrences or behaviors from their natural form to categories or numerical values. For example, exercise behaviors described by patients can be converted into levels of exercise by the data collector using precise definitions.

After the data are collected, they are summarized to produce a rather detailed composite picture of the phenomenon. The summary statistics used in descriptive research include counts, percentages, means, medians, ranges, and standard deviations. These descriptive statistics may be reported in tables, in the text, or in picture summaries, which include line and bar graphs, frequency distributions, and box plots. (These reporting techniques should be known to you from your statistics course.) The composite pictures often portray proportions and dispersion of the phenomena in the population and/or subpopulations, the different levels at which the phenomena is present, and which of its elements or features are most commonly present.

To get more real-world: a descriptive study examined the phenomenon of health-related quality of life in persons living with a urostomy, which is diversion of urine to a stoma and bag (Pazar, Yava, & Basal, 2015). Data were collected via mailed questionnaires from 24 patients 4 months after their having urostomy surgery. A 30-item quality of life questionnaire measured three aspects of quality of life: general wellness, daily function, and undesirable symptoms. In another questionnaire, associated issues including work status, feelings about changes in bodily appearance, sexual life, concerns about odor, and psychological health were scored as yes-no answers. The quality of life data was summarized by calculating the mean score and standard deviations for the total questionnaire and for each of the three sub-aspects. The associated issues were summarized as percentages who indicated the issue was a problem for them. The findings included the following:

1. In all three areas of health-related quality of life, persons with urostomies had lower mean scores than the population-based norms.
2. Most respondents stated that their urostomy affected their dressing habits (83.4%), sleep patterns (91.7%), family life (91.7%), participation in social activities (91.7%), and occupation (75.0%).
3. Although 41% of the patients worked outside their homes before urostomy surgery, the proportion of patients employed following surgery decreased significantly to 4%.

Study Variables

In the most basic form of descriptive research, there is one main variable of interest (i.e., the phenomenon of interest) and that is measured, sometimes using several different instruments that assign values to various aspects of it. In addition, several other contextual variables may also be examined. In the study just described, the phenomenon/variable of major interest was quality of life in persons with urostomy. Sleep patterns, family life, social activities, dressing ability, and sexual activity were some of the aspects of quality of life that were measured. The contextual variables of age, time since surgery, demographic information, body image, and employment status before and after surgery were also of interest—and quantified, even if just as yes/no.

By definition, a variable changes in amount, size, or level within a person over time, from person to person, and from situation to situation. In other words, it is not constant. In fact, most characteristics of human nature and of situations vary. Examples of variables are anxiety level, blood pressure, gender, weight, pressure ulcer rate, length of breastfeeding, attitudes toward birth control, family unity, and frequency of hand washing—quite a diverse list. To take just one: A person's level of anxiety varies over time depending on what is happening to him or her and not every person on the day of surgery has the same level of anxiety. Thus, anxiety varies across time in a person and across persons—it is a variable. *Home delivery* or *hospital delivery* is an example of a variable that usually has just two variations, whereas *ethnic identification* could have several categorical variations (Asian American, black or African American, Hispanic or Latino, white or Caucasian, and so on).

Measurement of Variables

In physiological studies, measurement is often made with a device:

- An adhesive pad with an embedded thermoelectric transducer attached to a transmitter measures body temperature continuously.
- A lab test measures serum 25-hydroxyvitamin D level.
- Blood flow to organs and extremities can be quantified with a probe and Doppler ultrasound flowmeter.

Alternatively, a measurement can be determined by an observer:

- Altered mental status can be quantified in the emergency department using a quick confusion scale (Stair, Morrissey, Jaradeh, Zhou, & Goldstein, 2007).
- Cervical dilation during pregnancy and labor can be assigned a centimeter value by determining how many fingers slip into the opening cervix.
- An edema grading scale assigns a numerical value to the degree of edema observed based on the depth of pitting (1+, 2+, 3+, 4+ as follows).

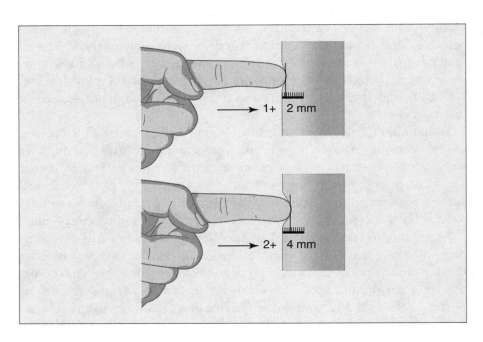

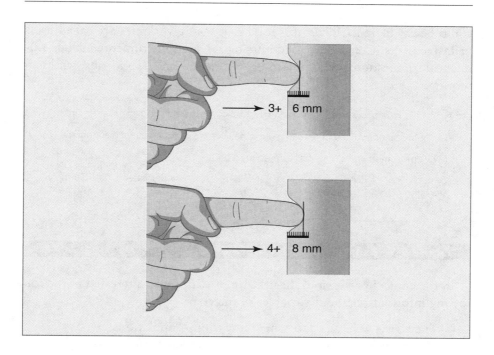

In psychosocial research, questionnaires are often used to quantify personality traits, emotional states, opinions, perceptions, and behaviors. A person's overall anxiety level at any point in time can be measured using a questionnaire with a scale that the responder uses to indicate to what degree each statement is true for him or her (see **Figure 5-1**). The scores for all the statements are then summed to produce a total score and often separate scores for subissues.

Measurement involves determining one or all of the following:

- Whether the variable is present or absent
- At what level it is present
- The aspects of the variable that are present
- At what level the aspects are present

Aspects of anxiety could include frequency, degree of perceived threat, physiological sensations, interference with functioning, and duration of the experience. A subscore for each of these aspects and a total anxiety score could be calculated. The devices used to measure variables are called tools or instruments. Commonly used nursing research instruments include rating scales, questionnaires, physiological measurement, and observational scoring.

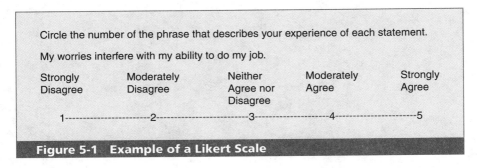

Figure 5-1   Example of a Likert Scale

In the clinical professions, healthcare providers are interested in the following information about variables of interest:

- Their level (average and range) in various populations.
  Example: How much knowledge do middle-age men have regarding the symptoms of heart attack?
- How they change over time.
  Example: How does hope fluctuate across time for women diagnosed with breast cancer?
- How they affect one another.
  Example: How does general health affect the exercise level of women in their 60s and 70s?

These interests stem from the nature of clinical practice, which uses information about expected levels, manifestations, and components to diagnose the problems of individual patients and plan preventive, therapeutic, and restorative care for them.

Good Data

In all quantitative research methods, data are considered good when the measurement of variables is consistent and true. Consistent means the measurement method obtains data values that are very close to each other across repeated testing in the same person, across several observers, and across various parts of a questionnaire. (Usually only one of these aspects of consistency is relevant to a particular measurement method.) A measurement method that is consistent is described in research terms as *reliable*.

A true measurement method captures the essence and attributes of what it is intended to measure. In other words, it really zeroes in on the variable of interest and accurately captures it in its totality. When a measurement method accurately captures to a high degree the totality of a variable of interest, researchers say the measure is *valid*. As you will learn, there are several ways of testing a measurement method's reliability and validity, and the results of these tests are often provided in research reports.

Reliability

Measurement is not as objective as one might think in that error and inconsistency can enter into measurement at many points. Consider the clinical situation in which two nurses obtain a blood pressure (BP) on a patient with a stable BP. Assume (1) when the first nurse meets the patient, he is standing at the doorway to the room; (2) the measurements are separated by a 5-minute interval; (3) the second nurse does not know the value the first nurse obtained. Most likely the two BP values obtained will not be exactly the same, even with digital machines. The difference is probably attributable to variations in their measurement methods more than it is to changes in the patient's BP. Differences in cuff size, improper application of the cuff, inconsistent patient body position, use of a different arm, arm position, failure to wait before repeating the measurement, and the calibration of the device used can contribute to variation in BP values. In research, differences in readings caused by the difference in measurement technique are considered measurement error because the two readings are not identical because of measurement technique as opposed to an actual difference in BP.

To the extent that the BP measurements are obtained using the correct technique each time, they will have less error and will more consistently reflect actual BP. When a measurement method consistently captures the actual value, or close to it, the measuring method is considered reliable. To increase the reliability of blood pressure measurements in research studies, researchers spell out in great detail the procedure for obtaining and recording a blood pressure measurement to ensure that all persons collecting data do so in the same way.

Specific tests of measurement consistency will be explained in detail as they are used in the exemplar study of this and later chapters.

Validity

A measuring instrument may be consistent but it may fail to fully capture the essence of the phenomenon of interest. In other words, the measure does not truly measure what it is supposed to measure. Often this is because the variable is difficult to define. For instance, coping with a stressful situation is difficult to define—in contrast to blood pressure, which is much easier to define.

First consider blood pressure. Conceptually, blood pressure is the pressure generated by the ejection of blood from the left ventricle into the aorta and dispersed throughout the arteries and capillaries. So, blood pressure is a combination of left ventricular ejection force, the elastic properties of the arterial system, and the location of the measurement relative to the level of the heart. The most direct measurement of blood pressure is achieved by placing a small catheter in a peripheral artery and connecting it to a transducer, which senses the pressure, converts it into a waveform, and eventually into a number value. Of course, blood pressure can also be measured indirectly by a blood pressure cuff and sphygmomanometer or nonmercury device. In most situations, indirect BP measurement captures the totality that makes up blood pressure, which is to say that it is a valid measure of what is generally defined as "blood pressure."

In everyday usage, the word *valid* means "true." This is similar to the meaning of the word when used to describe a measurement instrument. It is a true (or valid) measure if there is data supporting that it captures in essence and in full the concept it claims to represent. Over the years, a great deal of data supports the high validity of direct blood pressure measurement and the slightly lower validity of indirect BP measurement. The lower validity of indirect BP measurement is due to the fact that direct BP measurement produces accurate values under a wide range of conditions, including low cardiac output, high peripheral resistance, and patient obesity. However, indirect measurement is either difficult or inaccurate under these conditions. Thus, indirect BP measurement may be valid with some patient populations but have less validity with other populations.

The essence and features of coping are much more difficult to capture than BP. In part this is because coping is a complex, psychological, subjective response of a person over time. It has many features, contextual interactions, and manifestations, whereas blood pressure is made up of fewer, readily identified determinants that are very similar in everyone. Also, our understanding of coping is considerably less than is our understanding of BP. The result of the complexity, subjective nature, and limited knowledge of coping is that capturing its attributes and diverse manifestations is elusive.

Study participants can be asked to report their level of coping, but the word itself means different things to different persons. Alternatively, the researcher could ask participants to complete a questionnaire asking them to rate various aspects of their daily functioning, emotions, thought processes, sleeping, and eating. A total coping score for each participant could then be produced to reflect various levels of coping. This measurement process sounds comprehensive and straightforward, but the reality is that the questionnaire would have to be developed carefully over time to be sure that it truly captures the many features and manifestations of coping. It would also have to be tested in various populations because it could be valid with some groups of people and not with others. It could be valid with persons with chronic pain but not with persons in a stressful marriage. In short, the measurement of coping is much more complex and much less objective than is the measurement of blood pressure.

> **Reliability = Consistency of measurement**
> **Validity = Accurate capture of underlying concept**

Measurement of Psychosocial Variables

Measuring psychosocial variables is much trickier than measuring biophysical variables because psychosocial variables do not exist as physical realities. Rather, they exist in the minds, emotions, perceptions, experiences, and behaviors of individuals. They also exist conceptually as varying definitions that clinicians, researchers, and theorists assign to them. Thus, psychosocial variables are subjective and intangible—and thus hard to measure.

Often the content of the psychosocial questionnaires and scales used in quantitative research is influenced by earlier qualitative research that identified important issues. Researchers develop questionnaires, scales, and observation scoring guides to get at the features specified by a particular definition of the concept. To make questionnaires and scales reliable and valid, researchers revise, develop, and refine them over time, just as the indirect measurement of blood pressure was refined over the years.

It is all too easy for a questionnaire to include features of another psychosocial phenomenon that is similar to but slightly different from the phenomenon it is intended to measure. For example, self-confidence and optimism are concepts that have similarities to—even overlap with—coping. If the questionnaire items are not written carefully and the balance of items about various features of coping is not right, some questions might capture self-confidence or optimism instead of coping. Sometimes a physiological measure can be used as an indicator of a psychological state or behavior. Thus, instead of measuring a psychosocial variable by participant self-report, a physiological, trace indicator of that variable can be measured. For instance, salivary cortisol level is used as an indicator of stress and serum glycosylated hemoglobin (HbA1c), which reflects average blood sugar over the past 2 to 3 months (but is heavily weighted to the past 2–4 weeks), is used as an indicator of patient self-management of diabetes. In general, obtaining valid measurements of psychological states is more difficult than obtaining valid measurements of physiological states.

Establishing validity of a psychosocial instrument requires conceptual clarity, testing, comparison with other instruments, and revision. There are many ways of establishing validity of an instrument. You don't need to know them but you can be more confident about the validity of an instrument if the researcher reports that checks on the validity of the instrument have been performed. Rather than explain here how researchers test and report validity and reliability of instruments, I will explain it in the commentaries about the exemplar studies throughout the text. It is much easier to understand with a particular instrument and specific reliability and validity numbers in front of you.

> **Measurement instrument with high reliability and validity +**
> **Sound data collection procedures →**
> **Trustworthy data**

Extraneous Variables

Before leaving the topic of variables, I want to point out that when designing a study, the researcher decides which variables will be studied. Other variables may have influence in the situation but are not of interest in the particular study, and these are referred to as extraneous variables—*extraneous* meaning "outside the interest of the study." Even though they are not of interest, if they influence the data being collected, they can lead to wrong conclusions. To prevent this, researchers try to anticipate these variables in advance of doing the study by eliminating or controlling them. *Controlling* means "to isolate, eliminate, or hold steady their influence in the situation."

Let us say that a researcher is interested in studying whether women of different income levels have different levels of receptivity to TV spots about osteoporosis prevention. If the study involves collecting data from a random sample of women ages 15 to 50, age could act as an extraneous variable. Thus, even though the data may be analyzed so as to answer the questions about how income influences receptivity to TV health messages, any differences found could actually be from a combination of income and age (women with lower incomes might be younger than women with higher incomes). Thus, age is an extraneous variable. It is not of interest in the study, but it may be at work in the situation (e.g., younger women may watch more TV) and could confound the findings—meaning that it confuses, or muddies, the interpretation of the results.

Recognizing this problem in advance would allow the researcher to conduct the data analysis in a way that takes the effect of age into account. To do that, the researcher could control the age variable by studying only women in a narrower age range, say, 35 to 50 years. The research question would still be about income level and responsiveness to the TV spots, but the influence of age differences would be greatly reduced. However, in the process the researcher will obtain less information; depending on the research question, this may be okay. Alternatively, there are statistical methods of analysis that could be used to control the effect of age.

One extraneous factor that always must be kept in mind is that in most studies the participants are aware of the fact that they are being studied or that their responses will be examined in detail by the researchers. This may make them think more about issues than they would ordinarily, thus they may report differently than persons who are not in the study. Another possibility is that the questions asked on a questionnaire influence the person's thinking and change how they answer subsequent questions. Researchers try to minimize the effect of participation in a study, sometimes referred to as the Hawthorne effect, by considering the order in which data are collected and/or by giving equal attention to all groups from whom data are collected—so attention doesn't influence participants' responses.

Researchers design studies so as to gain control over extraneous variables and thereby produce findings regarding the variables that are of real interest. However, the world is complex, and it is almost impossible to control all the extraneous variables that are operative in a situation. Therefore, in the discussion section of the report, researchers often point out any extraneous variables that were not well controlled in their study and may have influenced the findings. Moreover, as clinicians read study reports, they often identify extraneous variables that may have influenced the results—and which the researcher was not aware of.

Target Population and Sampling

Ultimately, the aim of quantitative research is to create knowledge about a specified population of people, a population being a large group of persons with characteristics in common (e.g., they all have chronic bone pain after a complex leg fracture). However, data cannot be collected on all persons in the specified population—it is not possible for logistical and cost reasons. Instead, researchers collect data about the variables from a small group of people who are part of the larger population. This smaller group is the sample; the group to whom the researchers think their findings are applicable is the target population.

So, data are collected from the sample and descriptive statistics are calculated. Even though the statistical results are based on data from one sample, they are the best estimate of what the data might be in the target population. For instance, the mean of the sample is a single-point, best estimate of what the mean of the target population is. In research lingo, we say that the population mean is inferred from the sample mean (see **Figure 5-2**).

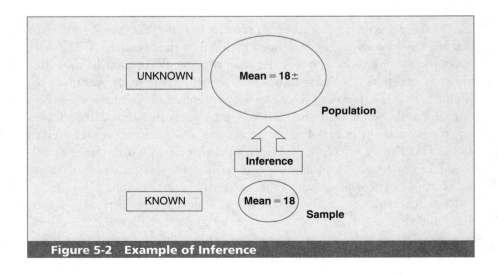

Figure 5-2 **Example of Inference**

The flaw in this method of estimating the population mean is that it is based on just one sample. We know that if the researcher obtained other samples from that same population, the mean of each of those samples would not be exactly the same, but chances are they would not vary widely. But, given the fact that data from other samples are not available, the best single-point estimate of the population mean is the mean obtained in the study.

However . . . there is a statistical way of estimating what the means of those other samples from the population might be. It is called a *confidence interval around the sample mean*. It is an interval with specified endpoints between which the means of many other samples from the population are likely to lie. Although it is based on the data from the sample at hand, this interval is highly likely to capture the true population mean. Thus, in **Figure 5-2**, there is a +/− sign indicating that the inferred population mean is an estimate and the population mean probably is not exactly that value. However, the amount of that +/− value can be estimated from the sample data.

Importantly, for an inference from a sample to a population to be legitimate, the sample must be representative of the population. This means that the sample must be like the population; the sample must match or accurately reflect the population. Any difference could make the inference to the population invalid.

Random Sampling

The very best way to ensure that a sample faithfully represents a population is to randomly select a specified number of persons to be in the sample from the entire population. *Randomly select* means that chance alone determines who is selected for the sample, thus every person in the population has the same chance of being in the sample. This is possible when a list of the entire membership of a defined population exists and a method that approximates drawing names out of a hat is used to select who will be in the sample; of course, computer programs, not names in a hat, are most often used to extract a random sample from a list. A sample that is randomly selected from a list of population members is known as a **simple random sample** and usually produces a sample whose profile is very similar to the characteristics of the actual population from which it was drawn. Generally speaking, however, the larger the sample size relative to the size of the population, the greater the likelihood that the sample will faithfully reflect

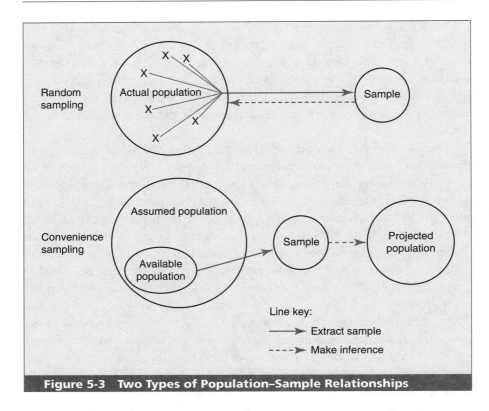

Figure 5-3   Two Types of Population–Sample Relationships

the population. This method of obtaining a sample and inferring results to the population from which it was drawn is shown graphically in the top diagram of **Figure 5-3**.

SIMPLE RANDOM SAMPLING

1. **Start with a list of all members of the actual population.**
2. **Randomly draw a sample of predetermined size.**
3. **Conduct the study with the sample.**
4. **Make statistical inferences and generalizations to the actual population.**

There are several more complicated ways of obtaining a random sample that is representative of a specified population.

- Stratified random sampling is used when the researcher wants to be sure to get data from subgroups of the population that are small and might not be present in sufficient numbers in a simple random sample. The researcher first identifies the relevant strata and their actual percentages in the population. Those percentages determine how many persons are randomly selected from each stratum. Let us say a researcher is interested in studying psychosomatic thinking in diabetics, prediabetics, and nondiabetics and has access to a health center's list of patients. First, the percentages of persons in each of the three strata would be determined. Then, from each stratum, as many persons as needed to maintain the population's strata percentages would be randomly selected to be recruited for the sample. See **Figure 5-4** for an illustration.

■ Cluster sampling is used when the target population is large and spread out and the researcher needs to concentrate data collection in a few locations. The population is divided into clusters, usually by geographical areas or practice setting, and a specified number of clusters are randomly selected. All persons (or other units of interest) within those clusters are sampled. For instance, if a researcher is interested in collecting data from home care agencies in a state but cannot go all over the state to collect data, five counties in the state could be

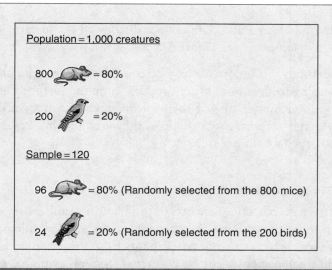

Population = 1,000 creatures

800 = 80%

200 = 20%

Sample = 120

96 = 80% (Randomly selected from the 800 mice)

24 = 20% (Randomly selected from the 200 birds)

Figure 5-4   Stratified Random Sampling

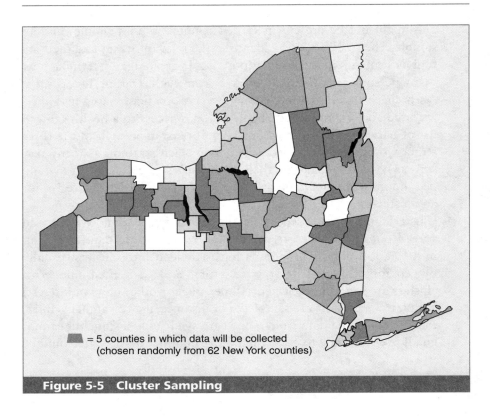

= 5 counties in which data will be collected
(chosen randomly from 62 New York counties)

Figure 5-5   Cluster Sampling

randomly selected and data collected from all home care agencies in those five counties (see **Figure 5-5**).

Other methods of random sampling are used but less frequently. So that is all I am going to say about other random sampling methods here. In the future, if you encounter one of them or an unknown (to you) sampling method in a study report, check out how they are done in a research methods book or via an online search.

Convenience Sampling

In healthcare research, complete lists of population members are quite rare; instead it is quite common to draw a sample from an available population. Many healthcare studies recruit participants from those available in one or two healthcare agencies. A sample extracted from an available population is referred to as a convenience sample. To avoid bias, recognized ways of selecting who from the available population will be asked to participate in the study are followed.

Convenience sampling starts with an assumed population that is defined by demographic, disease, functional, symptom, or wellness characteristics. Then, persons are identified who are (1) presumed to be in the assumed population and (2) accessible or available to the researcher; these persons may be accessible in the present or prospectively, i.e., going forward. When the study is reported, a detailed profile of the participants, i.e., the study sample, is provided; this profile becomes the basis for describing in detail the projected population to which statistical conclusions and generalizations can be inferred. Convenience sampling is graphically illustrated in the bottom diagram of Figure 5-3.

Convenience samples reduce the cost and effort of doing a study, but they also introduce the possibility that results of the study will not generalize to the target population. There may be something unique about the persons who made up the study sample or the setting in which the study was done that is different from other persons and settings in the assumed population. For this reason, it is important that studies done with a convenience sample be replicated in other settings to determine if the results do indeed generalize to others in the assumed population.

CONVENIENCE SAMPLING

1. Specify an assumed population.
2. Identify an available sample of present and/or future persons who are presumed to be members of the assumed population.
3. Conduct the study with the sample.
4. Develop a detailed profile of the sample's characteristics.
5. Make statistical inferences and generalizations from the study results to a projected population.

Erosion of Representativeness

An important caveat for both random sampling and convenience sampling is that even though the sample selected to be in the study may be representative of the target population, the representativeness of those who actually contribute data, i.e., the *actual* study sample, depends on a high level of consent to participate by those selected to participate and a low level of dropouts once the study is under way. Erosion of representativeness is particularly likely if those who were selected for the sample but decline participation or drop out have something in common, such as illegal immigration status, transportation difficulties, or language barriers.

Finally, sampling is a broad and complex topic. The preceding explanations just touch on it. Rather than discuss it further here, various methods of obtaining samples and the consequences of those methods are discussed in the commentaries of the studies you will read in this and later chapters.

A TARGET POPULATION CAN BE

■ **The actual population (with a random sample)**

or

■ **A projected population (with a convenience sample)**

Sample Size

There is no easy rule for determining how many participants should be in a descriptive study. Earlier, you learned that researchers conducting qualitative studies do not predetermine their sample size; rather they stop recruiting participants when no new information is forthcoming. In contrast, researchers conducting descriptive studies predetermine their sample sizes taking into consideration several factors:

- Whether a single group or two groups will be studied
- How the variables will be measured or categorized—that is, whether a mean or a proportion will be calculated
- How much variability is expected in measurements
- Resources available to conduct the study

Generally, the sample must be large enough that the statistics can precisely estimate the values that groups are likely to exist in the population.

Surveys

A common type of descriptive study is the survey. In surveys, self-reported data are collected by mail, Internet, telephone, or in person. Surveys are widely used because a lot of data can be collected from large numbers of people with minimal effort and expense. However, surveys are also widely misused—by persons who fail to recognize the various ways in which they can lead to erroneous conclusions (Dillman, Smyth, & Christian, 2009).

The main problems in surveys are the following:

- Failure to obtain a sample that is representative of the target population right from the start
- Difficulty in constructing questionnaires and interview questions that are clear to everyone who will complete the survey
- Low response rates, which make the respondents not representative of the target population (Dillman et al., 2009)

The response rate difficulties of surveys are revealed in a study of the cardiovascular risk factors and lifestyle habits of preventive cardiovascular nurses (Fair, Gulanick, & Braun, 2009). Emails ($n = 5,163$) were sent to all current and past members of the Preventive Cardiovascular Nurses Association using email addresses from the membership database. A total of 1,358 surveys were completed in the Survey Monkey database, which is a response rate of 26%. The low response rate occurred in spite of the use of participation enhancement strategies such as early notification, reminders, and incentives. The authors acknowledged the low response rate as a study limitation in their report. Unfortunately, the low response rate calls into question the generalizability of the findings to the larger population of preventive cardiovascular nurses. In fact, this level of response is not uncommon—it is even quite high—for mailed and email online surveys. Surveys present considerable challenges, but when conducted properly, they provide useful information. When conducted by the inexperienced, they often produce misleading information.

Results

Percentages

Descriptive studies report results in a variety of ways. Perhaps the most common way is as percentages. A study that explored the impact of implementing a care bundle with postcoronary artery bypass grafting (CABG) patients reported that the overall 30-day readmission rate decreased from 25.8% prior to implementing the care bundle to 12% following (Bates, O'Connor, Dunn, & Hasenau, 2014).

Center and Spread of the Scores

To convey the typical or representative score, the mean or median may be reported. Remember, the mean is the numerical average of the scores and is the best description of group average when the scores are evenly

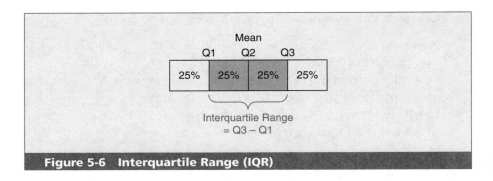

Figure 5-6   Interquartile Range (IQR)

distributed around the mean. Means are reported when most of the scores are near the mean with gradual decreases in frequency of scores on both sides farther from the mean. The median, which is the variable value of the middle case, is more typical when the distribution of scores is skewed (i.e., there are a few scores strung out on *one side* toward the end of the score continuum—away from the majority).

In a study of why elderly people delay responding to heart failure symptoms (Jurgens, Hoke, Byrnes, & Riegel, 2009), the median duration of various symptoms before hospital admission was reported. The median delay reported by patients experiencing dyspnea was 3 days. The authors reported the median because there were several persons who delayed for up to 90 days, and this skewed the data toward longer delay; those few cases elevated the mean so it was not representative of average or typical persons, so the delay reported by the middle case provided a better sense of the middle of the data.

To convey the variability or spread in the data, researchers often report the range of scores (actual low score and high score) or the interquartile range, which indicates the spread of the middle 50% of scores (see **Figure 5- 6**). Data with narrow ranges or interquartile ranges are less dispersed than are data with wide ranges. Sometimes data dispersion is of as much interest as is the average of the scores.

Wrap-up: Percentages, means, medians, and ranges are widely used in reporting the results of descriptive studies. This, plus the natural conditions under which data is collected, makes descriptive studies generally easy to read and understand. Thus, a descriptive study serves as the first quantitative design to be considered.

Beyond the Study Data

Most often the researcher conducting quantitative descriptive research aims to present a portrayal of the variables being studied as they occurred in the setting and sample in which the study was conducted. Other researchers, however, want to know if their study results would be likely to occur in other similar settings and populations, i.e., the larger group of which the sample is only a part. To do this they use inferential statistics—confidence intervals, chi square test, *t*-test, ANOVA, and others. However, these tests are not widely used in descriptive studies in nursing so they will not be discussed in this chapter. Inferential statistics will be explained at length in the chapters on correlational research (Chapter 6), experimental research (Chapter 7), and cohort research (Chapter 8).

Exemplar

Reading Tips

This research article is a description of the needed coordination between rapid-acting insulin administration and meals in an acute care setting. To fully understand the purpose and implications of this study, you should have a basic understanding of the pathophysiology involved in diabetes mellitus and the physiologic actions of rapid-acting insulin, particularly the time to onset of its action from administration.

Lampe, J., Penoyer, D. A., Hadesty, S., Bean, A., & Chamberlain, L. (2014). Timing is everything: Results to an observational study of mealtime insulin practices. *Clinical Nurse Specialist,* *28*(3), 161–167.

Abstract

Purpose: The purpose of this study was to evaluate the timing and practices of blood glucose testing and rapid-acting insulin administration around mealtimes.

Design: This study used an observational, descriptive design to assess the time between blood glucose testing and insulin administration and the time between first bite of the meal and insulin administration.

Setting: The setting was 4 cardiology units in 2 hospitals within a large community healthcare system.

Sample: Sixty-four mealtime practice events at breakfast, lunch, and supper were observed.

Methods: Investigators directly observed the timing of rapid-acting insulin administration at 3 mealtime periods an assessed timing of blood glucose testing, food intake, and method of glucose reporting.

Results: Overall, 14% (n = 64) of the patients received blood glucose testing within 1 hour prior to insulin administration and insulin administration within 15 minutes of the meal. As separate elements, blood glucose testing was done within the defined ideal range 35% (n = 63) of the time, and insulin was administered within range 40% (n = 58) of the time.

Conclusions: Timing for meals, blood glucose testing, and rapid-acting insulin administration varied significantly and was not well synchronized among the various patient caregivers with low achievement of ideal practices.

Implications: Results to this study revealed opportunities for better coordination of mealtime insulin practices. Lack of coordination can lead to medication errors and adverse drug events. Further study should include effect of mealtime coordination on glycemic control outcomes and testing the effect of interventions on timing of mealtime insulin practices.

Profile & Commentary

I will emphasize again that this Profile & Commentary will only make sense if you have read the exemplar article in full and have it in front of you.

STUDY PURPOSE

This study was conducted to improve the quality of care in two hospitals by examining the timing of subcutaneous, mealtime insulin administration in relationship to meals. The objectives of the study are stated more specifically on the bottom of page 162, and the background information provided is helpful. The takeaway is that because rapid-acting analog (RAA) starts acting within minutes of injection, the patient must start eating within 15 minutes of the injection or risk hypoglycemia. A second important factor in insulin administration is that the blood glucose (BG) testing that determines the dose of insulin to be given should be done close to the time the insulin is actually given to ensure the right dose for that meal.

Maintaining glycemic control in hospitalized patients with diabetes mellitus has always been challenging given the need for synchronization of BG testing, insulin administration, and meal delivery. However, with RAA insulin, also called mealtime insulin, the synchronization is even more demanding. In this study the researcher defined the ideal intervals as: (1) blood glucose (BG) testing is performed within 1 hour prior to insulin administrations, and (2) insulin administration is with 15 minutes (before or after) of the patient starting to eat. These two intervals are the variables of interest in this study. In the review of literature in the opening section, the authors note that surprisingly little published research has been conducted on nursing practices related to the timing of the recommended intervals of these three events.

METHODS

Design   These data were collected via direct observation of clinical activities, meaning that the data were obtained under natural conditions with no intent to manipulate the situation. The downside of direct observation is the potential for the Hawthorne effect, whereby participants may change their behavior due to being aware they are being studied. This effect was lessened in this study by the nurses on the units knowing that a study was being conducted but not being specifically informed about what was being studied.

Sample   At first reading, it may seem that the sample was nurses, however a careful reading reveals that the sample consisted of episodes of care consisting of the three interconnected activities that comprise the two timing intervals of interest. In support of episodes of care being the unit of analysis, note this sentence under *Data Collection*: "The investigators reviewed the census of each study unit to identify patients who were receiving subcutaneous RAA insulin" (p. 164). Thus, although the episodes were identified through patient records and nurses are the major players in insulin administration coordination, the data collected and results reported were about episodes of care, not patients or nurses. Assigning the nurse a code number served only to avoid observing a nurse more than once.

The authors note that cardiology patients are at high risk when the logistics fail because hyperglycemia and hypoglycemia have adverse effects on the cardiovascular system, thus the study focused on insulin administration events occurring on cardiology units. Three of the units had standard, scheduled meal delivery times while one had on-demand meal delivery.

Measurement and Quality of Data   Evaluation of the quality of observational data is often ignored because it seems straightforward—although often deceptively so. These authors are to be commended for paying attention to the reliability and validity of their measurement tools and procedures. The steps they took to assure the quality of their data are a bit difficult to ferret out in the report because the relevant information is not all in one place, so let's see if I can bring it together.

First, reliability. These researchers made considerable effort to make sure that they accurately and consistently captured the realities they were observing. In particular, they:

- Defined the activities of interest in observable terms
- Developed and improved their observational tool through a series of pilot tests
- Tested their observational procedures (e.g., where observers should stand; required that all stopwatches were timed to the network clock)
- Trained the observers in observing and recording
- Assessed interrater reliability

Interrater reliability is particularly important in this study. When two or more observers are using a data recording or scoring instrument, it is important that they are in sync; that is, they record or score the same activity in the same way. If they do not, the data will not be good because it is inconsistent, i.e., it is dependent on who did the recording. In this study, scoring requiring judgment was not required, just recording of the timing of activities was required, which is much less prone to differences of opinion. Eighty percent is considered the minimally acceptable level of agreement that must be established between two or more observers. The researchers in this study aimed at and achieved 100% interrater agreement. As result of the steps these authors took to assure the reliability of their data, we can be confident that the data consistently captured reality as it was playing out.

Validity of the measurement instruments is a bit more difficult to assess. First, it is important to recognize that the ideal intervals came from existing scientific literature, to the extent possible; the authors discussed these supporting studies in the opening section and in the *Discussion* section. So, the validity of these measurement instruments rests in prior scientific work that served as the basis for the ideal time frames.

To determine the validity of their observation tool, the researchers assessed its face validity. They did this by asking experts to look at the tool and determine whether the data that was to be recorded accurately and comprehensively captured the underlying concepts, i.e., ideal intervals between BG testing, mealtime insulin administration, and patient taking first bite of meal. Changes were made and a final observation test of the tool was conducted. Granted face validity is based on judgment and is not a rigorous test of whether the tool captures the underlying concept. However, the scientific foundations of the ideal time frames and the fact that the data related to them did not require interpretation is reassuring that the observation tool did capture the essential elements of these important timing issues.

Data collected by direct observation included the times the patient started to eat and the time insulin was administered. The result of BG testing was recorded in the electronic medical record at the point of care, and the researchers got the BG time data from there.

Data Analysis   The data was analyzed using descriptive statistics: means, medians, ranges, and proportions/percentages. The researchers were clearly only interested in capturing the reality of mealtime insulin practices in their settings and did not believe, as they stated, that results from their setting would be generalizable to other situations because of the considerable variability in how settings handle this issue. Thus, they did not conduct inferential analyses on their data.

Ethics Review   The study was reviewed and approved by the institutional review board (IRB) of the involved healthcare organization. An IRB is a group of people appointed by a university, hospital, or other healthcare organization who are charged with the responsibility of ensuring that the rights of human subjects are protected when a study is conducted under their auspices. Federal law requires that IRBs be nationally registered.

A researcher must receive IRB approval prior to beginning a study and provide reports to the IRB about the ongoing status of the research. In reviewing proposals, IRBs consider the following information:

- How participants will be protected from discomfort and harm and treated with dignity
- How informed consent (knowledgeable choice to participate or not) will be ensured
- Whether pressure or coercion to participate in the study is completely absent
- How participants in the study will be informed about the purpose of the study, the basis of subject selection, the experimental treatments, assignment to treatment groups, and risks associated with each treatment
- How privacy, confidentiality, and anonymity will be ensured

Normally the IRB requires an informed consent document to be signed and dated by the participant or the participant's legal guardian. The informed consent document must include a statement giving the researcher access to the participant's protected health information, if that is needed to conduct the study. In some cases a waiver of signed informed consent may be granted to the researcher due to low risk for discomfort or harm to the research subjects.

Some studies, by their very nature, involve minimal risk of violating human rights, whereas others are very sensitive. Studies involving infants, children, fetuses, prisoners, reproductive issues, imposed pain or distress, and risks are considered sensitive, and thus the procedures of the study must be spelled out in great detail (Department of Health and Human Services, 2009). Only individuals who are 18 years of age or older and legally competent can give their own informed consent. Parents or guardians must give permission for minors to participate. The capacity of persons with cognitive, developmental, and mental health limitations to give consent is considered carefully by IRBs.

Recognizing the great diversity of studies, an IRB chairperson or committee designates a study as (1) exempt from review, (2) eligible for expedited review, or (3) requiring complete review (Department of Health and Human Services, 2009). The criteria for exempt-from-review status are spelled out in a U.S. Department of Health and Human Services policy. If the risk is minimal, an expedited review can be carried out by the IRB chairperson or by one or more experienced reviewers. A study that has greater than minimal risk must receive full review by the entire IRB.

From the exemplar article, we do not know if this study underwent expedited review or full review; we do know that it was approved. Waiver of informed written consent of the participating nurses was approved because of the minimal risk for identification, discomfort, or harm to them. The nurses were assigned subject codes and their names were not used during data collection and analysis. The principal investigator was the only person with access to the code sheet and ensured its destruction following data collection.

 RESULTS

WHAT

Sample   The sample consisted of 64 episodes from breakfast, lunch, and dinner at 4 medical step-down units at 2 hospitals in a multihospital system in the southeastern United States. This sample was a convenience sample because no attempt was made to randomly select the episodes observed from all patients receiving RAA insulin on the study units. This is not a shortcoming of the study because the overall aim of the study was to understand mealtime insulin practices for the purposes of improving care in that healthcare system.

Findings   Descriptive statistical results pertaining to the two ideal timing intervals are reported in Tables 2, 3, and 4 of the report. Table 2 summarizes results of all the observations for both intervals of interest; the ideal standards and the *Note* under the tables. First, the left side of Table 2 informs us that BG testing was done on average 73 minutes before insulin was administered—greater than the recommended interval. The median tells us that 50% of the BG-insulin administration intervals were greater than 74 minutes (and 50% were less). The range indicates that the times ranged from 173 minutes to 4 minutes before insulin administration, which means that at least one person had his BG taken nearly 3 hours before insulin administration; this is a reminder to consider both average and variability/range. Overall, only 35% of the BG measurement to insulin administration intervals fell in the ideal range of 60 to 0 minutes; the fact that 65% of patients did not receive insulin based on a BG measured within an hour prior is a major care deficiency.

Then in the right column of Table 2 we see the data about the 2nd interval, insulin administration to first bite of food. The average time of insulin administration was 6 minutes before the patient took the first bite of food; this is within the ideal interval of 15 minutes before or after. However, again, the range indicates a problem; first, it is a quite wide interval, from 148 minutes before to 78 minutes after, and both extremes are of concern. The 148 minutes before is of particular concern because of the possibility of hypoglycemia resulting from receiving this fast-acting insulin and not taking in food. N.B.: The 2nd line of the lower right cell is a typo and should actually read "(23 [40%] in range)." (I contacted the corresponding author and confirmed this.)

Of greatest concern is that overall only 14% of the episodes observed resulted in all three activities occurring within the required intervals—this is a major quality deficiency.

In Tables 3 and 4, further breakdowns of the results by meal period and for just the on-demand/room-service food unit are provided in the form of the means, ranges, and percentages of observations that met the ideal care criteria. It was interesting to see that supper had the lowest percentage of ideal care for the BG testing–insulin administration interval (11%), while lunch was considerably better at 56%. The compliance rates for the insulin administration–first bite interval were different with lunch again being the best (57%), and breakfast being quite poor at just 5.3%. The authors offer some explanation for these wide differences in the *Discussion* section. The results for room-service food delivery as broken out in Table 4 indicate that coordination of insulin-related tasks was even more deficient than for the units as a whole.

Discussion　In this section, the researchers compare their results to those of two other studies and discuss shortcomings in practice that are likely to have serious ramifications for patients' well-being. Recommendations for practice based on the findings are also offered. Among the limitations of the study is the fact that the researchers did not directly observe amount of meal consumption rather relied on asking the nurses to recall this information. The fact that one-third of nurses reported they did not know the amount of food consumed by the patient during the meal is of concern because the insulin dose given assumes that the patient will eat at least 50% of their meal.

Patients who are not inclined, for whatever reason, to eat present a tricky issue since the insulin is often given before the patient starts the meal. However, one could envision the nurse asking the patient at the time of giving the insulin, "Do you think you will be able to eat at least half of your meal?" Care protocols should address what the nurse should do if the patient expresses doubts about eating. One possible solution is that insulin administration could be delayed for up to 30 minutes after the meal is delivered to see if the patient will actually eat half the meal.

Another limitation is that the observations were made in one healthcare system, which may not represent practice in other settings. Generalizability to other settings is limited because organization of nursing activities such as BG testing and insulin administration is unique to every setting. However, two other studies measuring BG testing and insulin administration times in hospital had similar results to this one. Thus, although the findings of this study are from one particular setting, in combination with results of the other studies cited they contribute to the body of knowledge about these practices. Also, the problems identified in this study undoubtedly are not unique to this health system, rather are widespread, making this a valuable contribution to quality improvement efforts beyond the health system in which it was conducted.

REFERENCES

Bates, O. L., O'Connor, N., Dunn, D., & Hasenau, S. M. (2014). Applying STAAR interventions in incremental bundles: Improving post-CABG surgical patient care. *Worldviews on Evidence-Based Nursing, 11*(2), 89–97.

Department of Health and Human Services. (2009). Code of Federal Regulations, Title 45, *Protection of Human Subjects*. http://www.hhs.gov/ohrp/policy/ohrpregulations.pdf

Dillman, D. A., Smyth, J. D., & Christian, L. M. (2009). *Internet, mail, and mixed-mode surveys: The tailored design method* (3rd ed.). New York, NY: John Wiley.

Fair, J. M., Gulanick, M., & Braun, L. T. (2009). Cardiovascular risk factors and lifestyle habits among preventive cardiovascular nurses. *Journal of Cardiovascular Nursing, 24,* 272–286.

Jurgens, C. Y., Hoke, L., Byrnes, J., & Riegel, B. (2009). Why do elders delay responding to heart failure symptoms? *Nursing Research, 58*(4), 274–282.

Pazar, B., Yava, A., & Basal, S. (2015). Health-related quality of life in persons living with a urostomy. *Journal of Wound Ostomy Continence Nursing, 42*(3), 264–270.

Stair, T. O., Morrissey, J., Jaradeh, I., Zhou, T. X., & Goldstein, J. N. (2007). Validation of the quick confusion scale for mental status screening in the emergency department. *Internal Emergency Medicine, 2*(2), 130–132.

CHAPTER SIX

Correlational Research

Another form of quantitative research goes beyond reporting basic facts about a variable of interest to explore how variables are related to one another. Questions such as: Is spousal or partner support associated with diabetics' blood sugar level? Are levels of hearing loss and levels of osteoporosis related? Do lung capacity levels predict exercise capacity? These questions ask, "Are variable *X* and variable *Y* related?" or "Do their levels move in sync to some extent?" These questions go beyond description of each variable separately to examine the relationship between them. They are the kinds of questions that can be answered by correlational research.

Defining *Relationship*

Just what does this word *relationship* mean in the research context? In simplest terms, relationship describes an association between two sets of scores. Let's say, from each person in a sample of 30–40-year-olds, the researchers collected two pieces of data: their heart rate after 5 minutes on a treadmill and their body mass index (BMI). If there was a strong trend for those with low 5-minute heart rates to have low BMIs and for those with high 5-minutes heart rates to have high BMIs, the two variables would be considered to be associated, i.e., correlated, in the sample. Importantly, the association says nothing about the dynamics that link them—just that they are connected in some way. Establishing the dynamics would require a persuasive theory and other research.

A relationship has two dimensions—direction and strength. The direction of change can be in the same direction or in opposite directions. In a positive relationship, as one variable's values increase, the other's values also increase, as in the example just given. In a negative relationship, as one variable's values increase, the other's values decrease; e.g., in a test situation, as anxiety levels rise, scores on the test decrease.

A relationship can also be characterized as strong, moderate, or weak, indicating the strength of the relationship between the two variables. A positive relationship is strong when:

1. Persons who score high on variable *A* also score high on variable *B* and
2. Persons who score low on variable *A* also score low on variable *B* and
3. Those who score intermediate on variable *A* also score intermediate on variable *B*.

Note that each of these statements could also be stated in the inverse, e.g., persons who score high on *B* also score high on *A*. By contrast, a weak relationship exists when:

1. Just a few persons who score high on *A* also score high on *B* but quite a few others score medium or low on *B and*
2. Just a few persons who score low on *A* also score low on *B* but quite a few others score medium or high on *B and*
3. Those who score intermediate on *A* have assorted scores on *B*.

In other words, the relationship is weak when there is very little connection between persons' scores on *A* and scores on *B*.

The opposite of *relationship* is *independence*, meaning that there is no association between scores on the two variables. There is no pattern in the scores of one variable with the scores on the other variable; both are scattered across the range of possible scores. A pattern or lack thereof is best seen by plotting the data points on a graph with values of *A* on one axis and values of *B* on the other axis—there will either be a degree of trend or a wide scatter, as you will see in the next section.

Measuring a Relationship

Statistical Perspectives on Relationship

The direction and strength of a relationship between two variables are quantified using one of several statistical tests. The actual statistic used depends on the scale that was used to quantify the variables. When both variables were measured on an interval level scale, the Pearson *r* coefficient is used; it is the most widely used correlation statistic (Grove, Burns, & Gray, 2012). An interval level scale is a measurement scale with a range of numerical values having equal distance between them, such as degrees on a thermometer or pounds on a weight scale. If either or both of the variables are measured using an ordered set of categories, for example, *freshman, sophomore, junior, senior*, the Pearson *r* coefficient is not used; rather another correlation coefficient would be used. There are several, but they all are interpreted similarly to the interpretation of the Pearson *r* coefficient.

The value of the Pearson *r* statistic varies from −1 to +1, which means that it can be: −1, a negative decimal, 0, a positive decimal, or +1. The sign indicates whether the two variables have a positive or negative relationship; if positive, they move in the same direction; if negative, they move in opposite directions. The closer the value is to −1 or +1, the stronger the relationship between the two variables. Zero means the two variables are completely independent of one another, and a value close to 0 (e.g., +0.2) indicates a very weak relationship.

			Interpretation of *r*				
r-Value	−1	−0.8	−0.5	0	+0.6	+0.8	+1
Relationship	perfect negative	strong neg	moderate neg	none	moderate positive	strong pos	perfect pos

Graph Perspectives on a Relationship

To illustrate relationship in the concrete, a hypothetical study (**Box 6-1**) and five possible data sets for the study are presented in the following figures (**Figures 6-1** through **6-5**). Each data set is accompanied by a scatter plot for the data, the Pearson *r* coefficient for the data, and explanations about what these two analytical tools tell us. The samples in the data sets were limited to five scores to make it easier to see the relationship between the two variables, although a real study would not have as few as five cases. If you are not up to speed regarding scatter plots, also called scatter diagrams, you should go back and read about them in your statistics reference text. You will not see many scatter plots in journal reports because

BOX 6-1   Hypothetical Correlational Study

STUDY PURPOSE: To examine the relationship between hope and adaptation in persons who have had multiple sclerosis for at least 3 years.

MEASUREMENT: On two short questionnaires, total hope scores can range from 0 to 5. A score of 0 = no hope and 5 = an abundance of hope; and total adaptation scores can range from 0 to 10, with 0 = not able to function independently in daily life and 10 = functioning without problems. Note that both variables are scored on continuous scales; this is a key requirement for using the Pearson r correlation coefficient to portray the relationship between the two variables. If one variable is continuous (e.g., adaptation) but the other is categorical (e.g., gender), the Pearson r statistic could not be used.

SAMPLE: Five persons

RESULTS: Several possible sets of scores are presented in Figures 6-1 through 6-6. To make the relationship between the variables stand out, the hope scores are the same from data set to data set, but the adaptation scores are different.

they take up too much room, but they are helpful in identifying trends in data.

Perfect correlations are, of course, a rare happening in the real world where variation and multiple influences are characteristic of reality, especially in the social, psychological, and behavioral realms. Instead, weak, moderate, and moderately strong correlations occur more often. These kinds of relationships are illustrated in the next three hypothetical data sets (Figures 6-3, 6-4, and 6-5).

In summary, a correlation coefficient indicates the direction (positive or negative) and strength (perfect, strong, moderate, weak, or none) of a relationship.

"There is zero correlation between IQ and emotional empathy . . . They're controlled by different parts of the brain."
—Daniel Goleman, author of *Emotional Intelligence*

Dataset 1	Person	Hope Score	Adaptation Score
	1	1	2
	2	2	4
	3	3	6
	4	4	8
	5	5	10

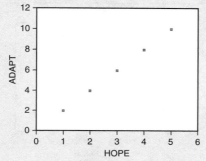

Note that for each increase of 1 point in hope scores, there is a 2-point increase in the adaptation scores. If you know a person's hope score, you can accurately predict that person's adaptation score; similarly if you know the person's adaptation score, you can accurately predict his or her hope score. When two variables change in lockstep with one another, we say that they have a perfect positive correlation. There is nothing magical about the 1-point-hope score to 2-point-adaptation score relationship. It could just as easily be that a 1-point change in hope is related to a 4-point change in adaptation; it depends on the scales used to measure the two variables.

Note that scatter plots provide the same information as the data set table. Each point on the scatter plot represents one score. For example, the person who scored 10 on hope scored 20 on adaptation and has a point on the scatter plot as does the person who scored 40 on hope and 80 on adaptation. Because the relationship between the two variables is in lockstep, a line drawn between all the data points is a straight line.

The Pearson *r* statistic for this data set is *r* = +1, which indicates a perfect positive relationship. The two variables move in lockstep with one another with high scores on one being paired with high scores on the other and low scores on one being paired with low scores on the other. The Pearson *r* statistic has possible values between +1 and −1.

Figure 6-1   Hypothetical Data Set 1

Caveat

Again, a strong relationship between two variables says nothing about the underlying dynamic that produces the relationship. Even a very high correlation (near −1 or +1) does not mean there is a cause-and-effect relationship between the variables. High correlation only conveys that there

Dataset 2	Person	Hope Score	Adaptation Score
	1	1	10
	2	2	8
	3	3	6
	4	4	4
	5	5	2

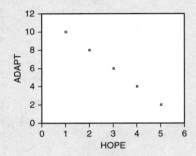

Note that for each increase of 1-point in hope score there is a 2-point decrease in adaptation score. Just as in data set 1, if you know a person's hope score, you can accurately predict that person's adaptation score; similarly if you know the person's adaptation score, you can accurately predict his or her hope score. However, instead of moving in the same direction as they did in data set 1, they move in the opposite direction. The variables in this data set have a perfect negative relationship: As one variable goes up, the other goes down in lockstep a specific amount. Again, a line drawn between all the data points is a straight line. The Pearson r-value for this data set is $r = -1$, indicating a perfect negative relationship.

Figure 6-2   Hypothetical Data Set 2

is a pattern in the relationship between the two variables. The relationship between the two variables could be much more complex than straightforward cause and effect.

For instance, look at **Figure 6-3** again. At first glance, the scatter plot and the Pearson r of 0.93 may seem to suggest that level of hope determines level of adaptation. However, identical data could be found if the reverse were true; that is, successful adaptation generates hope. Another possibility is that the relationship between the two variables is not a direct one. There could be another lurking variable in the background that has a strong effect on both hope and adaptation and causes them to move in concert with one another; that lurking variable could be something like prognosis or response to treatment. In any of the three dynamics just set forth, the data and the Pearson r-value could be the same as in Figure 6-3. The point

Dataset 3	Person	Hope Score	Adaptation Score
	1	1	2
	2	2	3
	3	3	6
	4	4	9
	5	5	8

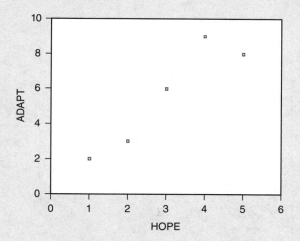

Note that an increase in hope is roughly related to an increase in adaptation. The two variables are strongly but not perfectly correlated. If you know a person's score on one variable, you can make a pretty good estimate of the person's score on the other variable.

A trend in the data is quite obvious, but all the data points are not in a straight line. If a straight line were drawn through the middle of the data, three data points would be on or very close to that line and two would be a bit farther away. The line is called the *trend line* and represents the middle of the data. Take a straight edge and add a trend line to this graph.

The Pearson *r* coefficient for this data set is +0.93, which is a strong, positive correlation.

Figure 6-3   Hypothetical Data Set 3

is this: Correlation sheds no light on the dynamic underlying the relationship—even when one precedes the other in time. Correlation analysis only detects a relationship. The dynamics of that relationship need to be ferreted out by further research using other research designs or justified by other knowledge about the two phenomena.

Dataset 4	Person	Hope Score	Adaptation Score
	1	1	2
	2	2	10
	3	3	6
	4	4	4
	5	5	8

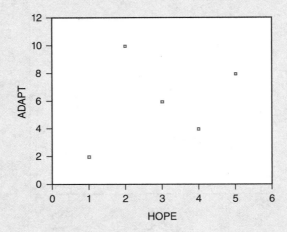

There is a bit of a linear trend in the relationship between hope and adaptation; as hope scores go up, there is a bit of a trend for the adaptation score to go up, but the relationship is weak. Any effort to base one score on the other score would have a low likelihood of being accurate.

A trend line drawn through the middle of the data would show that three data points are on or close to the trend line, but two are quite far from it. Thus, there is a trend, but a weak one. The Pearson r coefficient for this data set is +0.30, indicating a moderately weak positive correlation.

Figure 6-4   Hypothetical Data Set 4

Correlation ≠ Cause

When the relationship between ratings of perceived exertion and heart rates of young African Americans was studied in treadmill tests (Karavatas & Tavakol, 2005), the overall Pearson r was 0.58. The authors interpreted

Dataset 5	Person	Hope Score	Adaptation Score
	1	1	7
	2	2	3
	3	3	10
	4	4	5
	5	5	6

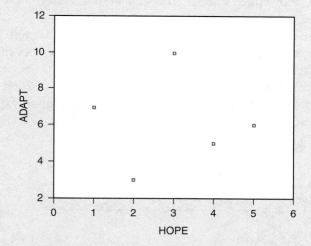

In this data set, there is no relationship between the hope score and the adaptation score; the two scores are independent of one another. Knowing one score will not enable you to predict the other one. All data points are quite far from a trend line drawn through the data. The Pearson *r* coefficient for this data set is 0, indicating no relationship between the two variables.

Figure 6-5   Hypothetical Data Set 5

this result as a moderately strong relationship in which heart rate influences perceived exertion. This directional interpretation was justified by physiological knowledge, not by the statistical result itself.

Outliers

When looking at scatter plots, the researcher looks for outliers, which are cases that have very atypical pairings of scores. An outlier's data point will lie very far from the trend line. Importantly, with small sample sizes, a single outlier can lower the Pearson r considerably. Consider the scatter plot in **Figure 6-6**. Note that most of the scores lie close to the positive correlation trend line, except for the person who scored 40 on hope and 10 on adaptation. This person's data is an outlier because it is very different from the other scores. The Pearson r for this data set is 0.50, which is a medium correlation. However, when this outlier is removed, reanalysis produces a Pearson r of 0.98 for the other four scores. The Pearson r calculated with the outlier left in is greatly influenced because the sample size is so small; still, studies with larger sample sizes can be moderately influenced by a single outlier.

An outlier can either understate or exaggerate the strength of the relationship between the two variables, depending on the values that make up the outlier. Removing an outlier or even several in a data set can uncover a trend that would be less clear if the outliers were left in. When researchers remove data for an analysis, they should do so with good rationale, and they should acknowledge that they did so. Removing data could be a form of bias, particularly when the study has a small sample size. Sometimes, a

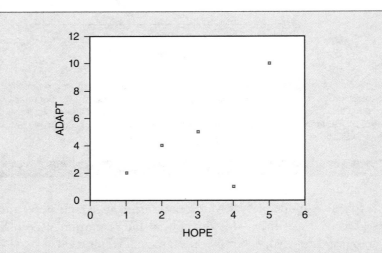

The Pearson r for this data set is 0.50, indicating a modest association. The outlier has lowered an otherwise high Pearson r-value. It pulls the r statistic down a lot because the data set is so small.

Figure 6-6   Example of Outlier

researcher will examine outlier cases in great depth because doing so can yield valuable insights that set the agenda for future research.

Practical Perspectives on r-Value

Even though an r of 1.00 indicates a perfect positive relationship between hope and adaptation in which the variables move in lockstep with one another, an r-value of 0.70 does *not* mean that 70% of the values of hope move in lockstep with adaptation; rather the r-value indicates the relative strength of the relationship on a scale from −1 to +1.

Huck (2011) points out that r exaggerates how strong the relationship really is between two variables. A more realistic and practical perspective is gained by squaring the value of r to produce r^2, which is called the coefficient of determination. The r^2 value indicates the percentage of variation in hope that is related to adaptation and the percentage of variation in adaptation that is related to hope (see **Figure 6-7**). When an r of 0.70 is squared, yielding an r^2 of 0.49, this tells us that about half the variation in hope is related to adaptation, and half of the variation in adaptation is related to hope. The other 51% of both variables is attributable to other, often unknown, influences. In short, r^2 provides a more practical sense of the strength of the relationship between the two variables than r itself does.

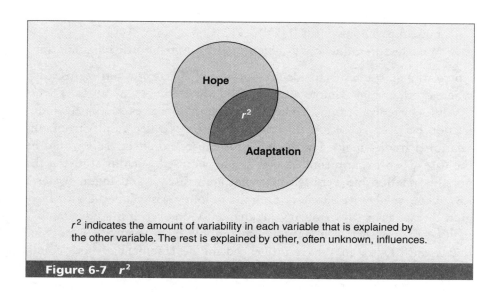

r^2 indicates the amount of variability in each variable that is explained by the other variable. The rest is explained by other, often unknown, influences.

Figure 6-7 r^2

Correlational Design

Bivariate Analysis

The most straightforward correlational design is when the relationship between two or more variables is studied in a sample of people. The researcher measures the participants on each of the variables of interest using instruments that have been established as reliable and valid with the population under study. No attempt is made to control or manipulate the situation. As with descriptive studies, good data are key to a good study; thus most researchers report information about the reliability and validity of the instruments they use. Analysis of the data consists of running correlational tests to determine if and how the variables are related. In basic correlational studies, the analysis consists of measuring the strength of the association between various combinations of two variables, which is called *bivariate correlation*. If there are three variables in the study, *A*, *B*, and *C*, bivariate analysis could be run on the relationship between *A* and *B*, *A* and *C*, and *B* and *C*, thus producing three correlation coefficients.

Some of the variables included in a study come from the hunches of clinicians practicing in the area; others come from theory or related academic work. Often, researchers conduct correlational studies to explore clinical issues that are murky, such as:

- What factors influence young women's positive adaptation to having human papilloma virus (HPV)?
- What factors influence a double amputee's motivation in rehabilitation?

Correlational studies help identify promising ideas for future research, whereas others may demote ideas that did not hold up.

Although correlational studies cannot by themselves establish a connection between cause and effect, there are times when results from correlational studies make a strong case for cause and effect. This would be the case when experimental design cannot be used, such as studying the possible relationship between maternal gum disease and infant preterm low birth weight. Researchers cannot randomly assign mothers to have gum disease prior to or during pregnancy. Moreover, if a study found a high correlation between gum disease and low birth weight, it is possible that a third factor may have influenced the development of both conditions—such as poor diet, smoking, or alcohol consumption. It would also be prudent to keep in mind that most health conditions are not caused by a single determinant and that several determinants often interact with each other to cause a condition. To make a claim that maternal gum disease causes infant low birth weight would require cohort studies and a credible theory regarding the causative mechanism—but a correlational study could be a starting point for examining the issue. Cohort studies are examined in Chapter 8.

Generalizing to a Population

Researchers can go beyond statistically estimating the relationship that exists among the variables in the sample studied to educated guesses about whether the relationships will also be found in a population with a similar profile. The statistical analysis that analyzes each bivariate relationship, in addition to producing an *r* statistic, also produces a data-based **p-value**. If this *p*-value is less than the preset, critical *p*-value (i.e., it is significant), this indicates that the correlation in the population is not zero. Importantly, it does *not* indicate that the correlation between the two variables in the population is of the same strength as was found in the sample. Nor does it indicate that the relationship is particularly strong. It just signals that the two variables are related to some degree (positively or negatively depending on the sign of *r*) in the population. If the data-based *p*-value produced by the analysis is greater than the critical *p*-level (i.e., not significant), it is likely that the correlation between the two variables in the population is zero. See **Figure 6-8**.

Further explanation of *p*-value interpretation is provided in the *Profile & Commentary* on the exemplar article of this chapter. Seeing it in context may make it clearer to you.

More Complex Designs

So far, this chapter has focused on the simplest type of correlational study, but there are more powerful ones. Complex correlational designs collect data on quite a few variables to determine the combination of variables that best *predict* the level of an outcome variable of interest. One such design uses multiple regression analysis to determine which *set* of predictor variables best predicts the level of an outcome variable. Using a statistical program, predictor variable values are entered into the analysis one at a time until the combination of variables that best predicts levels of the

Data-based *p*-value	< .001	.01	.025	**.05**	.08	.15	.42 >
Finding	Significant correlation			Nonsignificant correlation			
Conclusion	A correlation of zero may be found in the population.			A correlation of greater or less than zero would likely be found in the population.			

*Using a .05 level of significance decision point

Figure 6-8   Interpretation of *p*-Values Associated with Pearson *r*

outcome variable is found. The amount of variability among the scores of the outcome variable explained by the best set of predictor variables is quantified as the R^2 statistic.

For example, a study examined five variables that might predict functional recovery after a stroke (Hinkle, 2006). The Functional Independence Measure, which produces a functional score, was used to measure recovery. The major finding was that the predictor variables of age, cognitive status, and initial function had the highest correlations with recovery and were the best set of predictors of the level of motor recovery. $R^2 = 42\%$, meaning that together these three variables predicted 42% of the variability in functional recovery. Adding the other two predictor variables, lesion volume and motor strength, to the analysis did not increase the R^2.

Outcome Prediction   Other studies use predictor variables to distinguish between the prevalence of categorical outcomes (e.g., quit smoking/did not quit smoking; occurrence/nonoccurrence); a widely used statistical technique for this purpose is logistic regression. Whereas multiple regression is used when the outcome variable is a continuous one, logistic regression is used when the outcome variable is categorical. The results are reported using a measure called *odds ratio*.

An odds ratio (OR) compares the likelihood of two or more predictor groups being in the same outcome group. For example, it could be used to quantify the chances of women being admitted to graduate school to the chances of men being admitted. Women and men are the two groups of the predictor variable *gender* and being admitted and not being admitted are the two groups of the outcome variable *graduate school admission*. Using admission as the base outcome, an odds ratio of 1 or near 1 indicates that women and men have the same likelihood of being admitted. Using men as the base group and women as the comparison group (feminist alert: this analysis could be done in reverse with women as the base group), an odds ratio of 2 indicates that women have twice the likelihood of being admitted as men do. An odds ratio of 0.33 would indicate that women are one-third as likely to be admitted as men. Importantly, this OR does not mean women have a 33% admission rate; rather it is a likelihood of admission *relative to* the base group admission rate. OR = 0.33 could also be interpreted to mean that women have 67% less likelihood of being admitted as men. Is this difficult to get a handle on? That's understandable. Perhaps another example will help.

In a study of patient, environmental, and workforce factors that could contribute to patient falls during hospitalization, logistic regression was used to determine the factors that predicted the probability of a patient fall (Cox et al., 2015). So, fall/didn't fall are the groups of the outcome variable—*fall* being the base outcome of the analyses. Many predictor variables were analyzed but only eight of them were significant predictors of falls. To consider just two of their eight odds ratios:

■ Having narcotics or sedatives prescribed had an odds ratio of 16.64 (OR = 16.64) for a fall, which indicates that patients prescribed narcotics or sedatives were 16 times more likely to fall than patients who were not prescribed these medications.

■ Having a fall prevention strategy in place had an OR = 0.128 for a fall, which indicates that persons for whom a fall prevention strategy was in place had just a 13% likelihood of falling as persons who did not have such a protocol in place. An OR = 0.128 could also be interpreted as persons for whom a fall prevention strategy was in place had an 87% reduction in the likelihood of a fall compared to the likelihood of a fall for persons who did not have such a protocol in place.

$$\text{Odds ratio} = \frac{\text{Probability of occurrence in group A}}{\text{Probability of occurrence in group B}}$$

Studies using logistic regression as the main method of analysis are appearing with increased frequency. Because this is a basic text, an exemplar using it will not be included, but for those readers who anticipate getting involved in evidence-based practice in some way, it is essential knowledge. I refer you to a more advanced research methods book, a statistics book, or a website article. One of the clearest explanations I have found is in *Statistical Methods for Healthcare Research* (Munro, 2005). Also, several studies using multiple regression and logistic regression are posted on this text's student website.

In sum, multiple regression analysis and logistic regression are advanced forms of correlation in which the relationships among sets of predictor variables and an outcome variable are examined. However, the exemplar study you will be reading is a basic correlational study examining bivariate relationships.

Graven, L. J., Grant, J. S., Vance, D. E., Pryor, E. R., Grubbs, L., & Karioth, S. (2014). Factors associated with depressive symptoms in patient with heart failure. *Home Healthcare Nurse, 32*(9) 550–555.

Abstract

Home healthcare clinicians commonly provide care for individuals with heart failure (HF). Certain factors may influence the development of depressive symptoms in those with HF. This cross-sectional, descriptive, correlational pilot study (N = 50) examined interrelationships among HF symptoms, social support (actual and perceived), social problem-solving, and depressive symptoms. Findings indicated that increased HF symptoms were related to more depressive symptoms, whereas higher levels of social support were related to fewer depressive symptoms. The use of more maladaptive problem-solving strategies was also associated with more depressive symptoms. Study results have implications for home healthcare clinicians providing care for individuals with HF, indicating a need for programs that strengthen coping skills and resources (i.e., social support and problem solving) in an effort to decrease the risk of developing depressive symptomatology.

Profile & Commentary

STUDY PURPOSE

This study aimed to explore the relationships among social networks, problem-solving strategies, and depressive symptoms in persons who have congestive heart failure (HF). Note that it is a pilot study for a larger study that would explore these relationships in a more complex way (Graven et al., 2015). The study was preapproved by three ethics review boards because the participants were recruited across several settings.

METHODS

Study Design   The authors describe this study as "cross-sectional, descriptive, correlational design" (p. 551). Cross-sectional means that data was collected once; no attempt was made to study the issue over time. The study is descriptive because variables were not divided into predictor variables and outcome variables, and no attempt was made to determine how the social and problem-solving variables work together to predict depressive symptoms. Rather the bivariate relationships between the study variables were the focus.

Sample   The sample was composed of 50 persons from three outpatient clinics in northwest Florida. Potential participants were first contacted at home via telephone to obtain consent to participate, and completed four questionnaires when they came for their clinic visits. Thus, they were persons who were readily accessible to the researchers, i.e., a convenience sample; no attempt was made to randomly select them from a larger population. As a result, the confidence with which one can generalize the results of this study to a larger population is limited. Still, it provides insights that might be useful when giving care to patients with HF.

ASSUMED POPULATION: Outpatients with heart failure

SAMPLE: 50 patients from 3 outpatient clinics in northwest Florida

PROJECTED POPULATION: Mostly male, white, educated above high school level, with annual incomes below $50,000, and low levels of symptoms

Measurement   The report provides quite a bit of information about these instruments to assure the readers of their reliability and validity. Of note is that most of the questionnaires have been used previously and their reliability and validity have been established. This is what the authors mean, when, in the paragraph about the social problem solving instrument, they say, "Empirical evidence supports psychometric properties of the SPSI-R:S" (p. 552) and provide a reference. For the other instruments, information is provided about how well the questions/items hang together, i.e., the internal consistency of the questionnaire, in the form of factor analysis and Cronbach's alpha. Although you might not know anything about factor analysis and Cronbach's alpha, you should be reassured by the fact the instruments have been evaluated by these analyses. A brief comment about Cronbach's alpha: a value above 0.80 would indicate that together the items capture the physical symptoms of HF; a Cronbach's alpha below 0.7 introduces concern that some items of the instrument are not focused on the same concept as the others. So, Cronbach's alphas in the 0.90s indicate that the items are working together to measure different aspects of the same thing—in this study: physical symptoms of HF.

Beyond the data regarding the quality of instruments, you should take note of the possible range of scores and what a high score and a low score indicate. Unfortunately, in this report, the possible range of scores for each questionnaire is not provided, rather the actual range of scores obtained in this study is provided in Table 1, p. 553. However, in the report we learn that for all questionnaires, high scores indicate greater presence of the attribute being measured. Do be aware that is not always the case. For instance, in a study of fatigue in HF patients, a lower score on the Quality of Life questionnaire indicated a better quality of life (Evangelista et al., 2008).

Analysis   Descriptive statistics, Pearson r coefficients, and critical p-levels of 0.05 were used for the analysis.

 RESULTS

Sample   First, the characteristics of the sample and the scores on the questionnaires are reported in Table 1. Note that this sample is mostly male, white, well educated, and of modest income. On average, symptoms of HF were present at a fairly low level, as were depressive symptoms; "A cutoff of 16 indicates [the level above which] an individual is at risk for some degree of depressive symptoms" (p. 552).

Associations Then comes the correlational part of the results, i.e., the bivariate analyses, which are presented in table form (called a correlation matrix) and discussed in the text narrative. In Table 2, the variables are listed across the top of the matrix and down the left site. The number in the cell at each cross point of column and row is the Pearson r statistic for those two variables. Fifteen bivariate associations were measured. Note the bottom row, which shows that the depressive symptoms variable has moderate correlations with all the other variables. The highest association is with HF symptoms ($r = 0.627$), which indicates that persons who had high HF symptom scores tended to have high depressive scores. The lowest Pearson r in that row is a with adaptive problem solving ($r = -0.343$), indicating that adaptive problem solving and depressive symptoms are inversely associated. Several of the scores in the matrix are also inversely related. That is to be expected of some combination of variables such as depression and social support. The high positive correlation between social network and social support is to be expected as the two concepts are inherently very closely related; therefore it is a "knew that" result.

In the text, the authors commented on several of the associations. To gain further perspectives on the results, I would suggest calculating coefficients of correlation, i.e., r^2 for each r of interest. To take just one Pearson r, the one for depressive symptoms and maladaptive problem solving, the r of 0.549 translates to an r^2 of 0.30. That means that about 30% of the variability in depressive symptom scores is explained by its association with maladaptive problem solving scores and vice versa. Thus, maladaptive problem solving and depressive symptomatology are associated at a modest level, but other factors determine 70% of each. Chief among these other factors contributing to depressive symptoms is HF symptoms; we know this because of the high correlation between depressive symptoms and HD symptoms.

Don't Assume Unidirectionality The tendency is to first think that maladaptive problem solving contributes to depressive symptomatology, but thinking further, you can imagine how depressive symptoms could contribute to maladaptive problem solving. The same could be said for the negative relationship between social support and depressive symptoms. Yes, people with more social support would be expected to have fewer depressive symptoms than people with less social support. However, it may also be that persons who are depressed reach out less for social support than people who are less depressed do. I would have preferred the authors to consider these bidirectional possibilities more than they did. Nevertheless, these results exemplify how correlational research uncovers interesting associations that point the way to future studies that examine one or several of the associations more definitively.

Inference from Sample to Population Now, let's consider the symbols on the correlational matrix of Table 2. The authors ran tests of significance on the r statistics. The † and ‡ symbols indicate the levels at which the data-based p-values were significant. Remember p-values in the context of correlation statistics indicate whether or not the correlation is likely to be zero in a larger population. Based on the symbols, there are eight correlations about which we can have confidence that they are not just chance correlations; that is to say that for these eight combinations of two variables, some level of correlation is likely to exist in the larger population of similar persons. The data-based p-value for six of the correlation statistics were significant at the < 0.01 level and two were significant at the > 0.01 level, but not at the < 0.05 level. Therefore all eight combinations of variables are likely to have some correlation in the larger population.

Limitations Finally, the authors acknowledged the limitations of their study. The sample profile has been discussed, but the researchers' acknowledgment of the risk of type 1 error is worthy of explanation. Whenever a large number of statistical tests are run in a study, there is an increased chance that one or more of them will be statistically significant just by chance (Huck, 2011). To avoid accepting a correlation result as being likely in the population when it is actually just a chance resulting from multiple statistical tests being run, some experts advise that the critical p-level required for each statistical be lowered, i.e., made more demanding. That is often done using a procedure called **Bonferroni correction**. The amount of correction depends on the number of statistical tests run.

In this study, 15 correlation statistics were run, so applying the Bonferroni correction, the critical p-level would be changed from 0.05 to 0.003 $(0.05 \div 15)$. Thus, the data-based p-value produced by each bivariate statistical test would be considered to indicate an association in the population only if it were 0.003 or lower; this is much more demanding than a critical p of < 0.05 or even < 0.01. We don't know if any of the bivariate associations that achieved significance at the 0.01 level would have achieved significance after Bonferroni correction. Although the authors of this study did not do this correction, they are to be commended for calling our attention to the possibility that any of these correlations could actually be zero in the population (type 1 error) because of the large number of correlation statistics that were calculated.

REFERENCES

Cox, J., Thomas-Hawkins, C., Pajarillo, E., DeGennaro, S., Cadmus, E., & Martinez, M. (2015). Factors associated with falls in hospitalized adult patients. *Applied Nursing Research, 28,* 78–82.

Evangelista, L. S., Moser, D. K., Westlake, C., Pike, N., Ter-Galstanyan, A., & Dracup, K. (2008). Correlates of fatigue in patients with heart failure. *Progress in Cardiovascular Nursing, 23*(1), 12–17.

Graven, L. J., Grant, J. S., Vance, D. E., Pryor, E. R., Grubbs, L., & Karioth, K. (2014). Depressive symptoms in patients with heart failure. *Home Healthcare Nurse, 32*(9), 550–555.

Graven, L. J., Grant, J. S., Vance, D. E., Pryor, E. R., Grubbs, L., & Karioth, K. (2015). Predicting depressive symptoms and self-care in patients with heart failure. *American Journal of Health Behavior, 39*(1), 77–87.

Grove, S. K., Burns, N., & Gray, J. (2012). *Practice of nursing research: Conduct, critique, and utilization* (7th ed.). St. Louis, MO: Elsevier Saunders.

Hinkle, J. L. (2006). Variables explaining functional recovery following motor stroke. *Journal of Neuroscience Nursing, 38*(1), 6–12.

Huck, S. W. (2011). *Reading statistics and research* (6th ed.). Boston, MA: Pearson.

Karavatas, S. G., & Tavakol, K. (2005). Concurrent validity of Borg's rating of perceived exertion in African-American young adults, employing heart rate as the standard. *Internet Journal of Allied Health Sciences and Practice, 3*(1). Retrieved from http://ijahsp.nova.edu/articles/vol3num1/karavatas.htm

Munro, B. H. (2005). *Statistical methods for healthcare research* (5th ed.). Philadelphia: Lippincott.

CHAPTER SEVEN

Experimental Research

Chapter Map

This is a very long chapter; therefore it is divided into two main sections. The first section focuses on the methods used to conduct experimental studies testing the effectiveness of nursing interventions. The second section delves into the ways results of experimental studies are reported.

In the first section, the methodological characteristics of experimental studies are explained, followed by reprint of the exemplar study article in full. You should read only the *Introduction* and *Material and Methods* sections of the exemplar study, then read the *Profile & Commentary* about its methods. The second section opens with an explanation of the results of experimental studies. After reading that, you should read the *Results* section of the exemplar study and then the *Profile & Commentary* about its results. In other words, rather than ingest the whole research article at once, you will first consider the *why* and the *how*. Then you will delve into the *what*. When you see the amount of information in this chapter, you will understand why it is divided into two portions.

The explanations in this chapter will be limited to the classic two-group experiment, which is widely used in nursing research. Although in the future you will undoubtedly read three-group experimental studies, you should be able to understand them using what you know about two-group studies and reference to your statistics book. Other experimental designs that are used less often are not addressed in this text.

The classic experimental study discussed in this chapter is also referred to in healthcare research as a randomized clinical trial (RCT). Having said that, some people view an RCT more narrowly—in particular, as a definitive, late-stage test of an intervention's effectiveness, often in a large, diverse sample (Grove, Burns, & Gray, 2013).

CHAPTER LAYOUT

SECTION 1

Methods explained

Exemplar study: Read *Introduction* and *Material and Methods* sections only

Profile & Commentary: *Why* and *How*

SECTION 2

Results explained

Exemplar study: Read *Results* and *Discussion* sections

Profile & Commentary: *What*

Section 1: Experimental Methods

Determining the effectiveness of nursing interventions and treatments requires carefully designed studies. Assembling a group of willing participants and measuring them on a physiologic condition, psychological state, or knowledge level before and after receiving the intervention of interest is considered a weak design (Kerlinger & Lee, 2000). It is weak because if an improvement is found, the researcher cannot claim with certainty that the intervention produced the improvement. Natural recovery, natural fluctuations in condition, or influences in the environment may have caused the observed improvements. Adding a control group that is also measured before and after allows these extraneous influences to be taken into account.

Key Features of Experimental Studies

When researchers want to test the effects of a nursing intervention on patient outcomes, the ideal research design is an experiment. A sample is drawn from a target population, and participants are randomly assigned to one of two groups. One group receives the test intervention and the other group receives no intervention or another intervention. At an appropriate time after the intervention, the researcher measures an outcome variable, or

"Sameness" or designing SAME conditions allows for all "changes" seen to be the result of intervention and not any other influences.

several, in both groups to determine whether one group did better than the other (see **Figure 7-1**). In designing an experimental study, the researcher tries to create conditions in which all influences on the outcome of interest, other than the effects of the different interventions, are the same for both groups. This sameness is necessary to be certain that any difference found in the outcomes of the two groups can be attributed to the fact that they received different interventions, not to some other influence.

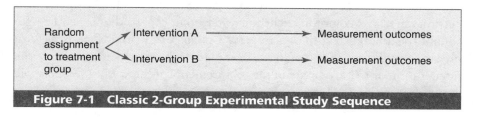

Figure 7-1   Classic 2-Group Experimental Study Sequence

The classic experimental study has six key features:

1. A well-defined target population
2. Adequate sample size
3. **Random assignment** of participants to intervention and **comparison** groups
4. Control of extraneous influences and bias
5. Low level of missing data
6. Consistent delivery of interventions

These features are key because they (1) control error, bias, and unwanted influences; and (2) determine to whom the results will apply. In so doing, they bolster confidence in the credibility and applicability of the findings.

Before explaining each of these key features, let's consider some of the terminology used in reports of experimental studies. The new intervention (frequently the intervention of greatest interest) may be called the *experimental intervention* or *test intervention*; however, the terms *experimental treatment* and **independent variable** are also used. When referring to both interventions, the terms *interventions* and *treatment groups* may be used. The researcher's control over the design and delivery of the interventions may be referred to as *manipulation of the intervention*. I will use all these terms to help you get accustomed to them.

RESEARCH LINGO: Intervention = Treatment = Independent variable

Well-Defined Target Population

When researchers first think about doing a study, they have a target population in mind. As study design proceeds, they need to be very clear about the criteria that define the target population, and in so doing they produce a list of inclusion criteria (also called *eligibility criteria*). Commonly used inclusion criteria are age range, gender, ethnic group, medical diagnosis, clinical or functional status, care setting, and geographical location. Sometimes, in addition to inclusion criteria, the researcher will also specify exclusion criteria. A common exclusion criterion in U.S. studies is people who cannot speak English. Other examples of exclusions would be persons with physical conditions that would make it inadvisable for them to receive the intervention or to participate in the requirements of the study. (See example in text box.)

> In a study testing the effects of music on postoperative pain relief after open-heart surgery during chair rest on the first postoperative day (Shu, 2010), the following eligibility criteria were used:
>
> 1. **First postoperative day after an open-heart surgery.**
> 2. **Stable condition and oriented.**
> 3. **Absence of hearing impairment.**
> 4. **Ability to follow commands and understand and read English.**
>
> Patients with a femoral artery sheath in place after surgery were excluded because 6–8 hours' bed rest is necessary to prevent hemorrhage after removal.

Inclusion and exclusion criteria serve four purposes:

1. Define the population to whom the findings will be generalizable.
2. Identify characteristics that must be present for a person to be included in the sample.
3. Control variables that will distort the results.
4. Make it feasible to actually conduct the study.

When it is known in advance that a particular patient characteristic has a strong influence on the outcomes of interest and that characteristic is not of interest in the study, the researcher may decide to remove its influence completely. This is done even though random sampling would even out the variable's influence across the two groups, because removing it all together allows the effect of the treatment being tested to stand out. One way to remove a very strong patient characteristic influence that is not of interest in the study is to include in the study only persons who do not have that characteristic.

To illustrate: If a study of persons with mild congestive heart failure examines the effects of two rehabilitation approaches on the distance they can walk in 6 minutes without stopping to catch their breath or rest, the researcher might exclude persons whose walking is affected by conditions other than their cardiac conditioning. This could be done by excluding all persons with preexisting physical disabilities that affect mobility, such as stroke, severe hip and knee arthritis, peripheral arterial disease, Parkinson's disease, lower extremity amputation, and neurological disease. From the research point of view, these exclusions make sense in that they control extraneous variables affecting mobility and thereby increase the likelihood that the analysis will identify differences in walking outcomes resulting from the two different rehab approaches. However, a long list of exclusion criteria can also create problems in finding eligible participants for the study.

From the clinical perspective, many persons who have mild congestive heart failure also have arthritis and other conditions affecting mobility. So, a study conducted with this many exclusions would apply only to a very narrow portion of the patients clinicians are likely to see, and we would say the study has limited generalizability in real-world practice. Thus, researchers have to use exclusion criteria with awareness regarding how they will affect the clinical usefulness of the findings.

Adequate Sample Size

An experimental study's sample size must be large enough to differentiate between a true difference and a chance difference in outcomes. A **true difference** is one that is large enough that a difference would likely be found in the population; it is indicated by a significant statistical result (that is a data based p-value less than the specified decision point p-level). A **chance difference** is one that just happened in the sample but would probably not be found in the population. Determining "large enough" requires taking the following into account:

1. The expected strength of the experimental intervention's impact vis-à-vis the impact of the comparison intervention. The strength of the intervention is often calculated using the smallest difference

between groups that would be considered a clinically meaningful impact on patient outcomes.

2. The amount of score dispersion that has been found in prior studies.
3. The desired level of significance (i.e., the *p* value that will be used as a decision point for statistical significance).

These values are entered into a calculation called a power analysis, which produces an estimate of the sample size required. You do not need to know how to do a power analysis, but you should know that doing a power analysis is the right way to determine sample size for correlational and experimental studies (Grove, Burns, & Gray, 2013).

Power analysis should be done when designing an experimental study to avoid doing a study that has a very low capacity for finding a statistically significant difference in the outcomes of the two groups. Insufficient sample size weakens the capacity of the statistics used to declare a difference in the outcomes of the two groups as significant. It is like using a microscope with weak magnification—you know something is there but it's not clear enough to know if it is something important or not. Researchers use the terms *low statistical power* and *underpowered* to refer to a study with low capacity to declare a significant difference in the outcomes of the two groups. A common reason for low statistical power is small sample size.

When there is good reason to expect that the intervention will have a very strong impact on the study outcomes, the power analysis usually indicates that a small sample size will be adequate. However, nursing interventions typically have modest impacts. The reality is that many nursing studies done with 30 persons in each group that find no statistically significant difference in the outcomes of the two groups would find one had they been done with 60 or 100 persons in each group. If the purpose of a study is to determine if one intervention is more effective than another, doing a study with too small a sample is a waste of time, effort, and resources on everyone's part (Grove, Burns, & Gray, 2013).

Random Assignment to Treatment Groups

Random assignment of enrolled participants to treatment groups is a defining feature of experimental studies. It is accomplished by assigning each person in the sample to either the experimental group or to the comparison group *based on chance determination*—not on the basis of patient preference for one treatment approach over the other, on physician request, or on the convenience of the research staff. Chance assignment requires that each participant have an equal chance of being assigned to either group. A flip of a coin is one way of randomly assigning each participant to one of the two study groups; more commonly today a computer-generated list of random numbers is used to determine each person's group assignment.

The contribution of random assignment to experimental design is that it controls differences in participant characteristics by distributing them evenly across both treatment groups, thus producing two groups that are similar before the interventions are given. Equivalent groups at the start are necessary in experiments because at the end of the study the researcher wants to be confident that the results were not influenced by different group compositions. When random assignment is not used, the possibility exists that some difference between the two groups that was present prior to giving the interventions may have produced the difference found in the outcomes. This possibility creates lack of confidence that any difference found postintervention was a result of the interventions they received.

The larger the sample size, the greater the chances are that random assignment will create treatment groups that are equivalent at baseline on important demographic and clinical variables (e.g., age, body mass index, disease severity). Nevertheless, even in large studies, researchers run comparison statistics on important demographic and clinical variables to make sure that random assignment worked effectively. A table profiling the two groups helps answer questions such as:

- Did the groups have similar mean ages?
- Did the groups have approximately equal proportions of men to women?
- Was the health status of the persons in both groups about the same?

In short, random assignment to treatment groups, sometimes referred to as *randomization,* is the most powerful way of ensuring that the two treatment groups are similar at the onset of the study; it works by evening out the presence of participant characteristics across both groups.

However, not all comparisons of treatment effectiveness can use randomization. It may be ethically or practically impossible to randomly assign persons to treatment groups. For instance, a comparison of the patient outcomes and costs associated with care of the frail elderly at home with support services versus nursing home living cannot create comparison groups by random assignment of persons to a care setting. The decision regarding how care will be provided to a frail elderly person is a highly personal one that hinges on many patient, family, and community factors.

As a result, the research done on this issue would have to use a cohort design (described in Chapter 8).

Do note that random assignment is different from random sampling. Briefly, random sampling is a way of obtaining a study sample that is representative of the target population, whereas random assignment is a way of determining the intervention each study participant will receive; what they share in common is the use of chance to control bias. (Random sampling was discussed in Chapter 5.)

The important point here is that certain patient characteristics can influence the outcomes being studied and thereby complicate comparing the effects of the two treatments. Random assignment controls the influence of patient characteristics by ensuring that the patient characteristics are present to the same extent in both treatment groups.

Having said that patient characteristics should be approximately equal in both treatment groups, it also should be noted that there are study designs that analyze how patient characteristics affect response to the intervention. These designs (called factorial designs) make important contributions to clinical knowledge because they provide valuable information about persons with whom the intervention is very effective, moderately effective, or not effective. I will not go there because factorial designs are complex and describing them here would lead us astray.

Control of Extraneous Variables and Bias

Even when patient characteristics that may have an influence on the outcome variable have been controlled through random assignment, they are still exerting their influence by increasing the variability in the outcome data. This variability makes it more difficult for any difference in outcomes between the two groups to be detected. To maximize detection of the relationship between the independent variable and the outcome variable, a potential extraneous variable may be eliminated altogether by exclusion criteria. Thus, exclusion and inclusion criteria serve the purpose of controlling extraneous variables and thereby giving prominence to the relationship between the independent and dependent variables of the study.

Study activities and the settings in which the study is conducted also give rise to extraneous variables that influence the outcome variables directly. Steps must be taken to control them because they mix with the situation and make it difficult to obtain a clear understanding of the relationship between the interventions and the outcomes. These influences can be persistent across the study setting or can influence one treatment group more than the other.

Sometimes the setting is the larger world of current events. For example, if during the time a study is being conducted to evaluate managing arthritis pain with the use of heat and cold, a new advertisement for a jazzy new whirlpool hits the TV waves big time, the advertisement could influence the results. Some persons in the heat group might be tempted to use the whirlpool instead of using heat according to the study protocol. In addition, some of those in the cold group might decide to abandon cold treatment all together. These changes in participant compliance with their assigned treatment method could result in persons in the treatment groups actually using different treatments than the study design indicates they are using. If the researcher is monitoring the study setting (immediate and more global), he may be able to detect such an extraneous influence and take steps to moderate it or check out its influence. To control extraneous variables originating in the study activities, researchers develop very specific study procedures or protocols. In advance of starting the study, they specify:

- Characteristics of persons who are eligible for the study
- How participants are to be recruited
- How consent to participate in the study will be obtained
- How participants will be randomly assigned to treatment groups
- The activities that compose each treatment
- The conditions under which the treatments will be delivered
- Training of data collectors
- How and when the outcomes will be measured

In studies where a research assistant observes and rates participants' responses, it is all too easy for well-intended data collectors to influence the outcome measurement even when they are trying to be neutral. Blinding the data collector controls this source of bias. Blinding is achieved by taking steps to ensure that the data collectors do not know which intervention the participant received. Obviously, blinding is not always possible. Consider a study comparing the effects of two positioning protocols on the comfort level of persons with fractured hips before they have surgery. It is almost impossible to blind data collectors as to which intervention the patient is receiving because the patient will be in a position associated with one or the other of the treatments when the data collectors obtain the comfort ratings.

Any important extraneous variable that is not controlled, eliminated, or taken into account statistically becomes a confounding variable; this means that its presence affected the variables being studied so that the results do not reflect the actual relationship between the variables under investigation. In other words, the researcher failed to recognize it and it was operative undetected in what was being studied.

Low Level of Missing Data

Another potential source of bias is missing data, also referred to as *lost to follow-up*. There are a variety of reasons for not having complete data on all participants who were entered into the study and were randomized to a treatment group, including:

- Some participants dropped out of the study (e.g., moved from the area, did not want to continue in the study).
- The condition of some participants worsened so that they could not continue in the study (e.g., transferred to ICU, too sick to answer questions).
- Some participants were not available for measurement of the outcome variable at one or several data collection times (e.g., missed an appointment, could not contribute a specimen).
- The data collector failed to obtain some data (e.g., she was sick, she overlooked something).
- The burden of participating in the study was too great.

Missing data is obviously more of a problem in studies that collect outcome data over weeks, months, or years—in contrast to an intervention being delivered and the outcomes measured just once shortly thereafter. Generally, the reasons for missing data and the pattern of missing data are more important than the amount, although 20% missing data is clearly of more concern than 2% missing data. Also, random missing data is of less concern than is a pattern of missing data (Polit & Beck, 2014). Random missing data consists of values missing here and there equally across both study groups. A pattern is present when more data is missing from one group than from the other, or when more data is missing from participants with a certain characteristic, such as the youngest or the oldest.

A high level or a pattern of missing data has the potential to change the results of the study because the equivalency between the groups that was created by randomization is altered; those who dropped out might have been different from those who stayed in on an unidentified characteristic, and that difference might have an association with the outcomes being studied (Altman, 2009). The actual effect of a high level or pattern of missing data are sometimes difficult to determine. The missing data can make the intervention look more effective than it was or make it look less effective than it actually was, depending on how those who dropped out are different from those who stayed in the study and how the different characteristic is associated with the study outcomes. A high level or pattern of missing data leaves us wondering: Would the outcomes of the study have changed significantly if all persons had completed the study and contributed data?

To illustrate the previous explanation of missing data, consider a hypothetical randomized study evaluating the effectiveness of a smoking cessation method: the study had a larger dropout rate in the test intervention group than in the comparison group. If only data from those who stayed in the study were analyzed, the results may have been biased because only the people who found the test intervention agreeable would be included in the analysis. This would make the test intervention look better than it would have been had all the persons randomized to that group contributed outcome data. The researcher of such a study should ask (1) Why did so many participants drop out of the intervention group? (2) How should I analyze or interpret the data to take this into account?

Because loss to follow-up is a potential source of bias in randomized studies, the CONSORT group (Consolidated Standards of Reporting Trials), a widely recognized organization composed of experts in clinical trial methodology and reporting, addressed loss to follow-up in its guideline for reporting of randomized clinical trials. It recommends that study reports include a flow chart displaying numbers of study participants from enrollment through data analysis, as shown in **Figure 7-2**.

Ideally, researchers put in place procedures to reduce loss of participants during the study, but when it occurs, there are several options: (1) run the data analysis using data only from those with complete data or (2) estimate the missing outcome data (Altman, 2009). When the first option is used, the researcher is obligated to try to understand why the data is missing and what impact it might have had on the results. An obvious way is to look at baseline data to see if those who dropped out are in any identifiable way different from those who stayed in until study completion. There are several ways of doing the second option but all involve assumptions

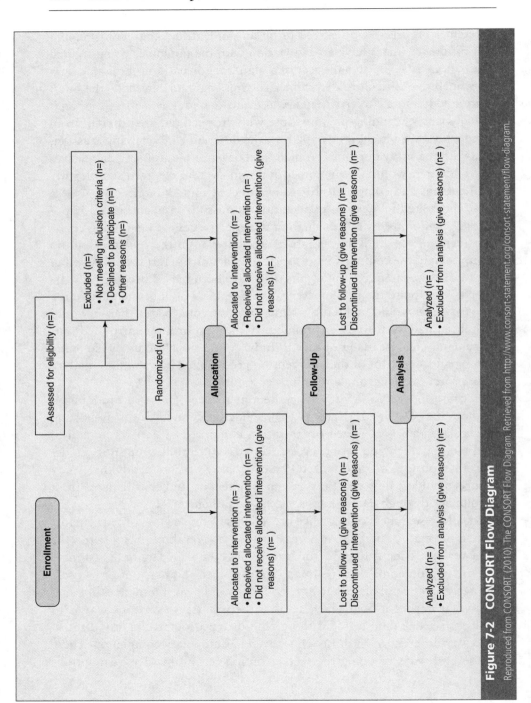

Figure 7-2   CONSORT Flow Diagram

about what scores or outcomes the lost-to-follow-up participants might have achieved. For those readers interested in the ways used to estimating values for the missing data, you could look for articles in the health literature about "intention to treat analysis."

Large numbers of dropouts and missing data also threaten the generalizability of the study's findings. For example, a randomized study of a new physical activity program for second- and third-grade inner-city children might find that the group who participated in the new program did better than those who received a placebo intervention. However, the study had a 26% dropout rate, which was evenly distributed across both treatment groups. Although the even distribution of dropouts may not have biased the study results, the benefit produced by the new program may not be realized if the program were given to all second- and third-grade inner-city kids. The high dropout rate could have produced a study sample that was not representative of the target population, and thus the generalizability of the study findings would be called into question.

While some researchers make a concerted effort to understand the impact of missing data, others, unfortunately, gloss over or ignore it. As a research consumer, you should expect the researcher to acknowledge large amounts or differential loss to follow-up proportions.

Consistent Delivery of Interventions

Two-group experiments involve actively doing something to half of the participants and something else to the other half. In research language, one group receives the experimental intervention and the other group receives a comparison intervention. The experimental intervention is usually a somewhat new intervention in that its effectiveness has not been thoroughly evaluated; however, there should be good reason to believe that it is safe and will have a meaningful impact on the outcomes of interest. The comparison intervention can take one of five forms (Kerlinger & Lee, 2000):

- No intervention at all
- A placebo intervention
- A usual care intervention
- A different intervention
- Same intervention but of different dose (i.e., intensity, frequency, or timing)

Placebo interventions are designed to look and feel similar to the intervention being tested but to not really have an effect on the outcomes being studied. At the very least, placebo interventions provide an attention activity for the comparison group to counterbalance the attention the intervention group receives. This is done because the attention involved in delivering an intervention, in and of itself, can have an impact on some outcomes. For this reason, studies of teaching or psychological support interventions often use a placebo group rather than a no intervention group.

Both the experimental and comparison interventions should be spelled out in considerable detail in advance of starting the study and consistently delivered throughout the study. Steps taken to ensure consistent delivery of the intervention include:

- Specific study protocols
- Training of those who will be delivering the intervention
- Checks on the delivery of the intervention to ensure compliance with study protocols

If either intervention morphs during the course of the study, the contrast between them will be lost. This loss of contrast will invalidate the results because the comparison the researcher set out to make will no longer exist.

Wrap-Up

In summary, an experimental study is usually sound when researchers do the following:

1. Specify the target population
2. Determine sample size by doing a power analysis
3. Use random assignment to ensure that groups are equivalent at the start of the study
4. Control extraneous influences and potential bias
5. Take steps to ensure that participants stay in the study and contribute data at all collection times
6. Ensure that interventions are delivered consistently

Use of these research methods ensures that any significant differences detected in the outcomes of the groups studied can be attributed with confidence to the difference in interventions the group received. And if no differences are found, use of these methods ensures that the lack of difference can be attributed to the fact that the two treatments do not have different impacts.

Measurement of the Outcome Variables

As the standard of "good data" (remember this from Chapter 5?) applies to experimental studies, the instruments used to measure the outcome variables should have high reliability and validity. The researcher should report the results of reliability and validity testing that has been done in prior research, particularly testing done in populations similar to the one being studied. Generally speaking, good data is produced by measurement instruments that have been rigorously developed through testing and thus have known reliability and validity levels. Instruments developed specifically for the study being reported often lack reliability and validity confirmation because they have no history.

Limitations of Randomized Experiments

The randomized experiment is the gold standard study design for determining if a healthcare intervention brings about desired outcomes. However, when clinicians read a study report of a randomized study, they often want to decide if they should use the intervention with their patients; in this regard randomized studies have limitations. The problem is that the findings of many studies often are reported as average outcomes of the two treatment groups. However, clinicians treat unique individuals, not average individuals, and thus the clinician does not know if the particular patient will respond like the average patient in the more effective study group or in a different way. Even if 80% of patients in a group respond favorably to an intervention, the clinician does not know if the patient he is treating will respond like the 80% or like the other 20%. One way used to address this is to compare the profile of those who responded favorably to the profile of those who did not and see if there are any differences.

A second limitation of randomized controlled experiments is that they may have weak generalizability resulting from the exclusion of patients with conditions other than the one of interest—as described earlier. Exclusions control extraneous variables and thereby afford more certainty about the effectiveness of the intervention. However, they pose a dilemma for clinicians in that the patients in the study may have fewer health problems (i.e., comorbidities) than do patients seen in everyday practice. As a result, the intervention itself may be difficult to use, or similar results may not be realized.

Another issue limiting the generalizability of the findings of randomized controlled experiments is that the interventions are delivered in a controlled manner, whereas in everyday practice an intervention is delivered by a diverse group of clinicians. Often it is not clear how much variation can be introduced into the delivery of an intervention and still retain its effectiveness.

These limitations do not mean that randomized controlled experiments are not useful; however, they do point to the need for multiple studies regarding an intervention—under different conditions and with diverse groups of people. The limitations also require that researchers explore deeply why some people responded very positively to an intervention, others responded in a moderately positive manner, and still others responded negatively or poorly.

Quasi-Experimental Designs

Although experimental design is the gold standard for evaluating the cause–effect relationship between an intervention and an outcome, sometimes it is *not* possible to (1) use random assignment to intervention groups; (2) have tight control over the delivery of the intervention; or (3) have a comparison group (Grove, Burns, & Gray, 2013).

Studies that lack one or more of these features are described as quasi-experimental. They are enough like experiments to retain the word *experiment* in their description, but because they lack one of the important features of experiments, they leave open the door to uncontrolled extraneous variables and wrong conclusions to an extent that experimental designs do not.

To illustrate, if two methods for preventing heel pressure ulcers were studied on one unit of a long-term care facility, the staff might have difficulty keeping the two methods pure. So, the researchers might decide to use method A with at-risk patients on one unit and method B with at-risk patients on another similar unit. This would be a quasi-experimental study because individual participants are members of intact groups (patients on a particular unit) and the unit determines which intervention they receive, not random assignment. Even when the two patient groups seem similar, there is concern that they might be different in unidentified ways or that the quality of care on the two units is different. Any difference could act as an extraneous variable giving statistical results indicative of an intervention effect on the outcome, when in actuality it was a patient or unit difference that produced the results, not the intervention. The researcher conducting such a study could take steps to identify, control, or take into account extraneous influences. These steps would include comparing the characteristics of the patients on the two units and comparing the two units on variables such as staffing pattern, years of experience of the staff, and their educational levels. Taking any differences into account in the analysis would build confidence in study results indicating that one intervention was more effective than the other in preventing heel ulcers.

Another example of a quasi-experimental design is a study in which the first 100 participants receive treatment A and the second 100 receive treatment B. This would be a consecutive series method for assigning individuals to treatment groups; thus patient-participants are not randomly assigned to treatment groups. This design also raises concerns that the two treatment groups might not be equivalent at the start. Something may have changed in the environment during the time that lapsed between the beginning of one series and the beginning of the second series, such as a seasonal difference in patients, a change in staffing, or a change in work flow. Thus, an extraneous variable could be at work and produce a difference in patient outcomes.

Generally, quasi-experimental study designs are considered weaker than randomized experimental designs because there is lack of certainty that the two groups actually were equivalent at baseline or that they received exactly the same treatment. The reader of a report of a quasi-experimental study needs to be alert to nonequivalent groups, inconsistent treatment delivery, or the presence of extraneous variables because they could distort the results and study conclusions.

Exemplar

Reading Reminder

At this point, read just the *Introduction* and *Material and Methods* sections (up to *Results*).

Canbulat, N., Ayhan, F., & Inal, S. (2015). Effectiveness of external cold and vibration for procedural pain relief during peripheral intravenous cannulation in pediatric patients. *Pain Management Nursing, 16*(1), 33–39.[1]

Original Article
Effectiveness of External Cold and Vibration for Procedural Pain Relief During Peripheral Intravenous Cannulation in Pediatric Patients

Nejla Canbulat, PhD,* Fatma Ayhan, MSc,[†] and Sevil Inal, PhD[‡]

From the *Nursing Department, Karamanovglu Mehmet Bey University, Karaman, Turkey; [†]Selcuk University, Institute of Health Science, Surgical Nursing, Konya, Turkey; [‡]Istanbul University, Health Science Faculty, Midwifery Department, Istanbul, Turkey.

Address correspondence to Nejla Canbulat, PhD, Department of Nursing, Karamanovglu Mehmet Bey University, Karaman 70100, Turkey. E-mail: ncanbulat @gmail.com

Received October 6, 2012; Revised March 12, 2014; Accepted March 17, 2014.

The authors report there are no conflicts of interest.

Abstract

The aim of this study was to investigate the effect of external cold and vibration stimulation via Buzzy on the pain and anxiety level of children during peripheral intravenous (IV) cannulation. This study was a prospective, randomized controlled trial. The sample consisted of 176 children ages 7 to 12 years who were randomly assigned to two groups: a control group that received no peripheral IV cannulation intervention and an experimental group that received external cold and vibration via Buzzy. The same nurse conducted the peripheral IV cannulation in all the children, and the same researcher applied the external cold and vibration to all the children. The external cold and the vibration were applied 1 minute before the peripheral IV cannulation procedure and continued until the end of the procedure. Preprocedural anxiety was assessed using the Children's Fear Scale, along with reports by the children, their parents, and an observer. Procedural anxiety was assessed with the Children's Fear Scale and the parents' and the observer's reports. Procedural pain was assessed using the Wong-Baker Faces Scale and the visual analog scale self-reports of the children. Preprocedural anxiety did not differ significantly. Comparison of the two groups showed significantly lower pain and anxiety levels in the experimental group than in the control group during the peripheral IV cannulation. Buzzy can be considered to provide an effective combination of coldness and vibration. This method can be used during pediatric peripheral IV cannulation by pediatric nurses.

Introduction

The simple insertion of a needle has been shown to be one of the most frightening and distressing medical procedures for hospitalized children (Baxter et al., 2011; Cohen 2008; Kolk, van Hoof, & Fiedeldij Dop, 2000). It is well known that even minor and frequently performed procedures, such as peripheral intravenous (IV) cannulation, invoke significant pain in children and increase fear and anxiety in children and their caregivers (Smith, Shah, Goldman, & Taddio, 2007). Thus, interest in the management and study of pain in children has increased in recent years. Nurses should be able to manage painful procedures to reduce their emotional and physical effects in children (Rogers & Ostrow, 2004). Various approaches to manage pain, including pharmacologic and nonpharmacologic methods, have been described (Taddio et al., 2010). Pharmacologic options, such as 5% lidocaine-prilocaine cream, 4% tetra caine gel, 4% lidocaine cream, needle-free powder lidocaine (S-Caine Patch) and iontophoresis, provide adequate cutaneous analgesia for a variety of clinical situations. However, most of these formulations have limitations, and there have been reports of adverse reactions (Pershad, Steinberg, & Waters, 2008; Sethna et al., 2005; Zempsky et al., 2008). To date, no single formulation or physical means of improving the permeation of local anesthetics has gained universal acceptance because of the aforementioned limitations (cost and duration of this application) (Sethna et al., 2005). Additionally, most current options are time consuming, costly, and require staff training (Fein & Gorelick, 2006; Leahy et al., 2008). This is a problem for busy medical settings, such as emergency departments or immunization departments (MacLean, Obispo, & Young, 2007). Nonpharmacologic techniques are generally divided into physical and behavioral techniques. Physical techniques include, but are not limited to, injections, massage, and counter-stimulation. Behavioral techniques include music distraction, cartoon distraction, communication, the valsalva maneuver, and blowing into sphygmomanometer tubing (Dutt-Gupta, Brown, & Mycama, 2007; Sinha, Tandon, & Singh, 2005).

Despite anecdotal evidence of the efficacy of these techniques, there has been very limited evaluation of these interventions for procedural pain in children (MacLaren & Cohen, 2007). An easy-to-use, inexpensive, and rapid method is needed that can ameliorate procedural pain and anxiety in busy medical settings. External cold and vibration via Buzzy (MMJ Labs, Atlanta, GA, USA) is a method that combines cooling and vibration (www.buzzy4shots.com) (Fig. 1). Buzzy was applied in an adult population during cannulation attempts and found to be effective for pain relief (Baxter, Leong, & Matthew, 2009). The Gate Control Theory may offer an explanation for the effect of cold stimulation and vibration (Melzack & Wall, 1965). This theory suggests that pain is transmitted from the peripheral nervous system to the central nervous system, where it is modulated by a gating system in the dorsal horn of the spinal cord. The afferent pain-receptive nerves (A-δ fibers carrying acute pain and unmyelinated slower C fibers carrying chronic pain messages) are blocked by fast non-noxious motion nerves (A-β) (Kakigi & Shinbasaki, 1992). Prolonged cold stimulates the C fibers and may block the A-δ pain signals. Cold also may result in enhanced activation of supraspinal mechanisms, raising the body's overall pain threshold (Nahra & Plaghki, 2005).

Only two published studies have investigated the application of the Buzzy method in pediatric populations during venipuncture (Baxter et al., 2011; Inal & Kelleci, 2012). There have been no published studies of the application of this method in pediatric populations during peripheral IV cannulation. The aim of this study was to investigate the effects of external cold and vibration via Buzzy on pain and anxiety levels during peripheral IV cannulation in children aged 7 to 12 years.

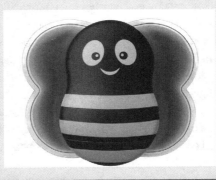

Figure 1   Buzzy

Courtesy of MMJ Labs. Retrieved from www.buzzy4shots.com.

Research Hypotheses

Hypothesis 1: Buzzy reduces procedural pain felt during peripheral IV cannulation in pediatric patients.

Hypothesis 2: Buzzy reduces procedural anxiety felt during peripheral IV cannulation in pediatric patients.

Material and Methods

The study was conducted in the Pediatric Surgical Department of the Maternal and Child Hospital in Karaman, Turkey, between July and September 2012. This was a randomized clinical trial. Informed consent was obtained from each child's parents.

During the peripheral IV cannulation, the nurse used the dorsum of the child's left or right hand, depending on whether the child was left or right handed. In left-handed children, the peripheral IV cannulation was inserted in the dorsum of the right hand. In right-handed children, it was inserted in the dorsum of the left hand. External cold and vibration stimulation were applied with Buzzy. Buzzy is a reusable $8 \times 5 \times 2.5$-cm plastic bee containing a battery and vibrating motor. Buzzy was designed especially for pain control in children and adults. An ice pack is placed under the device. The combination of coldness and vibration with Buzzy is considered more effective than the use of cold or vibration. In Turkey, routine nonpharmacologic methods are not used to reduce the pain and anxiety associated with peripheral IV cannulation.

Sample

The inclusion criteria were patients aged 7 to 12 years who required peripheral IV cannulation. Potential participants were excluded if there was a break or abrasion on the skin where the device would be placed. Additional exclusion criteria were nerve damage in the affected extremity, critical or chronic illness or poor health, neurodevelopmental delays, verbal difficulties, use of an analgesic within the last 6 hours, or a history of syncope due to blood specimen collection or immunization. None of the children had any prior experience of peripheral IV cannulation.

Ethical Considerations

This study was approved by the Ethical Commission of Selcuk University Selcuklu Medical. Faculty, Konya (06. 26.2012/115). The aim and the method of the study were explained to the children and their parents, and they were informed that if they did not want to continue, they could withdraw from the study without stating a reason.

Procedure

This study was conducted with one volunteer nurse trained by the researcher. The nurse had 5 years of experience in pediatric patient care and peripheral IV cannulation. The nurse had no monetary interest. The nurse was informed about the study at the beginning. The preprocedural and procedural fear and anxiety levels of the children were assessed via self-parental and observer reports. The data were obtained by interviewing the children, their parents, and the observer. The Children's Fear Scale (CFS) was used for this purpose. The CFS is a well-established method for evaluating pediatric fear and anxiety. It rates fear and anxiety on a 5-point scale and consists of five cartoon faces that range from a neutral expression (0 = no anxiety) to a frightened face (4 = severe anxiety) (McMurtry, Noel, Chambers, & McGrath 2011). The responses of the children, their parents, and the observers were scored blindly.

The children's pain levels immediately after the peripheral IV cannulation procedure were also assessed via self-reports using the Wong-Baker Faces Scale (WBFC [sic]) and the visual analog scale (VAS) (Hockenberry & Wilson, 2009; Wewers & Lowe, 1990). The WBFC [sic] is a scale ranging from 0 to 10, consisting of six cartoon faces that range from a neutral expression (0 = very happy/no pain) to a screaming face (10 = hurts more than you can imagine) (Hockenberry & Wilson, 2009). The VAS is a measurement instrument that tries to measure a characteristic or attitude that is believed to range across a continuum of values and cannot easily be measured directly. For example, the amount of pain that a patient feels ranges across a continuum from none to an extreme amount of pain. The VAS is usually a horizontal line, 100 mm in length, anchored by word descriptors at each end. The child marks on the line the point that he or she feels represents his or her perception of the current state. The VAS score is determined by measuring in millimeters from the left-hand end of the line to the point that the child marks (Wewers & Lowe, 1990).

The same nurse conducted the peripheral IV cannulation procedure in all cases. The same researcher applied the external cold and vibration stimulation via Buzzy (Fig. 2).

The children (N = 220) and their parents were informed about the purpose and the content of the study and asked if they would volunteer to participate in the study. Of the 220 children, 176 children and their parents agreed to participate. All the parents signed a research consent form. Background information about demographics, medical history, recent analgesics, and body mass index (BMI) were collected via self-report forms. Before randomization, the researcher read a standard script to explain the pain and anxiety measures. The parents and the observer (the researcher) assessed the children's anxiety levels. The 176 children were randomized using a computer generated table of random numbers into two equal groups:

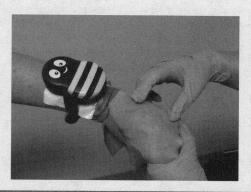

Figure 2   An example of the use of Buzzy

Courtesy of MMJ Labs. Retrieved from www.buzzy4shots.com.

an experimental group and a control group (n = 88 for each group). The control group received no intervention. The experimental group received external cold and vibration stimulation via Buzzy. The dorsum of the child's hand area was cleaned and cannulated with Buzzy. Buzzy was administered about 5 cm above the application area just before the procedure, and the vibration was continued until the end of the procedure.

Data Analysis

Data were analyzed with SPSS version 15.00 (SPSS, Inc., Chicago, IL, USA). A *p* value < .05 was considered significant. Parametric data, such as the pain and anxiety levels of the children, were compared with the Student's t test. Nonparametric data, such as sex and mother's and father's education, were compared with frequency and χ comparisons.

Results

The study was conducted between July and September 2012. One hundred seventy-six children aged 7 to 12 years (8.43 ± 1.61 years) and their parents volunteered to participate in the study. There were no differences between the two groups in terms of age, sex, BMI, and preprocedural anxiety according to the self, the parents', and the observer's reports (*p* > .05) (Table 1).

When pain and anxiety levels were compared with an independent sample *t* test, consistent with hypothesis 1, the children in the external cold and vibration stimulation group had significantly lower pain levels than the control group according to their self-reports (both WBFC [*sic*] and VAS scores; *pp* < .001) (Table 2).

Table 1   Comparison of Groups in Terms of Variables that May Affect Procedural Pain and Anxiety Levels

Characteristic	Buzzy (n = 88)	Control (n = 88)	χ^2 p
Sex			
Female (%) n	11 (12.5)	13 (14.8)	.82
Male (%) n	77 (87.5)	75 (85.2)	.41

Characteristic	Buzzy (n = 88)	Control (n = 88)	t p
Age (mean ± SD)	8.25 ± 1.51	8.61 ± 1.69	−1.498 .136
BMI (mean ± SD)	25.41 ± 6.74	26.94 ± 8.68	−1.309 .192
Preprocedural anxiety			
Self-report (mean ± SD)	2.03 ± 1.29	2.11 ± 1.58	−0.364 .716
Parent report (mean ± SD)	2.11 ± 1.20	2.17 ± 1.42	−0.285 .776
Observer report (mean ± SD)	2.18 ± 1.17	2.24 ± 1.37	−0.295 .768

BMI = body mass index

Consistent with hypothesis 2, the external cold and vibration stimulation group had significantly lower fear and anxiety levels than the control group, according to the parents' and the observer's reports ($p < .001$) (Table 3).

Table 2   Comparison of Groups' Procedural Pain Levels During Peripheral IV Cannulation

	Buzzy (n = 88)	Control (n = 88)	tp
Procedural self-reported pain with WBFS (mean ± SD)	2.75 ± 2.68	5.70 ± 3.31	−6.498 0.000
Procedural self-reported pain with VAS (mean ± SD)	1.66 ± 1.95	4.09 ± 3.21	−6.065 0.000

IV = intravenous; VAS = visual analog scale; WBFS = Wong-Baker Faces Scale

Table 3 Comparison of Groups' Procedural Anxiety Levels During Peripheral IV Cannulation

Procedural child anxiety	Buzzy (n = 88)	Control (n = 88)	*tp*
Parent reported (mean ± SD)	0.94 ± 1.06	2.09 ± 1.39	−6.135 0.000
Observer reported (mean ± SD)	0.92 ± 1.03	2.14 ± 1.34	−6.745 0.000

IV = intravenous

Discussion

Pain experienced during medical procedures that are routinely performed in hospitals, such as phlebotomy, immunization, and IV cannulation, can cause stress, fear, and anxiety in children (Cassidy et al., 2001; Razzaq, 2006). These procedures also may cause anxiety and fear in the family members of these children (Cohen, 2008; Shavit & Hershman, 2004). Although procedural pain and anxiety levels may be influenced by the type of procedure applied (Rawe et al., 2009), they also are associated with a number of individual factors, including the child's and parents' emotional status, previous experiences, and physicians' skills. The American Society for Pain Management Nursing recommends that optimal pain control before and during painful procedures be provided (Czarnecki et al., 2011). Therefore, pharmacologic and nonpharmacologic approaches are recommended to control pain and the resulting future anxiety behavior (Schechter et al., 2007).

The results of this study suggest that external cold and vibration stimulation via Buzzy are effective for reducing pain and anxiety in children during peripheral IV cannulation. Studies reported that children who had frequently experienced needlesticks reported less pain than children who had experienced few needle-sticks (Inal & Kelleci, 2012; McCarty & Kleiber, 2006). In this study, the children in both groups were similar in terms of the factors that might influence pain perception, such as age, sex, BMI, and levels of preprocedural anxiety.

This supports the efficiency of the external cold and vibration stimulation method via Buzzy in reducing pain and anxiety levels of children. Previous research has shown the long-term negative effects of early pain experiences in children (Thurgate & Heppell, 2005). Another study demonstrated that reduction increases patient satisfaction during needle procedures (Magaret, Clark, Warden, Magnusson, & Hedges, 2002). Although a large number of pharmacologic and nonpharmacologic methods have been used for pain relief during medical procedures in the past, and many methods are employed in the present, there is no single integrated intervention to optimize pain relief. A widely used pharmacologic method for pain relief is topical anesthetics (O'Brien, Taddio, Ipp, Goldbach, & Koren, 2004) during peripheral IV cannulation. In a pilot study conducted by Baxter et al. (2009), external thermo-mechanical stimulation via cold application and vibration was applied to adults during cannula placement. The researchers compared pain reduction with external cold and vibration stimulation with that of the Vapocoolant spray. Compared with a control group, where no means of pain reduction was used, both methods were found to be effective. There was no statistically significant difference between the Vapocoolant spray and the external cold and vibration stimulation in terms of pain reduction. In another randomized controlled study conducted by Baxter et al. (2011), external cold and vibration stimulation were found to be as effective as the Vapocoolant spray (the standard procedure) for pain relief in children during IV access. Inal and Kelleci (2012) reported that the application of external cold and vibration stimulation via Buzzy are effective in relieving pain and anxiety in children during blood specimen collection. In our study, the pain and anxiety levels of the Buzzy group were lower than those of the control group. It is widely accepted that most children who previously experienced a painful medical procedure also perceive fear and anxiety in future procedures. Therefore, decreasing the emotional effects of painful procedures in clinical practice with better pain control is essential in children. To avoid future undesirable effects of painful medical procedures, successful pain control should be the objective in all procedures.

Conclusion

The application of external cold and vibration stimulation were effective in relieving pain and anxiety in children during peripheral IV cannulation. Therefore, it can be concluded that this method may be routinely used during peripheral IV cannulation in children. Nurses need to be aware of procedural anxiety and pain during peripheral IV cannulation. Interventions should be implemented to decrease anxiety and pain in children. Nurses can use external cold and vibration stimulation for pain and anxiety relief in children during peripheral IV cannulation. This study contributes to the literature on quick-acting and effective non-pharmacologic measures for pain reduction.

Limitations

There are three significant limitations in the current investigation. First, this study was not double-blind. Researchers had information on which child was in which study group. To correct researcher bias, the pain and anxiety levels were not assessed by the researchers.

Second, the parents may have anticipated specific results because they were informed about our hypothesis. Thus, placebo effects were not controlled. This could have biased our results by affecting the reports of the parents and the observer reports. Third, the nurse who participated in the study was not selected randomly. This could have influenced the usual care process.

Acknowledgments

The authors acknowledge the participating children and their parents of this study.

References

Baxter, A. L., Cohen, L. L., McElvery, H. L., Lawson, M. L., & von Baeyer, C. L. (2011). An Integration of vibration and cold relieves venipuncture pain in a pediatric emergency Department. *Pediatric Emergency Care, 27*(12), 1151–1156.

Baxter, A. L., Leong, T., & Matthew, B. (2009). External thermomechanical stimulation versus Vapocoolant for adult venipuncture pain: Pilot data on a novel device. *The Clinical Journal of Pain, 25*(8), 705–710.

Cassidy, K. L., Reid, G. J., McGrath, P. J., Smith, D. J., Brown, T. L., & Finley, G. A. (2001). A randomized double-blind, placebo-controlled trial of the EMLA patch for the reduction of pain associated with intramuscular injection in four to six-year-old children. *Acta Paediatrica, 90*(11), 1329–1336.

Cohen, L. L. (2008). Behavioral approaches to anxiety and pain management for pediatric venous access. *Pediatrics, 122*(3, Suppl.), S134–S139.

Czarnecki, M. L., Turner, H., Collins, P. M., Doellman, D., Wrona, S., & Reynolds, J. (2011). Procedural pain management: A position statement with clinical practice recommendations. *Pain Management Nursing, 12*(2), 95–111.

Dutt-Gupta, J., Brown, T., & Mycama, M. (2007). Effect of communication on pain during intravenous cannulation: A randomized control trial. *BJA, 99*(6), 871–879.

Fein, J. A., & Gorelick, M. H. (2006). The decision to use topical anesthetic for intravenous insertion in the pediatric emergency department. *Academic Emergency Medicine, 13*(3), 264–268.

Hockenberry, M. J., & Wilson, D. (2009). *Wong's Essentials of Pediatric Nursing,* (8th Edition). St. Louis: Mosby.

Inal, S., & Kelleci, M. (2012). Relief of pain during blood specimen collection in pediatric patients. MCN. *The American Journal of Maternal Child Nursing, 37(5), 339–345.*

Kakigi, R., & Shinbasaki, H. (1992). Mechanisms of pain relief by vibration and movement. *Journal of Neurology, Neurosurgery & Psychiatry, 55, 282–286.*

Kolk, A. M., van Hoof, R., & Fiedeldij Dop, M. J. (2000). Preparing children for venepuncture. The effect of an integrated intervention on distress before and during venepuncture. *Child: Care, Health and Development, 26*(3), 251–260.

Leahy, S., Kennedy, R. M., Hesselgrave, J., Gurwitch, K., Barkey, M., & Millar, T. F. (2008). On the front lines: Lessons learned in pediatric hospitals. *Pediatrics, 122*(3, Suppl), 161–170.

MacLaren, J. E., & Cohen, L. (2007). Interventions for paediatric procedure-related pain in primary care. *Paediatrics and Child Health, 12*(2), 111–116.

MacLean, S., Obispo, J., & Young, K. D. (2007). The gap between pediatric emergency department procedural pain management treatments available and actual practice. *Pediatric Emergency Care, 23*(2), 87–93.

Magaret, N. D., Clark, T. A., Warden, C. R., Magnusson, R., & Hedges, J. R. (2002). Patient satisfaction in the emergency department—a survey of pediatric patients and their parents. *Academic Emergency Medicine, 9*(12), 1379–1388.

McCarty, A. M., & Kleiber, C. (2006). A conceptual model of factors influencing children's responses to a painful procedure when parents are distraction coaches. *Journal of Pediatric Nursing, 21*(2), 88–98.

McMurtry, C. M., Noel, M., Chambers, C. T., & McGrath, P. J. (2011). Children's fear during procedural pain: Preliminary investigation of the Children's Fear Scale. *Health Psychology, 30*(6), 780–788.

Melzack, R., & Wall, P. D. (1965). Pain mechanisms: A new theory. *Science, 150*(3699), 971–979.

Nahra, H., & Plaghki, L. (2005). Innocuous skin cooling modulates perception and neurophysiological correlates of brief CO_2 laser stimuli in humans. *European Journal of Pain, 9,* 521–530.

O'Brien, L., Taddio, A., Ipp, M., Goldbach, M., & Koren, G. (2004). Topical 4% amethocaine gel reduces the pain of subcutaneous measles–mumps–rubella vaccination. *Pediatrics, 114,* e720–e724.

Pershad, J., Steinberg, S. C., & Waters, T. M. (2008). Cost-effectiveness analysis of anesthetic agents during peripheral intravenous cannulation in the pediatric emergency department. *Archive of Pediatric and Adolescent Medicine, 162*(10), 952–961.

Rawe, C., Trame, C. D., Moddeman, G., O'Malley, P., Biteman, K., Dalton, T., & Walker, S. (2009). Management of procedural pain: Empowering nurses to care for patients through clinical nurse specialist consultation and intervention. *Clinical Nurse Specialist CNS, 23*(3), 131–137.

Razzaq, Q. (2006). The underuse of analgesia and sedation in pediatric emergency medicine. Annals of Saudi Medicine, *26(5), 375–381.*

Rogers, T. L., & Ostrow, C. L. (2004). The use of EMLA cream to decrease venipuncture pain in children. *Journal of Pediatric Nursing, 19,* 33–39.

Schechter, N. L., Zempsky, W. T., Cohen, L. L., McGrath, P. J., McMurtry, C. M., & Bright, N. S. (2007). Pain reduction during pediatric immunizations: Evidence-based review and recommendations. *Pediatrics, 119*(5), 1184–1198.

Sethna, N. V., Verghese, S. T., Hannallah, R. S., Solodiuk, J. C., Zurakowski, D., & Berde, C. B. (2005). A randomized controlled trial to evaluate S-Caine Patch™ for reducing pain associated with vascular access in children. *Anesthesiology, 102,* 403–408.

Shavit, I., & Hershman, E. (2004). Management of children undergoing painful procedures in the emergency department by non-anesthesiologists. *The Israel Medical Association Journal: IMAJ, 6*(6), 350–355.

Sinha, P. K., Tandon, A. A., & Singh, S. D. (2005). Evaluating the efficacy of valsalva manuever on venous cannulation pain: A prospective randomized study. *Anaesthesia and Analgesia, 101*(4), 1230–1232.

Smith, R. W., Shah, V., Goldman, R. D., & Taddio, A. (2007). Caregivers' responses to pain in their children in the emergency department. *Archives of Pediatric and Adolescent Medicine, 161*(6), 578–582.

Taddio, A., Appleton, M., Bortolussi, R., Chambers, C., Dubey, V., Halperin, S., Hanrahan, A., Ipp, M., Lockett, D., Macdonald, N., Midmer, D., Mousmanis, P., Palda, V., Pielak, K., Riddell, R. P., Rieder, M., Scott, J., & Shah, V. (2010). Reducing the pain of childhood vaccination: An evidence-based clinical practice guideline. *Canadian Medical Association Journal, 182*(18), 43–55.

Thurgate, C., & Heppell, S. (2005). Needle phobia-changing venepuncture practice in ambulatory care. *Paediatric Nursing, 17*(9), 15–18.

Wewers, M. E., & Lowe, N. K. (1990). A critical review of visual analogue scales in the measurement of clinical phenomena. *Research in Nursing and Health, 13,* 227–236.

Zempsky, W. T., Bean-Lijewski, J., Kauffman, R. E., Koh, J. L., Malviya, S. V., Rose, J. B., Richards, P. T., & Gennevols, D. J. (2008). Needle-free powder lidocaine delivery system provides rapid effective analgesia for venipuncture or cannulation pain in children: Randomized, double-blind comparison of venipuncture and venous cannulation pain after fast-onset needle-free powder lidocaine or placebo treatment trial. *Pediatrics, 121*(5), 979–987.

Profile & Commentary: Why and How

STUDY PURPOSE

As the authors of this study note, various methods have been tried to control pain in children during venipuncture, including distraction and topical anesthetics. Buzzy is a commercial product that uses a small frozen ice pack and vibration to block pain sensations from the area where the IV cannula will be placed. It probably also provides an element of distraction for some children. "The aim of this study was to investigate the effect of external cold and vibration via Buzzy on pain and anxiety levels during peripheral IV cannulation in children aged 7 to 12 years" (p. 34). Two more specific research hypotheses are then stated. So, the purposes of this study are quite straightforward.

METHODS

Ethical Review   First the date and the site of data collection is noted as is the fact that the study was approved by the university Ethical Commission, presumably similar to an institutional review board (IRB) in the United States. As this study involved collecting data from children, there may have been special conditions that had to be met for approval by the ethical commission. In the United States, when children age 7 or older are involved in research, IRBs generally require the assent of the child as well as the written permission of the parent(s). The child's assent is required when the child has the capacity to comprehend what the study will require of her or him; parents must give permission before the researcher contacts the child for assent (U.S. Department of Health and Human Services, n.d.).

In this study, having the IV cannula placed was not a research variable as all participants had an IV cannula placed as part of their treatment plan; thus the need for IV cannula placement was one of the inclusion criteria. The study required the child and the parents to (1) answer several questions before and after the procedure; (2) agree to randomization; and (3) allow the Buzzy device to be put in place if assigned to the experimental group. So the study itself did not do anything to the child that was hurtful, invasive, or risky and imposed only a very low burden of effort on child and parent. Thus, it was a low-risk study. We don't know exactly how all this was handled, but the authors inform us that before randomization, the researcher read a standardized script to the parent and child. Presumably that script explained randomization and what was involved in participating; it was undoubtedly required or at least reviewed by the Ethical Commission.

Sample   The inclusion criteria were children 7 to 12 years old whose care required peripheral IV cannulation and who had not had prior experience of IV cannulation. The latter is important because prior experience (good or bad) could be an extraneous variable in that it could affect the child's level of preinsertion anxiety and reaction to having the IV inserted. So, the researchers controlled its potential influence by eliminating it all together. The list of exclusion criteria was fairly long, but understandable in that they excluded children who might have an unusual reaction to the IV insertion procedure and thereby affect the outcomes that were evaluated. The children were recruited in the pediatric surgical department of a maternal and child health hospital. From the information provided, we can't determine if they were same-day surgery patients or inpatients or a combination thereof, but the exclusion criteria would seem to limit the sample to basically healthy children.

I would note that there is no information pertaining to how the sample size of 176 was arrived at. As explained earlier, generally it is desirable to determine sample size by doing a power analysis. We don't know why this was not done, but the sample size is large, and given the results, the study was not underpowered.

Interventions   The experimental treatment involved placing the Buzzy device prior to starting the placement of the IV cannula. The placement of the Buzzy device is well-described in the report. The control group received usual care, which consisted of no pain control intervention. Importantly, the same nurse did all the IV placements and the same researcher applied the device in all cases.

Data Collection and Measurement   Before the IV procedure started, the researcher collected a few pieces of information and obtained ratings of the child's preprocedure anxiety using the Children's Fear Scale (CFS) from the child, parent, and an observer. Then the Buzzy device was placed (or not) and the IV cannula was inserted. Immediately after the procedure, the child was asked to rate his pain during the procedure using two measures, the Wong-Baker Faces Scale (WBFS) and a visual analogue scale (VAS). The parent and the observer (the researcher) then rated the child's anxiety during the procedure.

SEQUENCE OF MEASUREMENTS

Preprocedure	After Procedure
	Pain (by child)
	WBFS (0–10) and VAS (0–10)
Anxiety (by child, parent, and observer)	Anxiety (by parent and observer)
CFS (0–4)	CFS (0–4)

The authors do not provide information about the reliability and validity of the CFS; rather, they describe it as "a well-established method for evaluating pediatric fear and anxiety" (p. 35). This claim is easily checked out by a search for information pertaining to it. And, indeed, it is widely used. In addition, I was able to quickly identify several studies evaluating its reliability and validity. One of these, which actually was cited in the article (McMurty, Noel, Chambers, & McGrath, 2011), found that the CFS had a high positive relationship with several other measures of children's fear (validity); a high correlation between children's rating at the time of an event and their rating of it 2 weeks later (test-retest reliability); and a moderate correlation between child and parent ratings (interrater reliability). So, the CFS produces good data. Do note that the CFS is a 5-point scale (0 to 4).

The Wong Baker Faces Scale (WBFS), with scores from 0 to 10, is also widely used. Wong and Baker (1988) tested the scale with 150 hospitalized children and found acceptable levels of validity and test-retest reliability. More recently, its validity was established by its high correlation with a visual analogue scale in older children in an emergency department (Garra et al., 2009).

Visual analog scales (VASs) are widely used to evaluate pain in clinical practice. In a review of the theoretical and empirical studies of single-item measures (which VASs are), the reviewer concluded that single-item measures in general can be valid and reliable measures of multidimensional concepts, which pain is (Patrician, 2004). Just a bit of a heads up: In the description of the VAS in the Buzzy article, it says that it is "a horizontal line 100 mm in length, anchored by word descriptors at each end" (p. 35). First we aren't informed about what the word anchors used were, and secondly one needs to remember that 100 mm = 10 cm. The latter point is important because in Table 2 the VAS mean scores are reported in centimeters (possible scores being 0 to 10).

All in all, I would conclude that the instruments used in this study have been found to have acceptable reliability and validity.

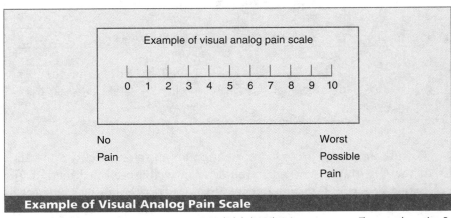

Example of Visual Analog Pain Scale

Reproduced from Portenoy, R.K., & Kanner, R.M. (Eds.). (1996). Pain management: Theory and practice. By permission of Oxford University Press.

Section 2: Study Results

More Effective?

In most two-group experimental studies, the researcher's goal is to determine if one intervention is more effective than the other. Effectiveness is defined as impact or influence on the outcome variable(s), and more effectiveness is a greater degree of positive impact or influence. There are two ways of thinking about effectiveness: from the clinical perspective and from the statistical perspective. At the center of both perspectives is a comparison of the size of the effect each intervention had on the outcome variable of the two groups. From the clinical perspective, the bottom line question is, "Is the difference in the outcomes of the two groups large enough to be clinically meaningful to patients or to how I practice?" This perspective on the data is also referred to as the *importance* or *practical significance* of the results. From the statistical perspective the bottom line question is, "Is the difference found a true difference that is likely in the target population or a chance difference unique to this sample?" When reading a report of an intervention study, too many people get hung up in the results of the statistical analysis (e.g., *p*-values, statistical significance). I suggest that you start by first considering at the results from a clinical perspective and then proceed to considering the meaning of the statistical tests of significance.

Generally speaking, the results of 2-group experimental studies are reported in one of two ways:

1. As the mean scores of the two groups on the outcome variable
2. As the percentage of persons in each group who achieved a clinical outcome or milestone

Some studies report just mean scores and no percentages attaining particular clinical outcomes; whereas other studies report attainment of clinical outcome attainment percentages and no mean scores. A few studies report both.

Outcome Reported as a Mean

When the outcome variable of a study is measured on an interval-level scale, a score is obtained for every patient, and group means and/or medians are calculated for the control group and for the intervention group. The term *score* refers to the numerical values obtained by all forms of measurement, be it physiological measurement, questionnaires, or rating scales. The explanations below will focus on means although the general principles could also be applied to medians, the other measure of central tendency. If you are not sure when medians are used instead of means and the inferential tests used in analyzing them, you should consult a basic statistics book.

Clinical Perspective on Mean Differences

To make clinical sense of the results, you should first note the difference between the means of the two groups by subtracting one from the other—keeping in mind the range of the scale that was used to measure the variable. Then ask: Is this difference large enough to have clinical importance? For example:

- Is a mean difference 950 cc per day difference between the mean fluid intakes of two groups large enough to make a difference in patients' hydration status?
- Is a mean 8 mm difference between mean diastolic blood pressure levels of two groups large enough to represent better blood pressure control and lowered risk of complications?
- Is a mean 10-meter increase in distance walked in 6 minutes after a 12-week exercise program compared to a control group mean increase of 5.6 meters (increase over control = 4.4 meters) enough of a difference to have an impact on patients' daily functioning (Li, Xu, Zhou, Li, & Wang, 2015)?

Consideration of the size of the difference between the means of the two groups provides some clinical sense of whether the difference in the impact of the two treatments is large, small, or somewhere in between. Do remember that the size of the difference is a point estimate based on the sample and that the difference found in the population could be a somewhat lower or higher. If the researcher provides a confidence interval (**Figure 7-3**) around the difference in the means, that would give you a better sense of the high and low of that might be realized in the target population (DiCenso, Guyatt, & Ciliska, 2005).

The take-away: Thinking about the difference in means between the two groups from a clinical/practical perspective is a useful starting point for making practical sense of results.

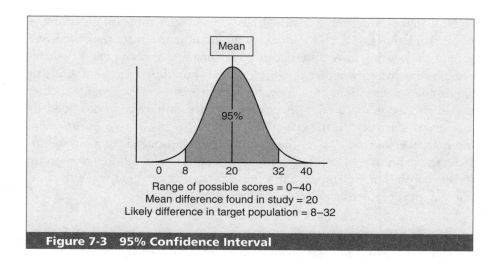

Figure 7-3 95% Confidence Interval

Statistical Perspective on Mean Differences

When an outcome variable of a study is measured on an interval level scale and the results are reported as the means of each group, the statistical analysis provides information useful in answering the question: *Is the difference between the means of the two groups a true difference or a chance difference?* A true difference between the mean scores of the two groups is a difference that is robust enough that a difference is also likely to occur in the target population, not just in the study sample; the difference found in the population could be higher or lower than what was found in the study, but it is likely a difference will be found. A chance difference is caused by the normal variation in outcomes one would expect when measuring an outcome in two samples drawn from the same population; it is unlikely that a difference would be found in the target population.

In an experimental study, the two groups received different treatments; therefore a difference in outcome scores is of interest. A treatment effect is present when one treatment produces a larger effect on the outcome than the other treatment does. The larger the difference found between the outcome mean of the two groups, the greater the chance that the difference is caused by one group receiving a treatment that was truly more effective than the other. Moreover, the larger the difference in the means of the two groups, the greater the likelihood that a difference would be found if the whole target population had been studied.

Note that even for the statistical question, your starting point is common sense. Sometimes, just by looking at the outcome mean scores of the two groups and noting how different or close they are, you can get a first impression regarding whether the difference is caused by treatment effect or is just chance variation. However, the definitive answer regarding whether the difference is a true difference or a chance difference is provided by inferential statistics. In the comparison of the scores of two groups with interval level outcome data, the *p*-value result produced by a *t*-test provides the definitive answer regarding interpretation of a difference in group mean scores. (Do remember that different statistics are used when the outcome data is reported as group median scores.)

> **The *t*-test results provide the definitive answer regarding whether a difference in mean effectiveness is likely in the target population.**

t-Test and *p*-Value   The *t*-test is used to compare scores of two groups when the outcome variable is measured using an interval level scale and the mean is the average being analyzed; it should not be used when the data are skewed or when the outcome variable is a proportion or a categorical variable. The *t*-test analyzes the size of the difference between the means of two groups while taking into account the sample size and the spread of the scores across the possible range of scores (i.e., the standard deviation). It essentially asks: Even though a difference in means was found in this sample, what are the chances that *no* difference would be found in the target population?

The *t*-test analysis produces a *p*-value indicating the probability that the difference found between the means is just a chance occurrence. This data-based *p*-value probability is then compared to a previously chosen level of significance *p*-level decision point. A *p*-value at or lower than the decision point represents low probabilities that the difference found is just a chance difference; a *p*-value higher than the decision point represents high levels of risk that the difference found is a chance difference. Thus, if the data-based *p*-value is equal to or lower than the decision point *p*-level, the researcher will conclude that the difference found is a true difference; i.e., a difference would likely be found in the population as well as in this sample. In contrast, if the data-based *p*-value is higher than the decision point *p*-level, the researcher will conclude that the difference found is a chance difference, i.e., no difference is likely to occur in the population.

The researcher does not want to wrongly conclude that a difference is a true difference when in reality it is a chance difference; by only accepting a low level of probability that the difference is a chance difference, he or she can be quite confident when saying, "This is a true difference." Often, but not always, the level of significance decision point is set at 0.05. By setting it there, the researcher is accepting a 5% or less risk of being wrong when he or she says the difference found is a true difference.

So, let's say the researcher set the level of significance decision point at $p = 0.05$ and the data-based p-value comes in at 0.03. The researcher had decided in advance that she would be willing to accept a 5% chance of being wrong when concluding that the difference found is not just a chance occurrence, and the result of $p = 0.03$ indicates there is just a 3% chance that she would be wrong. So, the researcher says, "Okay, I'm confident in concluding that the difference found between the two groups is a true difference. I so conclude because there is only a 3% chance that I am wrong in doing so." In research lingo, a result like this would be reported as, "The difference found was statistically significant at the $p \leq 0.05$ level."

In contrast, consider the situation in which the researcher also sets the level of significance decision point at $p = 0.05$ but the data-based p-value comes in at 0.08. This result means that the researcher was willing to accept a 5% chance of being wrong when concluding that the difference found was a true difference, but the difference found results in an 8% chance that she would be wrong in concluding that the difference found is a true difference. In this situation, the researcher will think, "If I conclude this is a true difference, there is too high a probability of being wrong. Therefore, I am going to conclude that the difference found could be a chance occurrence and no difference would likely be found in the population." A result like this would be reported as not significant (ns). The contrasting types of statistical results just described are portrayed graphically in **Figure 7-4**. Hopefully, it will make these complex issues a bit clearer.

Scenario   A hypothetical study tested the effects of two different methods of reducing discomfort in adults while freezing a precancerous lesion on the lower leg with liquid nitrogen (method A and method B); the person's pain experience during the freezing was determined immediately after the procedure using a scale with a value range of 0 to 10 (0 being no pain, 10 being a great deal of pain). Group A ($n = 42$) had a mean score of 3.6 and group B ($n = 40$) had a mean of 4.6, indicating that those in the method A group had on average less pain. A t-test was run on the difference

Data-based p-value	< .001	.01	.025	**.05**	.08	.15	.59 >
Finding	Significant difference				Not significant difference		
Conclusion	A difference would likely be found in the population.				A difference would *not* likely be found in the population.		

*Using a .05 level of significance decision point

Figure 7-4   Interpretation of p-Values Produced by t-Tests

between the means (1 point), and the result was $p = 0.02$. This is the data-based probability value; it indicates there are only 2 chances in 100 that a difference this large would occur because of chance variation. Said differently, if the researcher concluded that method A was more effective than method B, there would be 2 chances in 100 that his or her conclusion is wrong. When this data-based probability is compared to the decision point level of significance probability ($p = 0.05$), the conclusion would be that it is a true difference in outcome, because there is an acceptably low probability that the difference is just chance variation. See the Scenario 1 summary in **Table 7-1**.

Consider a different result for this same study: Group A had a mean of 3.6, group B had a mean of 3.8, and $p = 0.14$ (Scenario 2 in Table 7-1). Now, the difference is just 0.2 and there are 14 chances in 100 that the difference was a chance result. With this result, *if* the researcher concluded that the difference is a true difference, there would be 14 chances in 100 that his conclusion would be wrong. Based on the researcher's chosen level of significance decision point ($p \leq 0.05$), this is too high a chance of being wrong, so the researcher would conclude the two methods of comforting are essentially equivalent; i.e., a difference in effectiveness is doubtful, the difference found is not significant.

Summary of p-Values   A difference in means associated with a low p-value (i.e., a data-based p-value that is equal to or below the decision

TABLE 7-1   Statistical Conclusions

Scenario 1	Group A	Group B	
Mean pain level	3.6	4.6	
Difference in the means	1		
Level of significance p-level			0.05
Data-based $p =$			0.02
Conclusion		→	True difference
Probability that conclusion is wrong			2%

Scenario 2	Group A	Group B	
Mean pain level	3.6	3.8	
Difference in the means		.2	
Level of significance p-level			0.05
Data-based $p =$			0.14
Conclusion		→	Chance difference
Probability that conclusion is wrong			Not easily calculated

point p-level) is considered statistically significant; it is a true difference in treatment effectiveness, meaning that a difference would likely be found in the population as well. A difference with a high p-value (i.e., a data-based p-value that is above the decision point p-level) is considered to be a not significant difference, meaning the probability that it is a chance difference is high; a difference would most likely not be found in the population. In study reports, the statistics just described are reported in a variety of ways. The absolute difference between the means of the two groups' outcomes may or may not be stated, but it can be easily calculated by subtracting the mean of one group from the mean of the other. The t-value may or may not be reported, but in and of itself, it is not of importance to the clinical reader. However, the p-value associated with a t-test or an indication of whether the difference is statistically significant will almost always be provided in the text or indicated by a symbol in a table.

BOX 7-1   Example of *p*-Value Interpretation

In a randomized controlled trial of the efficacy of a breathing training program on depression in patients on hemodialysis (Tsai et al., 2015), the participants who received breathing training showed a mean reduction 3.69 points on their depression score whereas the control group had a 1.48 mean reduction. The difference was significant at the $p = 0.01$ level. Thus, there is just 1 chance in 100 that a difference in depression would not be found in the larger population.

Reporting of *p*-Values   Researchers aim to present their results in ways that are both honest and favorable. For that reason, you will see a variety of adjectives used to describe the significance of results. When the researcher had preset the level of significance *p*-level at 0.05 and the data-based *p*-value comes in at 0.02 or 0.03, the researcher may connote this with a symbol or superscript letter indicating that the result was *significant at* $p \leq 0.05$. If, however the data-based *p*-value came in at 0.002, the researcher may describe the result as *highly significant.* This communicates that there is an even lower probability of the difference found being a chance event—much lower than the decision point he had set—thus he is very confident that the difference found is a true difference.

Another scenario is that the data-based *p*-value comes in just above the decision point *p*-level, with say $p = 0.06$ or 0.07. In this situation, the researcher might say that the result was "marginally significant" or "approached significance." This conveys that the *p*-value was close to the level of significance decision point; i.e., the difference in the two means was almost large enough to have confidence that it is a true difference. Reporting marginal results is justified when the study is an early test of an intervention because it may indicate a promising intervention that warrants another study.

Did I lose you in the last six to eight pages? If so, you need to go back to your statistics book and read about hypothesis testing, the *t*-test, and *p*-values. I offer the observation that the meaning of *p*-values will become clearer as you read more study reports. You will, however, have to pay attention to the *p*-values provided in reports and note how the researchers interpret them. This way, your understanding of them will increase over time. Understanding the meaning of *p*-values is crucial to understanding reports of quantitative studies. It is a concept that you must master.

Attainment of an Outcome

When attainment of an outcome or milestone is reported as a "yes" or "no," it is called a dichotomous outcome. Examples of dichotomous variables are these:

- Complication/no complication
- Increased self-care knowledge/did not increase self-care knowledge
- Gained the ability to walk 50 feet without assistance/did not gain this ability
- Smoking at 1 year after intervention/not smoking at 1 year

Clinical Perspective on Proportions

In experimental studies with dichotomous outcomes, the proportions of persons in each treatment group who attained the yes/no outcomes are determined. Obviously, you can look at the two proportions and determine whether the difference in proportions is large or small. This difference can be clarified a bit further. When the outcome is a good event, the difference in these two proportions is called the absolute benefit increase (ABI). It is one of several measures of treatment effect used to portray the relative impact of two treatments (Sackett, Straus, Richardson, Rosenberg, & Haynes, 2000). The other one explained next is number needed to treat (NNT).

Let's start with a concrete example: a study in which a new program to encourage physical activity in second- and third-grade inner-city kids is evaluated. (Focus on the results, not the study design, and assume a low rate of dropout.) Two hundred children were randomly assigned to attend the new once-a-week after-school exercise program for 3 weeks or to receive a placebo treatment in which a study assistant played electronic, card, and board games with them once a week for 3 weeks. The milestone outcome being considered is actively exercising for 8 hours or more outside of school each week when measured 3 months after the program; this is a dichotomous outcome that is either achieved or not achieved. The results showed that 26% of the kids in the program attained the milestone outcome, whereas 12% of those in the placebo group attained it; stated as proportions, these percentages are 0.26 and 0.12. So, the difference between the proportion of those in the program who met the milestone and the proportion in the placebo group who met it is 0.14 (0.26 minus 0.12); thus the

ABI produced by the exercise intervention over the placebo intervention is 14%. The clinical ramifications of this measure of clinical significance should be considered: Is this a sizable enough difference to justify saying that the new program has a success rate that is clinically important?

The NNT provides an even better take on this question. It is the number of kids who would have to be given the more effective treatment rather than the less effective treatment for one additional kid to achieve the milestone outcome. In our fictional study, the NNT is 8. This means that for every eight kids entered into the exercise program, rather than just getting attention, one kid will achieve the milestone exercise level who would not have had s/he just received attention. This provides a practical sense of how much benefit the exercise program would produce over just attention. Note that the NNT is easily calculated from the ABI; it is the inverse (reciprocal) of the ABI. That is: 1/ABI rounded up to a whole number—we do not treat 0.1 of a person. These measures of benefit are portrayed in Table 7-2.

NNT is useful for two reasons. First, it provides a clinical perspective on how many more people are likely to benefit at a meaningful level from the exercise program compared with no program. If the NNT were 3 or 4, it would mean that the exercise program is very effective, whereas an NNT of 20 or 30 would mean that quite a few would have to receive it for one additional person to benefit. Second, NNT can be considered in the context of the cost of the program, risks of exercise, and long-term risks of not developing an exercise habit. Combining NNT, the costs of implementing the program and the costs of the kids not developing an exercise habit, the NNT of 8 benefit could be good value.

TABLE 7-2 Exercise Program for Kids: Measures of Clinical Effect	
Measures of Clinical Effect (dichotomous data)	
Milestone attained with program	26% (0.26)
Milestone attained without program	12% (0.12)
Absolute benefit increase (ABI)	14% (0.14)
Number needed to treat (NNT)	$1 \div .14 = 7.1$ rounded up to 8

Statistical Perspective on Proportions

Often researchers also want to know whether the difference in the proportions that attained the clinical outcomes in the two groups is large enough to be likely in the larger population, so they will run chi square statistical test or a binomial test. These statistical tests produce a *p*-value indicating whether the difference in the proportion in the two groups is large enough to be statistically significant, i.e., a difference in proportions between the two groups would be likely in the population. Thus, the data-based *p*-value of these tests is interpreted in the same way as the *t*-test's *p* result even though the data consisted of proportions and a different statistical test was run.

> ### Example of *p*-value for a Difference in Proportions
>
> **Two strategies for teaching inhaler use at the time of discharge from acute care hospitals were compared; the control group received a brief intervention and written instruction and the other group received teach-to-goal education, also known as teach-back (Press et al., 2016). Patients who received teach-to-goal education were less likely to report having required acute care at 30 days compared with the brief instruction group (17% vs. 36%; *p* = .03) but there was no significant difference at 90 days (34% vs. 38%, *p* = 0.6). (Do note that the latter *p*-value is 0.6, not 0.06.) The researchers concluded that teach-to-goal has short-term benefits but ongoing instruction regarding inhaler technique is required to achieve long-term skill retention and improved health outcomes.**

Both Perspectives

Having explained both the clinical perspective and the statistical perspective for both types of study results, I want to point out that statistical significance and clinical significance do not necessarily equate; rather, their relationship can take different forms:

1. The difference between the outcomes of the two treatment groups can be *clinically significant* and *statistically significant*. This would occur when the difference between means is large—of course, large is relative to the nature of the outcome being studied and to the scale used to measure it.

2. The difference can be *clinically not significant* and *statistically not significant*. This would occur when the difference between the means of the two groups is very small.

3. The difference between the two group means can be *clinically significant* but *statistically not significant*. This occurs most frequently in studies with small sample sizes, which are common in nursing. The clinician sees promise in the results, even though statistically they could be due to chance, and is of the opinion that the intervention needs to be studied with a larger sample.

4. The difference between two group means can be *clinically not significant* but *statistically significant*; that is, from a practical clinical perspective it is trivial or unimportant. Statistically significant but clinically not significant results occur most frequently in studies with very large sample sizes.

POSSIBLE RESULT COMBINATIONS

- Clinically Significant and statistically Significant CS-SS
- Clinically not significant and statistically not significant Cs-Ss
- Clinically Significant and statistically not significant CS-Ss
- Clinically not significant and statistically significant Cs-SS

The results of a fictional randomized study comparing a new weight loss program to a program that has been around for a while are displayed in **Table 7-3**. First, note that the mean difference in weight lost by the two groups is 2.4 pounds and that this difference is statistically significant

TABLE 7–3 Weight Loss Example		
	New Program Group $n = 50$	Old Program Group $n = 50$
Mean lb lost at 6 months	13 lbs (sd = 4.9)	10.6 lbs (5.3)
Difference in the two means = 2.4 lbs		
95% CI of the difference: 0.37 to 4.4 lbs		
t-test *p*-value: 0.02		
% achieved a 10 lb loss or more	52%	30%
ABI = 22%		
NNT = 5 (1 ÷ 0.22 = 4.5 rounded up)		

($p = 0.02$). But do you think it is clinically significant? Note that the ABI and the NNT are more impressive than the mean difference. Based on the NNT of 5 for a weight loss of 10 pounds or more, I am inclined to say that the new program achieves a weight loss that is clinically significant for more people than what the old program achieves. However, this is an opinion and others may look at these results and say that the effectiveness of the two programs is not different enough to make a meaningful change in weight over time. Ultimately, this call must be made with the details of the full report and within the context of participants' feelings about the demands and cost of the two programs.

In many nursing studies, consideration of the clinical significance of the difference between outcomes is as important, if not more important, than consideration of whether the results are statistically significant. Unfortunately, the size of the clinical impact of the better intervention is not always discussed in a useful way in reports of nursing intervention studies—even though it should be. Once again, I would advise you not to obsess over the statistical results in a report; rather, think about the size of the difference between the outcomes of the two groups from a clinical perspective before moving on to thinking about them from the statistical perspective.

Opinion Regarding Reporting of Outcomes

Dichotomous (attained or didn't attain) clinical outcomes and their associated measures of effectiveness, ABI and NNT, are widely reported in the medical research literature but less often in the nursing literature. Hopefully, reporting dichotomous clinical outcomes will increase in nursing research because they add relevancy for clinicians. This is so because attainment of clinical outcomes and milestones are often important to patients—and memorable for clinicians. In contrast, mean scores on a scale or test are often indirect measures of outcomes important to patients and clinicians. I am of the opinion that reporting attainment of dichotomous patient outcomes adds clarity and clinical relevance to study reports.

Consider a fictional study in persons facing a risky medical procedure who were taught different ways of controlling anxiety in the days prior to the procedure; anxiety was measured on the morning of the procedure using a scale in which a low score indicated low anxiety and a high score indicated high anxiety. If the results reveal that the group taught method A had a mean anxiety score of 3 and group taught method B had a mean anxiety score of 7, we could say that clearly method A produced better anxiety prevention/relief, but we do not get a practical sense of how using method A actually improved *patients' experiences* of anxiety. In contrast, if the results were also reported as 11% of the persons in group A reported enough anxiety that it interfered with their sleep during one of the two nights before surgery and 24% of those in group B reported sleep disturbance during those nights, the difference in treatment effectiveness has immediate clinical relevance.

Exemplar

Reading Tip

You should now reread the *Introduction* and *Material and Methods* sections of the exemplar article about pediatric pain and anxiety during peripheral IV cannula insertion and then carefully read the *Results*, the *Discussion*, and the *Conclusions* sections. The *Profile & Commentary: Results* section that follows will focus on the results, discussion, and conclusions.

RESULTS

WHAT

Profile & Commentary: Results

The results are reported in the text and in the three tables provided; I will focus on the tables. Note that both outcomes, children's pain scores and parents' assessment of anxiety scores during the procedure, are measured on interval level scales and reported as means plus standard deviations.

Comparison of Groups Preintervention In Table 1, the two treatment groups are profiled. From it we learn that randomization created two very similar treatment groups because on all the variables (sex, age, BMI, and preprocedural anxiety), the difference between the groups is small and the data-based *p*-values for the differences are high. Thus, the differences are just chance variation that one would expect in drawing two samples from the same population. It is important that we know that the BMI and the anxiety levels of the two groups are essentially equal because both of these variables could be extraneous variables if they were not equal in both groups. A high BMI, i.e., overweight/obesity, could affect the difficulty of getting the cannula inserted, and in turn the pain experience. These equivalencies along with the fact that the same nurse inserted the cannulas in all the children maximize the likelihood that the insertion process was as similar as possible in both groups of children.

Children's Scoring of Their Pain   In Table 2, we see how the children scored the pain they experienced during the procedure. From the clinical perspective comparing the mean values of the two groups on both the WBFS (1 to 10) and the VAS (0 to 10), we see there is quite a difference between groups (almost 3 points on the WBFS and 2.43 points on the VAS). From the statistical perspective, the far right columns tells us that the t-test analysis indicates that there is essentially no chance ($p = 0.000$) that the differences between the two groups could just be due to chance; rather they are different because the two groups received different pain interventions—with the Buzzy group reporting significantly lower pain. Thus a difference in the target population would likely occur under similar conditions.

Parent and Observer Scoring of Anxiety   In Table 3 we see how the parent and the observer scored the child's anxiety during the procedure. First, the mean scoring of the parent and the observer are quite close together, which supports the validity of the measures used. Then the difference between the Buzzy group mean and the control group mean by both parent and observer was over a point—remember this is just a 5-point scale. So from a clinical perspective that seems sizeable. From the statistical perspective, the difference was significant at the 0.000 level. Again, the difference is not chance; rather is inferred to be the result of receiving the pain intervention or not.

Limitations   The authors acknowledge limitations of their study. The authors acknowledge that the parents and the observer who rated the child's anxiety at two times were not blind to whether the child received the Buzzy intervention or not, thus there is potential for expectation bias. This could have been overcome by placing a Buzzy device which was neither cold nor vibrated on children in the control group—as a placebo intervention, rather than usual care.

REFERENCES

Altman, D. B. (2009). Missing outcomes in randomized trials: Addressing the dilemma. *Open Medicine, 3*(2), 51–53. Retrieved from http://www.openmedicine.ca/article/view/323/233

Canbulat, N., Ayhan, F., & Inal, S. (2015). Effectiveness of external cold and vibration for procedural pain relief during peripheral intravenous cannulation in pediatric patients. *Pain Management Nursing, 16*(1), 33–39.

DiCenso, A., Guyatt, G., & Ciliska, D. (2005). *Evidence-based nursing: A guide to clinical practice*. Philadelphia, PA: Elsevier Mosby.

Garra, G., Singer, A. J., Taira, B. R., Chohan, J., Cardoz, H., Chisena, E., & Thode, C. (2009). Validation of the Wong Baker Faces Scale in pediatric emergency department patients. *Academic Emergency Medicine, 17,* 1750–1754.

Grove, S. K., Burns, N., & Gray, J. R. (2013). *Practice of nursing research: Conduct, critique, and utilization* (7th ed.). St. Louis, MO: Elsevier Saunders.

Kerlinger, F. N., & Lee, H. B. (2000). *Foundations of behavioral research* (4th ed.). Fort Worth, TX: Harcourt College.

Li, X., Xu, S., Zhou, L., Li, R., & Wang, J. (2015). Home-based exercise in older adults recently discharged from the hospital for cardiovascular disease in China. *Nursing Research, 64*(4), 246–255.

McMurtry, C. M., Noel, M., Chambers, T., & McGrath, P. J. (2011). Children's fear during procedural pain: Preliminary investigation of the Children's Fear Scale. *Health Psychology, 30*(6), 780–788.

Patrician, P. A. (2004). Single-item graphic representation scales. *Nursing Research, 3*(5), 347–352.

Polit, D. F., & Beck, C. T. (2014). *Essentials of Nursing Research: Appraising Evidence for Nursing Practice* (8th ed.). Philadelphia, PA: Lippincott Williams & Wilkins.

Press, V., Arora, V. M., Trela, K. C., Adhikari, R., Zadravecz, F. J., Liao, C., et al. (2016). Effectiveness of interventions to teach metered-dose and diskus inhaler techniques: A randomized trial. *Annals of the American Thoracic Surgery Society, 13*(6), 816–824. doi: 10.1513/AnnalsATS.201509-603OC

Sackett, D. L., Straus, S. E., Richardson, W. S., Rosenberg, W., & Haynes, R. B. (2000). *Evidence-based medicine: How to practice and teach EBM*. Edinburgh, Scotland: Churchill Livingstone.

Shu, T-T. (2010). *Effects of duration of selected music as an intervention on postoperative pain in open-heart surgery patients during chair rest on the first postoperative day*. (Master's thesis, paper No. 321). Eastern Michigan University, Ypsilanti, MI. Retrieved from http://commons.emich.edu/theses/321

Tsai, S-H., Wang, M. Y., Miao, N. F., Chian, P. C., Chen, T. H., & Tsai, P. S. (2015). The efficacy of a nurse-led breathing training program in reducing depressive symptoms in patients on hemodialysis: A randomized controlled trial. *American Journal of Nursing 115*(4), 24–32.

U.S. Department of Health and Human Services. (n.d.). *Research with Children FAQs*. Retrieved from http://www.hhs.gov/ohrp/policy/faq/children-research/index.html

Wong, D. L., & Baker, C. M. (1988). Pain in children: Comparison of assessment scales. *Pediatric Nursing, 14*(1), 9–17.

CHAPTER EIGHT

Cohort Research

S tudying the cause–effect relationship between risk factors and health outcomes presents unique challenges. Random assignment of participants to a risk factor exposure that could result in disease or a poor health outcome ethically is not an option. Thus, cohort studies evolved as a way of studying risk factors associated with heredity, environment, behavior, a particular life experience, or a medical treatment. For instance, a cohort design could be used to compare the cognitive health of urban elderly persons who were living in senior versus nonsenior housing.

Design

In a cohort study, a sample is drawn from a larger population and classified into two distinct groups—those with the risk factor and those without it. The two groups, called cohorts, are followed over an appropriate length of time to determine how often the outcomes of interest occur in both groups. Cohort studies are like experiments in that they involve comparison of outcomes in contrasting groups of a specified population; however, they are unlike experiments in that the contrasting groups are not created by random assignment. Rather, two naturally occurring groups are observed; the groups are defined based on whether or not they have had exposure to a particular risk factor. Most often, the cohorts are identified after exposure to the risk factor and before the outcomes of interest develop; they are then followed to determine the rate at which the outcome of interest occurs.

In a study of a little more than 11,000 Danish nurses over age 44, one of the issues studied was use of estrogen therapy and subsequent development of breast cancer during 6 years of follow-up (Hundrup, Simonsen, Jørgensen, & Obel, 2011). At the time of enrollment, the participants had been classified into two groups: using estrogen therapy and never used estrogen therapy, and the outcome was development of breast cancer during the 6-year follow-up. The using-estrogen-therapy group was found to have almost twice the risk of breast cancer during the 6-year follow-up as the never-used-estrogen-therapy group did.

A 2 × 2 matrix, which is used to portray the results of a cohort study, is helpful in understanding the logic of cohort design (**Table 8-1**). The first division of the sample is into the exposed or not exposed group. Later, when the outcome is measured, everyone in the sample is classified into one of the four groups (a, b, c, or d), which becomes the basis for the comparison of the outcomes of the two original groups.

Cohort studies often use information in health system databases to reconstruct the presence of a risk factor at a point in time or over time and the subsequent development of a particular outcome. A cohort study looked at adverse drug reactions among frail elderly persons after discharge from hospital (Hanlon et al., 2006). Data were collected from patients' healthcare records regarding various risk factors for adverse drug reactions, and patients were followed to determine those who experienced an adverse drug reaction. The main finding was that the number of medications the patient took and the use of the drug warfarin increased the risk of adverse drug events.

TABLE 8–1 Logic of a Cohort Study				
		Adverse Outcome		
		Present	Absent	Totals
Exposed to	Yes	a	b	a + b
Risk Factor	No	c	d	c + d
Totals		a + c	b + d	

Exposed Cohort
   a = exposed to risk factor and develop adverse outcome
   b = exposed to risk factor but do not develop adverse outcome
Unexposed Cohort
   c = not exposed to risk factor but develop adverse outcome
   d = not exposed to risk factor and do not develop adverse outcome

Data Analysis and Results

In cohort studies, data analysis is often done by comparing the risk of the outcomes for the two groups being compared; this analysis produces a relative risk (RR) measure, which I will explain shortly. Chi-square analysis is also used to determine whether the difference in risks found is statistically significant. Logistic regression analysis is also used to determine whether any of the identified potential confounding variables could have influenced the occurrence of the outcomes of interest. This combination of analyses allows the researcher to:

1. Compare the risk of two groups for the outcomes of interest
2. Determine whether the risks of the two groups are significantly different
3. Check for the effect of possible confounding variables

Reading Tip: You might want to reread the sections about logistic regression and odds ratio in Chapter 6 under the *More Complex Designs* section heading.

Confounding

The major concern in cohort studies is that the two groups could be different in some way other than the presence or absence of the risk factor, and that difference may produce different outcomes for the two groups. For instance, they may have different biophysical characteristics, lifestyles, or experiences. The difference could be something as easy to identify as an age difference or something as buried as different levels of nutrition during youth. If the difference is a determinant of the outcomes being studied and is unequally distributed in the two groups, it is called a confounding variable (Mamdani et al., 2005). Recognizing confounders in advance of doing a study allows researchers to collect data about them and run analyses to check on their influence on the outcome variable. In the study you will read later in this chapter, you will learn about the techniques researchers take to rule out confounding. However, even when the analysis has ruled out suspected confounders, cohort studies are still vulnerable to unknown confounders.

Other Limitations

Cohort studies that follow participants for long periods of time often suffer from high dropout rates. High dropout rates can bias the incidence of the outcome in either or both groups, thus confounding the results. Another limitation of cohort design is that it does not work well if the outcome being studied occurs rarely. A rare outcome would require following a very large number of people to detect a connection between the risk factor and the outcome. Therefore, when the outcome being studied is rare, researchers may use another design: case-control design.

Case-Control Studies

In a sense, a case-control study is the opposite of a cohort study. Remember, a cohort study starts by identifying cohorts of persons and then follows them forward to determine if they develop certain outcomes. In contrast, a case-control study starts by identifying persons with and without a particular outcome, for example, a disease, and then looks backward in their history to identify how the two groups were different in regard to suspected causes of the outcome. The logistics of the two types of studies are shown in **Figure 8-1**.

Generally, cohort studies are used to study exposures and outcomes that occur rather frequently and outcomes that develop or occur not too long after the risk factor or exposure, whereas case-control studies are used to study outcomes that are rare or take a long time to become evident (e.g., osteoporosis fracture, lung cancer). Case-control studies are even more prone to confounding by unknown factors than are cohort studies. They are highly prone to confounding because the study involves looking back in time, and important data may not be available or may be forgotten or distorted by memory.

A case-control study was conducted to determine the association between unplanned extubations in a pediatric intensive care unit and several patient, staffing, and care variables (Marcin, Rutan, Rapetti, Rahnsmayi, & Pretzlaff, 2005). During a 4-year period, 55 patients with unplanned extubations were identified. They were matched for age, intubation duration, and severity of illness with 165 control patients who did not experience unplanned extubation. Looking back at data from both groups' records of their time in ICU, they determined that patient agitation and nurse-to-patient assignment ratios of 1:2 were associated with unplanned extubations, whereas nurses' years of experience in pediatric intensive care nursing, patient restraints, and method of sedation delivery were not associated. Thus, by looking back after the event at possible risk factors, this case-control study identified two that put patients at risk.

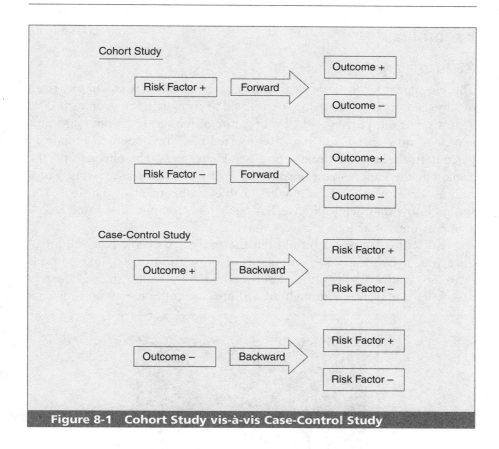

Figure 8-1 Cohort Study vis-à-vis Case-Control Study

Wrap-Up

Cohort studies provide a way of evaluating risk factors for health conditions or events; they do so by comparing groups with and without exposure to a preidentified risk factor. Because random assignment is not used to form the comparison groups, cohort studies are prone to confounding, which threatens the validity of study conclusions about the relationship between the risk factor and the outcome of interest. However, cohort studies do provide control over follow-up and diagnosis of the outcome. An alternative design that is used to study risk factors when the outcome of interest is rare is the case-control study, but this design has even greater potential for confounding.

Exemplar

Reading Tips

The big phrase in the title of this article, *hemicallotasis technique*, is an orthopaedic surgical procedure performed to straighten knees deformed by arthritis. For our purposes, the exact nature of the surgery is not important except to note that metal pins are inserted into the bone and remain in place until the realigned bones fuse (see **Figure 8-2**). The pins go into the bone, but the ends remain outside the skin where they are attached to a rigid external frame, which is what enables realignment of the tibia. You should know that hemicallotasis has fairly high complication rates, which is in part due to the long recovery time.

I realize this study is a bit old but the analysis is classic and will introduce you to frequently used measures of association: risk ratio and odds ratio. So, read it for learning about methodology, rather than as current orthopaedic evidence, although an orthopaedic colleague assures me that

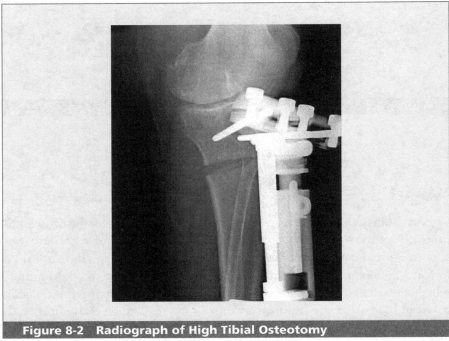

Figure 8-2   Radiograph of High Tibial Osteotomy

Reproduced from W-Dahl, A., Toksvig-Larsen, S., & Roos, E. M. (2009). Association between knee alignment and knee pain in patients surgically treated for medial knee osteoarthritis by high tibial osteotomy. A one year follow-up study. BMC Musculoskeletal Disorders 2009, 10, 154. doi:10.1186/1471-2474-10-154. Creative Commons license available at http://creativecommons.org/licenses/by/2.0

the hemicallotasis procedure is still being done in much the same way as described in this study (personal communication Annette Dahl, December 2015).

Dahl, A W., and Toksvig-Larsen, S. (2004). Cigarette smoking delays bone healing: A prospective study of 200 patients operated on by the hemicallotasis technique. *Acta Orthopaedica Scandinavica, 75*(3), 347–351.

Background: Cigarette smoking is known to impede bone healing. The hemicallotasis technique is based on an external fixation and delayed healing prolongs treatment and increases the risk of further complications.

Patients and methods: 200 patients, 34 smokers and 166 nonsmokers, operated on by the hemicallotasis technique in the proximal tibia for deformities of the knee (knee arthrosis in 186 patients) were consecutively studied. We recorded their preoperative smoking habits, postoperative complications and the duration of treatment with external fixation.

Results: Half of the smokers and one fifth of the nonsmokers developed complications. Their mean time in external fixation was 96 (SD 20) days. Smokers required an average of 16 days more in external fixation. Delayed healing and pseudoarthrosis were commoner in smokers than nonsmokers. The risk ratio for smokers to develop complications was 2.5, as compared to nonsmokers.

* * *

Tibia osteotomy by the hemicallotasis technique (HCO) is based on external fixation. Delayed healing and nonunion prolong the treatment and increase the risk of further complications.

Studies on rabbits have shown delayed bone healing and decreases in bone mineral density (BMD) and strength in the lengthened tibia caused by cigarette smoking (Ueng et al., 1997, 1999). Smoking was the single most important risk factor for the development of serious postoperative complications after elective arthroplasty of the hip and knee (Møller et al., 2003).

We studied whether smokers had longer healing times and more complications than nonsmokers who underwent HCO.

Methods
Patients

In a prospective study, 200 consecutive patients (119 men), mean age 53 (18–75) years, were operated on by HCO for knee deformities (Tables 1 and 2).

The patients' smoking habits (smoker or nonsmoker) were noted preoperatively. They were called *nonsmoker* if, at the preoperative examination, they stated that they had never smoked or had stopped smoking more than 6 months previously. Thirty-four (17%) were smokers and 166 (83%) nonsmokers. Seven patients underwent simultaneous bilateral surgery (1 smoker and 6 nonsmokers).

Table 1 Patient Characteristics of the Study Group	Nonsmokers n = 166	Smokers n = 34
Gender		
Men	102 (61)	17 (50)
Women	64 (39)	17 (50)
Age		
Mean	53	53
SD	10	6
< 50	47 (28)	9 (26)
50–59	77 (46)	22 (65)
60+	42 (25)	3 (9)
Preop HKA-angle in medial cases		
Mean	170°	170°
SD	5°	4°
≤ 189°	17 (11)	2 (3)
> 190°	5 (5)	3 (12)
BMI		
< 25	25 (16)	12 (35)
25–29	77 (48)	13 (38)
30+	58 (36)	9 (27)

Percentages within parentheses
Preop HKA-angle = Preoperative hip-knee-ankle-angle
BMI = Body mass index

Table 2 Indication for Surgery in 200 Patients Who Underwent HCO		
	All n = 200	Nonsmokers/Smokers n = 166/34
Knee osteoarthrosis	186	153/32
Medial	163	134/29
Lateral	20	15/5
Pre[a]	2	2/0
Fracture sequelae	8	6/2
Knee deformity	4	4/0
Osteonecrosis	1	1/0
Sequelae of tibia osteotomy	1	1/0

[a]Arthroscopic osteoarthrosis with symptoms but no osteoarthrosis, according to radiographic Ahlback grade I.

Hemicallotasis Osteotomy

Four conical pins were inserted, 2 hydroxyapatite-coated in the metaphyseal bone and 2 standard pins (Orthofix®, Bussolengo, Italy) in the diaphyseal bone. The Orthofix® T-garche was used. The patients were allowed free mobilization and full weight bearing after the operation.

The distraction started 7–10 days postoperatively. Eight weeks after surgery, the fixation was dynamised to stimulate healing of the bone. The first evaluation of bone healing was done 12 weeks postoperatively. If healing of the osteotomy was deemed satisfactory on both the radiographic and ultrasound examinations, the patient did a weight-bearing test—i.e., walked for a few hours or even some days without the instrument, but with the pins in situ. If no symptoms developed, the pins were removed in the outpatient clinic, but if the patient developed symptoms, the T-garche was applied again for 2–4 weeks.

Outcome

We recorded the duration of external fixation (from surgery until the external pins were removed) and the complications, such as delayed healing (> 16 weeks in external fixation), pseudoarthrosis, septic arthritis, deep venous thrombosis, nerves injury, and interrupted treatment (i.e., loose pins due to a pin site infection).

Statistics

The analysis of variance (ANOVA) test, t-test and Chi-square test were used for the statistical analysis, and the statistical significance was set at $p < 0.05$. A multiple logistic regression analysis (checked for potential confounder) was used to estimate the odds ratio (OR) of complications, delayed healing and pseudoarthrosis.

The study was approved by the Ethics Committee, Lund University, Sweden.

Results

More complications occurred among the smokers than the nonsmokers. Fifty-one patients had one or more complications (delayed healing, pseudoarthrosis, septic arthritis, deep venous thrombosis, nerves injury or interrupted treatment) (34/166 [Table 3] nonsmokers and 17/34 smokers, $p < 0.001$). 12/51 patients had two or more complications (7 nonsmokers and 5 smokers, $p = 0.02$). The risk ratio for the smokers who developed complications, as compared to the nonsmokers, was 2.5 (95% CI 1.5–3.9).

Delayed healing and pseudoarthrosis occurred more often among the smokers. The risk ratio for delayed healing was 2.7 (95% CI 1.5–4.7) in the smokers. Eight patients with delayed healing developed pseudoarthrosis. The risk ratio for smokers to develop pseudoarthrosis was 8.1 (95% CI 1.8–42.0) (Table 3). Six of the patients who developed pseudoarthrosis required additional surgery for healing (5 smokers and 1 nonsmoker) and 2 patients (nonsmokers) healed after low intensity ultrasound stimulation (Exogen®, Tuttlingen, Germany).

In the 3 patients who developed septic arthritis (2 nonsmokers and 1 smoker), the treatment was interrupted and in one patient (nonsmoker), the treatment was interrupted due to loose pins. The mean time in external fixation was 96 (SD 20) days in all patients. The mean time in external fixation for nonsmokers was 94 (SD 18) days and 110 (SD 25.2) days for smokers ($p < 0.001$). The smokers had 16 days ($p < 0.001$, 95% CI 7.0–25) longer mean time in external fixation than the nonsmokers. In patients with a frame time > 112 days, the smokers had a mean of 17 days more ($p = 0.004$, 95% CI 5.5–26) in external fixation than the nonsmokers (Table 4). Among the 7 patients who underwent bilateral HCO in one

Table 3 Complications in 200 Patients Operated On by HCO				
			Relative Risk	
	Nonsmokers	Smokers	(RR)	(95% CI)[a]
Delayed healing[b]	25	14	2.7	(1.5–4.7)
Pseudoarthrosis	3	5	8.	(1.8–42)
Septic arthritis	2	1	2.4	(0.1–34)
Deep venous	3	2	3.3	(0.4–23)
Nerve injury	1	0	0	(1.0–84)
Interrupted treatment	3	1	1.6	(0.1–17)

[a](95% CI) = 85% confidence interval.
[b]Includes 5 patients who developed pseudoarthrosis after removal of external fixation.

Table 4 Frame Time > 112 days in Patients Operated On by HCO			
	Nonsmokers	Smokers	P-value
Mean (days)	126	143	0.004
SD	13	16	
n	23	11	

séance, 3 patients had complications—i.e., 2 had delayed healing, 1 smoker and 1 nonsmoker. And 1 (nonsmoker), with osteonecrosis after treatment for leukemia, developed pseudoarthrosis (rapid loss of correction) in one of the osteotomies.

The multivariate analysis, used to detect potential confounder, showed that cigarette smoking was the greatest preoperative risk factor for complications OR 5.1 ($p = 0.001$, 95% CI 2.2–12), delayed healing OR 4.0 ($p = 0.004$, 95% CI 1.7–9.5), and pseudoarthrosis OR 8.9 ($p = 0.02$, 95% CI 1.7–47.1) (Table 5).

Discussion

Smokers operated on by HCO for knee deformities needed a longer time in external fixation and had more complications, such as delayed healing and pseudoarthrosis than nonsmokers. Half of the smokers developed complications. The risk for the smokers developing complications was 2.5 times higher than in the nonsmokers.

A recent study by Møller et al. (2003) on patients operated on for arthroplasty of the hip and knee confirmed our findings—i.e., smoking is the greatest risk factor for developing postoperative complications.

The number of smokers (34 of 200 patients) in our material is similar to the percentage of smokers in the Swedish population, 19% (18% men and 20% women) (Mackay and Eriksen, 2002).

The mean time in external fixation in patients operated on by HCO has ranged from 79 to 91 days in various studies (Magyar et al., 1998; Klinger et al., 2001, Gerdhem et al., 2002), as compared to our 96 days. These differences may be due to the time when the first examination for healing was done, the methods used to assess healing, the experience in evaluating the healing on radiographs and perhaps the use of ultrasound. The size of the correction and whether bilateral osteotomies were done in one séance could also account for a longer treatment time. We found no differences between unilateral and bilateral osteotomies or the preoperative HKA-angle, as regards the longer healing time.

Cigarette smoking has been shown to cause slower healing and pseudoarthrosis in tibial fractures, both after closed (Kyro et al., 1993) and surgical treatments (Adams et al., 2001). In closed and grade I open tibial shaft fractures,

Table 5   Relationship of Risk Factors to Complications, Delayed Healing and Pseudoarthrosis in Patients Operated On by HCO

	Complications Adjusted OR[a]	Delayed healing Adjusted OR[a]	Pseudoarthrosis Adjusted OR[a]
Gender			
Men[b]	1.0	1.0	1.0
Women	1.4 (0.7–2.9)	1.8 (0.8–4.1)	5.0 (0.8–31)
Age			
< 50[b]	1.0	1.0	1.0
50–59	0.9 (0.4–2.3)	1.0 (0.4–2.6)	0.5 (0.09–3.3)
60+	1.4 (0.5–3.9)	0.9 (0.3–3.0)	1.4 (0.2–12)
BMI			
< 25[b]	1.0	1.0	1.0
25–29	0.7 (0.3–1.8)	0.7 (0.3–2.1)	0.9 (0.1–6.0)
30+	1.2 (0.5–3.1)	1.1 (0.4–3.1)	0.5 (0.06–3.6)
Preop HKA-angle[c] medial/lateral			
> 171/< 189[b]	1.0	1.0	1.0
< 170/> 190	1.8 (0.9–3.7)	1.7 (0.8–3.8)	3.6 (0.6–21)
Smoking			
Nonsmokers[b]	1.0	1.0	1.0
Smokers	4.1 (1.8–3.7)	3.7 (1.5–8.9)	7.5 (1.4–41)

[a]Odds ratio (OR) adjusted simultaneously for all other risk factors listed and 95% confidence interval in parenthesis.
[b]Reference category.
[c]Hip-knee-ankle-angle preoperatively (varus or valgus).

Schmitz et al. (1999) found statistical differences in clinical and radiographic healing rates in smokers and nonsmokers in patients who underwent intramedullary or external fixation.

Cobb et al. (1994) reported that the relative risk of nonunion after ankle arthrodesis was 4 times higher in smokers. When patients had no known risk factors for nonunion, the risk of nonunion was 16 times higher in smokers.

Examination after a laminectomy and fusion showed more pseudoarthrosis among smokers than nonsmokers (Brown et al., 1986). After ulna-shortening osteotomy, the smokers had longer healing times and nonunion than the nonsmokers. The mean union rates were 7 months in smokers and 4 months in nonsmokers (Chen et al., 2001). Our study of patients who underwent HCO can be added to the list of treatments showing that smoking is an important risk factor for the development of complications in orthopaedic surgery.

In a preoperative smoking intervention study, cessation of smoking from 6–8 weeks preoperatively and 10 days postoperatively reduced the postoperative complications in patients undergoing hip and knee replacement. The smoking cessation group was compared to one with an at least 50% reduction in smoking. The patients who reduced their smoking did not differ from the smoking group in other respects (Møller et al., 2002). Patients undergoing arthroplasty of the hip and knee who smoked previously had a better short-term outcome than those who were smoking (Lavernia et al., 1999). Glassman et al. (2000) showed that the cessation of smoking after surgery helped to reverse the effects of cigarette smoking on the outcome of spinal fusion.

These studies indicate that smoking cessations both preoperatively and postoperatively decrease the risk for complications, whereas smoking reduction is not enough to decrease the risk.

The conclusions of the present study were that information about smoking cessations prior to surgery should be an important part of the preoperative information as well as cigarette smoking should be a factor to consider when selecting patients for callus distraction.

References

Adams C I, Keating J F, Court-Brown C M. Cigarette smoking and open tibial fractures. *Injury* 2001; 32 (1): 61–5.

Brown C W, Orme J T, Richardson H D. The rate of pseudoarthrosis (surgical nonunion) in patients who are smokers and patients who are nonsmokers: a comparison study. *Spine* 1986; 11 (9): 942–3.

Chen F, Osterman A L, Mahony K. Smoking and bony union after ulna-shortening osteotomy. *Am J Orthop* 2001; 30 (6): 486–9.

Cobb T K, Gabrielsen T A, Campbell D C, Wallrichs S L, Ilstrup D M. Cigarette smoking and nonunion after ankle arthrodesis. *Foot Ankle Int* 1994; 15 (2): 64–7.

Gerdhem P, Abdon P, Odenbring S. Hemicallotasis for medial gonarthrosis: a short-term follow-up of 21 patients. *Arch Orthop Trauma Surg* 2002; 12 (3): 134–8.

Glassman S D, Anagnost C S, Parker A, Burke D, Johnson J R, Dimar J R. The effect of cigarette smoking and smoking cessation on spinal fusion. *Spine* 2000; 25 (20): 2608–14.

Klinger H M, Lorenz F, Harer T. Open wedge tibial osteotomy by hemicallotasis for medial compartment osteoarthritis. *Arch Orthop Trauma Surg* 2001; 121 (5): 247–7.

Kyro A, Usenius J P, Aarnio M, Kunnamo I, Avikainen V. Are smokers a risk group for delayed healing of tibial shaft fractures? *Ann Chir Gynaecol* 1993; 82 (4): 254–62.

Lavernia C J, Sierra R J, Gomez-Marin O. Smoking and joint replacement: resource consumption and short-term outcome. *Clin Orthop* 1999; (367): 172–80.

Mackay J, Eriksen M. *The Tobacco Atlas.* Myriad Edition Limited. Brighton 2002.

Magyar G, Toksvig-Larsen S, Lindstrand A. Open wedge tibial osteotomy by callus distraction in gonarthrosis. Operative technique and early results in 36 patients. *Acta Orthop Scand* 1998; 69 (2): 147–51.

Møller A M, Pedersen T, Villebro N, Munksgaard A. Effect of smoking on early complications after elective orthopaedic surgery. *J Bone Joint Surg Br* 2003; 85 (2): 178–81.

Møller A M, Villebro N, Pedersen T, Tonnesen H. Effect of preoperative smoking intervention on postoperative complications: a randomised clinical trial. *Lancet* 2002; 359 (9301): 114–7.

Schmitz M A, Finnegan M, Natarajan R, Champine J. Effect of smoking on tibial shaft fracture healing. *Clin Orthop* 1999; (365): 184–200.

Ueng S W, Lee M Y, Li A F, Lin S S, Tai C L, Shih C H. Effect of intermittent cigarette smoke inhalation on tibial lengthening: experimental study on rabbits. *J Trauma* 1997; 42 (2): 231–8.

Ueng S W, Lin S S, Wang C R, Liu S J, Tai C L, Shih C H. Bone healing of tibial lengthening is delayed by cigarette smoking: study of bone mineral density and torsional strength on rabbits. *J Trauma* 1999; 46 (1): 110–5.

Profile & Commentary

STUDY PURPOSE

This study was conducted to determine if cigarette smokers and nonsmokers had the same rates of healing and complications after having an orthopedic surgical procedure called tibial hemicallotasis osteotomy. In brief, then:

- Population: Persons having this orthopedic surgical procedure
- Risk cohorts: Smokers and nonsmokers—note the definition of smoker
- Outcome variables: Complications, delayed bone healing, infection, loose pins

METHODS

Design   The design of this study is a consecutive series, prospective cohort design. Consecutive series indicates that the sample was created by asking a series of patients who were having the surgical procedure to participate in the study. *Prospective* indicates that the participants were entered into the study and followed to determine how many developed complications after the surgery. In fact, this study design is the only way to compare complication rates in smokers and nonsmokers after surgery because random assignment to a smoking or not smoking group is not logistically possible.

Risk Factor of Interest Prior research indicates that a history of recent smoking and current smoking slow, and in some cases prevent, bone healing after orthopedic surgeries. This is the first study examining the effects of smoking with this particular procedure. Note that the definition of who was considered a nonsmoker depended on the patient's report. Many cohort studies rely on patient reports regarding exposure to the risk factor, although some cohort studies use a very rigorously applied set of criteria to classify patients into one risk group or the other. I assume from the definition of nonsmoker that persons who were categorized as smokers preoperatively continued to smoke postoperatively—although this was not explicitly stated.

Sample The target population was persons having a particular knee reconstruction procedure. The researchers obtained a sample of this population by studying 200 consecutive patients in one Swedish hospital. Enrolling consecutive patients is a reasonably unbiased way of obtaining a sample because it does not allow anyone on the research team to pick and choose who is in the study. In this study, consecutive enrollment of patients does not present any obvious concerns about the sample being different from persons who have the surgery at other times.

Outcomes Note how the outcomes were measured and the timing of the measurements. The main outcomes (various complications) were measured as dichotomous outcomes; that is, the complication either occurred or did not occur. The overall complication rate (one or more complications) was measured as well as the rate of each of six complications. The outcome of time in external fixation was measured using an interval scale (days).

Potential Confounders It wasn't clear to me that all cases were done by the same surgeon so I contacted the lead author who told me that *yes they were*. This was important because *if* different surgeons had performed the surgeries, that would have been a potential confounding variable; as it was just one surgeon: no issue. I also asked about the length of time over which patients were entered into the study; the answer: 3½ years. That too could have been a confounding variable if the enrollment had taken place over a long period of time because the surgeon's technique or skill could have changed and influenced the outcomes; as it was, it is a bit of a concern but not a lot.

RESULTS
WHAT

Sample   In a cohort study, the first table often profiles the two cohorts as a first step in identifying potential confounders. Accordingly, Table 1 provides a profile of the smoker and nonsmoker groups with specifics about variables the researchers think could have an influence on the occurrence of complications. First note that the smokers' cohort comprised 17% of the sample and the nonsmokers cohort made up the rest (83%). Then, there are differences between the composition of the two groups, particularly in terms of gender and proportion of persons over age 60. This raises a concern that perhaps these differences influenced the occurrence of complications and contributed to the differences found. At this point, the differences just send up a red flag and remind us to note whether the researchers deal with them during data analysis.

Dichotomous Outcomes   In the text, the researchers tell us that 20% of nonsmokers (34/166) and 50% of smokers (17/34) had one or more complications; thus, the absolute difference in the complication rates of the two groups is 30% (50% minus 20%). Further, the p-value associated with this difference indicates that this is a real difference, not a chance difference ($p < 0.001$).

To provide additional clinical perspective on the risk of one or more complications, the risk for smokers to develop a complication was compared to the risk for nonsmokers. This was reported as relative risk (RR), which is the ratio between risk in the smoker group and risk in the nonsmoker group.[1] The risk of the smoker group was 50% and the risk of the nonsmoker group was 20%, thus the relative risk was 0.50:0.20 = 2.5.

---

[1]Risk $= \dfrac{\text{Number in the group who have the complication}}{\text{Total number in group}}$

Relative risk $= \dfrac{\text{Risk of smoker group}}{\text{Risk of nonsmoker group}}$

To understand the meaning of this RR, you need to know that if the two groups had equal risk, the RR would be 1.0., whereas an RR greater than 1.0 indicates that the smoker group had a higher risk of a complication than did the nonsmoker group. A RR of less than 1.0 would mean that the smoker group had a lower risk of a complication than did the nonsmoker group. Thus, the RR = 2.5 for smokers having at least one complication means that the risk for smokers developing complications was 2.5 times the risk for nonsmokers— keeping in mind the absolute risk level of the nonsmokers (which was 20%).

Relative risk (RR) was also used in Table 3 to portray the risk of smokers in relation to nonsmokers for six poor outcomes. From this table, you can tell that being a smoker puts persons at much higher *relative risk* (8.1) of developing pseudoarthrosis and a lower level of *relative risk* of delayed healing (2.7). This means that the risk of smokers developing pseudoarthrosis was 8 times that of nonsmokers and their risk of developing delayed healing was 2.7 times that of nonsmokers. When interpreting RR, the operative word is *relative*—glossing over it can easily lead to misinterpretations of RR. Generally, the group that is unexposed to the risk is used for the denominator.

RR allows a comparison of smokers' relative risks for several outcomes. Comparing smokers' RRs for delayed healing (2.7) and pseudoarthrosis (8.1) tells us that being a smoker increases the risk of pseudoarthrosis more than it increases the risk of delayed healing (note the relative word *more*). When looking at smokers' RRs for delayed healing and pseudoarthrosis, *do not* make the mistake of interpreting it to mean that smokers are at a higher risk of pseudoarthrosis than they are of delayed healing. Again, you have to keep in mind the risk rate of the baseline/unexposed group.

Because this can be confusing, I like to see the absolute rates and the RRs together, so I did my own fiddling with the data in Table 3; the data

TABLE 8–2	Reformulation of Results to Clarify Risk			
	Risk Nonsmokers	Risk Smokers	Absolute Difference	Relative Risk
Outcome	*n* = 166	*n* = 34		
Delayed healing	25 (15%)	14 (41%)	26%	2.7
Pseudoarthrosis	3 (1.8%)	5 (14.6%)	12.8%	8.1

Modified from Dahl, A. W., & Toksvig-Larsen, S. (2004). Cigarette smoking delays bone healing: A prospective study of 200 patients operated on by the hemicallotasis technique. *Acta Orthopaedica Scandinavica, 75*(3), 347–351.

used were obtained from Table 3 of the report. This display reminds me that the absolute risk rate of a complication in a group and its relative rate when compared to another group are quite different takes on the data. Essentially, delayed healing is a more common complication than pseudoarthrosis in both groups, but smoking increases the risk of pseudoarthrosis more than it increases the rate of delayed healing.

One last point related to Table 3 concerns the far right column, *95% CI for Relative Risk*. To take just one line, *Delayed healing*, the sample had an RR of 2.7. This value is also the best single number for estimating what might occur in the larger population of persons having the HCO surgery. However, the 95% confidence interval (CI) provides additional information about what might occur in the population. It tells us that in the population the RR for delayed healing could be anywhere from 1.5 to 4.7. First off, 1 is not in the CI interval, so smokers are likely to be at greater risk of a complication in the population, not just those in this sample. Then, the CI is fairly narrow, so it gives us a pretty precise estimate of what would be found in the population. Also, note that the RR confidence intervals for septic arthritis, deep vein thrombosis, and interrupted treatment include 1, so no difference in the RR of smokers is possible in the population for those outcomes.

Interval Level Outcomes   Switching to the analysis of days in external fixation, which is an interval level outcome, the mean days in external fixation for smokers and nonsmokers were compared. In the text of the *Results* section, we learn that smokers spent 16 more days than nonsmokers in external fixation (110 minus 94). From a clinical perspective, this difference in means is clinically significant because it represents on average 2 more weeks of having the fixation in place. From a statistical perspective, the *t*-test comparing the two means was statistically significant at the $p < 0.001$ level. This means that there is less than 1 chance in 1,000 that a difference as large as the one found could have occurred just by chance—thus a difference is likely to exist in the larger population as well as in this sample.

Note in the text that, although the mean *difference* of days in external fixation for the two groups was 16 days (110 versus 94), the 95% confidence interval for the days in external fixation is 7.0–25.0. This means that in the target population, smokers could spend as much as 25 days or as few as 7 days more in external fixation than nonsmokers do. This wide CI probably is the result of wide variability in how long fixation was required.

Still, the CI provides a better sense of what might occur in the population than does the sample mean all by itself.

At this point, if you do not understand confidence intervals, you should go back to your statistical text because you are likely to encounter them when reading research reports and SRs. They are of practical, clinical value because they provide good estimates of the likely results that will be realized when applying the study's intervention in everyday practice.

Looking for Potential Confounders   The researchers were aware that smoking was not the only risk factor for complications and that the smoking and nonsmoking groups could be different in ways other than just their smoking status. And we remember that Table 1 revealed some of those differences; for example, a greater percentage of women in the smoker group and a greater percentage of people over age 60 years in the nonsmoker group. To more definitively address the possibility that differences between smokers and nonsmokers on these other risk factors could have influenced the occurrence of complications, the researchers ran a multiple logistic regression analysis.

The results, shown in Table 5, were reported using a statistic called odds ratio. The analysis had to be done with odds ratios rather than risk ratios because of the technical requirements of logistic regression, which analyzes several risk factors at once. First, let us consider the concept of odds and how it compares to risk. Odds of a complication are similar to risk of a complication but slightly different. A risk is the likelihood (i.e., probability) of something occurring in relation to the number of times it could have occurred. You roll a die (just one) and are hoping to roll a five. There is one chance in six that you will get a five; thus, the risk of a five is one in six, which is 0.17 when converted to a decimal ($1/6 = 0.166$) and rounded up. In contrast, odds are the chances of something occurring in relation to the chances of it not occurring; thus, the odds of rolling a five are one to five ($1/5$) or 0.20. The numerator is the same in both calculations, but the denominator is different (compare the formulas in the footnote[2] to the one given earlier for risk).

---

[2]$$\text{Odds} = \frac{\text{Number in group with complication}}{\text{Number in group without complication}}$$

$$\text{Odds ratio} = \frac{\text{Odds of complication in smokers}}{\text{Odds of complications in nonsmokers}}$$

Like relative risk, an odds ratio is a ratio, specifically the odds of a particular outcome occurring in the exposed group (the numerator) relative to the odds of it occurring in the unexposed group (the denominator).[2] For practical purposes, they can be interpreted similarly as they both are ratios representing the association between the frequency of an outcome occurring in two groups. An RR or OR of 1 means the two groups had the same risk or odds of experiencing the particular outcome. A value greater than 1 means the exposed group had a greater likelihood of the outcome than the baseline group and a value less than 1 means the exposed group had a lesser likelihood. Therefore, an RR or OR of 4.0 means that the exposed group had four times the risk of the unexposed group, i.e., were 4 times as likely to experience the outcomes as those in the unexposed group. An RR or OR of 0.75 means the exposed group had 0.75 times the risk of the outcome compared to those who had no exposure. Said differently, the exposed group had a 25% reduction in risk compared to those without the exposure.

Because of the different denominator, RR and OR of an outcome will not be identical. In the exemplar study the RR of the smoker group for a complication was 2.5 but the OR was 4.1. Importantly, RRs are more intuitive than OR because they represent the relative likelihood of an event occurring in one group relative to its likelihood in the other group. As a clinical reader, you are not expected to know when one or the other should be used. The researcher and the peer review team are responsible for getting this right.

> **For practical purposes, RRs and ORs can be interpreted similarly as both are ratios representing the association between the frequency of an outcome occurring in two groups.**

Getting back to Table 5 in the report, we notice that the smokers were the only subgroup having an odds ratio (actually adjusted OR)[3] significantly larger than 1.0; their confidence intervals were the only ones that did not include 1.0. Therefore, being a smoker is the only possible risk

---

[3]An adjusted OR is an OR that takes into account the other variables in the analysis; the adjustment essentially holds the other variables constant while calculating the OR of each variable.

factor that determined whether each of the complications occurred. This analysis in essence ruled out the other risk factors as confounders, leaving smoking as the best explanation for why complications occurred at different rates in the smoker and nonsmoker groups.

Wrap-up of RR and OR   To sum up the RR and OR explanations, you don't have to know how to calculate RRs and ORs or the even technical difference between them, but you should know how to interpret their meanings. Hopefully, from their use in this article you know how to do that. You may find that RRs and ORs have a commonsense meaning if you just remember that:

1. The key word to understanding RRs and ORs is the word *relative*.
2. You need to note which group is the baseline/unexposed group, i.e., the denominator.
3. An RR or OR with 1 in the confidence interval means that the two groups have the same frequency of having the outcome.
4. A value greater than 1 means that the numerator group has a greater likelihood of the outcome than the baseline group and a value less than 1 (and 1 is not in its confidence interval) means a lesser likelihood of the outcome.

Discussion   Importantly, the researchers placed their findings in the context of other work that has been done on the subject and concluded that the findings of this study add to the list of studies showing that smoking is a risk factor for postoperative complications after orthopedic surgery.

References

Dahl, A. W., & Toksvig-Larsen, S. (2004). Cigarette smoking delays bone healing: A prospective study of 200 patients operated on by the hemicallotasis technique. *Acta Orthopaedica Scandinavica, 75*(3), 347–351.

Hanlon, J. T., Pieper, C. F., Hajjar, E. R., Sloane, R. J., Linblad, C. I., Ruby, C. M., & Schmader, K. E. (2006). Incidence and predictors of all preventable adverse drug reactions in frail elderly persons after hospital stay. *Journals of Gerontology. Series A, Biological Sciences and Medical Sciences, 61*(5), 511–515.

Hundrup, Y. A., Simonsen, M. K., Jørgensen, T., & Obel, E. B. (2011). Cohort profile: The Danish nurse cohort. *International Journal of Epidemiology,* 1–7. doi:10.1093/ije/dyr042

Mamdani, M., Skyora, K., Li, P., Normand, S. L., Streiner, D. L., Austin, P. C., . . . Anderson, G. M. (2005). Reader's guide to critical appraisal of cohort studies: 2. Assessing potential for confounding. *British Medical Journal, 330*, 960–962.

Marcin, J. P., Rutan, E., Rapetti, P. M., Rahnsmayi, R., & Pretzlaff, R. K. (2005). Nurse staffing and unplanned extubation in the pediatric intensive care unit. *Pediatric Critical Care Medicine, 6*(3), 254–257.

CHAPTER NINE

Systematic Reviews

O nce several, or many, studies have been conducted on an issue, clinicians or researchers will feel the need to pull together the findings of the various studies into a summary so as to see the big picture. This pulling together is called a systematic research review, most often shortened to systematic review. When done well, a systematic review (SR) helps clinicians and researchers identify what is known with certainty, what is tentatively known, and what the gaps in knowledge are regarding an issue. Not infrequently, SRs serve as a link between individual studies and clinical decision making and between individual studies and clinical practice guidelines.

Sometimes a well-conducted systematic review calls into question a widely used clinical practice method. Other times it confirms the effectiveness of existing practice. For instance, a systematic review of studies examining the effectiveness of rapid response systems included 29 eligible studies (Maharai, Raffaele, & Wendon, 2015). The results for adults were a reduction in cardiopulmonary arrests outside intensive care units and a reduction in hospital mortality outside of ICUs. The reduction in adult hospital mortality was in contrast to an earlier systematic review that found no reduction in this outcome (Chan et al., 2010).

Types of Systematic Reviews

First, a definition of systematic review:

> "The purpose of a systematic review is to sum up the best available research on a specific question. This is done by synthesizing the results of several studies. A systematic review uses transparent procedures to find, evaluate and

synthesize the results of relevant research. Procedures are explicitly defined in advance, in order to ensure that the exercise is transparent and can be replicated" (The Campbell Collaboration, http://www.campbellcollaboration.org/what_is_a_systematic_review/).

There are three ways of summarizing results across studies:

1. Systematic review with narrative synthesis
2. Systematic review with statistical synthesis
3. Systematic review with qualitative synthesis

Just to clarify: synthesis in this context is the combining of the results of multiple individual studies to produce conclusions that represent the body of results—said differently, it is a new whole (group of conclusions) that is produced from the parts (results of individual studies). Although the goal of all three methods of SR is to use rigorous methods to produce integrated conclusions about what is known and not known about an issue, their methods of analysis and synthesis are different. The differences are necessary because the essential nature of clinical issues varies widely, and therefore are studied using different study designs which produce results in different forms.

- Systematic reviews with narrative synthesis are used to analyze and summarize the findings of studies with various types of quantitative data. The adjective *narrative* refers to the fact that the analysis and synthesis are done using logical reasoning and text (in contrast to statistics).
- Systematic reviews with statistical synthesis, widely called meta-analysis, are used to combine the results of experimental studies of treatments and interventions by statistically pooling data to produce an estimate of the direction and size of the treatment effect.
- Systematic reviews with qualitative synthesis aims to identify trends in the findings of qualitative studies so as to develop deeper and more complete understandings of social, psychological, and experiential phenomenon. As the newest method of systematic review, criteria for how to do qualitative synthesis are still evolving and several approaches are in use (Whittemore, Chao, Jang, Minges, & Park, 2014).

Although all three types of SRs produce important knowledge for practice, systematic reviews with narrative synthesis (SRwNS)[1] are more commonly

---

[1]SRwNS are also called state-of-the-science summaries, narrative reviews.

found in clinical nursing journals. Thus, they will be the focus of this chapter and again later in the text. Examples of the other two types of SRs are posted on the student website.

Close and Distant Relatives of SRwNS

A related matter is that you will find articles in the nursing literature called integrative research reviews. The use of this term is quite variable. Some reviews that self-identify as integrative research reviews would qualify as systematic reviews with narrative synthesis whereas others would not. Integrative research reviews are more likely than SRwNS to include both qualitative and quantitative studies, and many integrative reviews incorporate conceptual and theoretical sources; this is not a negative, rather it serves to integrate research and theoretical perspectives. Generally speaking, to qualify as a SRwNS, an integrative research review report should explicitly and transparently describe the review methods used, appraise study quality, and summarize findings (Whittemore et al., 2014).

Before heading into a description of how SRs are produced, I also want to point out that all three types of systematic reviews are different from literature reviews in several ways (see also **Table 9-1**), including:

- Prescribed criteria regarding how an SR should be done have been established. Additionally, SR reports include detailed descriptions about each step in the production process. In contrast, no production process is prescribed for literature reviews; rather they are done according to the reviewers' predilections. And there is no expectation that the production process be described. The lack of a prescribed process for literature reviews and the lack of detailed reporting about how they are done increase the likelihood that they are prone to bias.
- Systematic reviews incorporate only research reports. Literature reviews typically include a wide variety of types of articles including essays, anecdotal accounts, and opinion.
- Systematic reviews are based on a wide and diligent search for studies, whereas literature reviews can be, and often are, selective in what they report.
- Systematic reviews use a quality filter either to exclude poor quality studies or to categorize the quality of studies included; literature reviews do not do this.

TABLE 9-1   Differences Between Systematic Reviews and Literature Reviews

Feature	Systematic Review (SR)	Literature Review
Purpose	Thorough examination of a specific issue	Highlights of an issue; varying degrees of thoroughness
Production process	Standards exist and the process used is described in report	No standards; process not described
Search	As exhaustive as possible	Often limited
Inclusion	Original study reports, previous SRs, information from large databases	Original study reports, theoretical literature, essays, opinion articles
Selection	Should use a quality appraisal filter	Quality filter not used
Report	Inclusive of all qualifying studies	Often selective based on purpose (cherry picking)

The SR Production Process

To be able to judge whether the conclusions of an SR are a sound basis for care, you need to be aware of the standards for producing them. The steps taken to produce all three types of SRs are as follows:

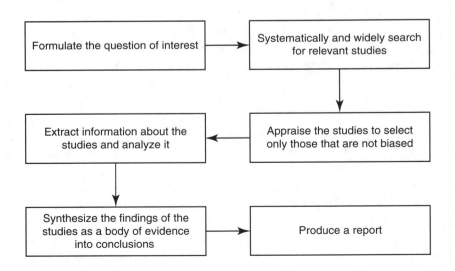

These steps are in accordance with the more detailed process standards set by internationally recognized organizations: Cochrane Collaboration (Higgins & Green, 2011); Institute of Medicine (2011); Joanna Briggs Institute (2011); PRISMA Group (2009). These standards have been set forth in detail to control error and bias. The early steps are similar in all SRs but data extraction, analysis, and synthesis are different for each type of SR.

Formulate the Topic and Assemble a Panel

Panels or individuals with expertise in the issue of interest conduct systematic reviews. The word *conduct* is used because doing an SR is a demanding and rigorous undertaking. A panel has greater potential to conduct an SR that is free of error and bias than does an individual because the panel members act as checks and balances to each other's work and uncover unconscious bias.

Scope

Typically a professional organization identifies the topic, issue, or problem its members think need summarization. The scope of SRs varies; sometimes, the topic is broad; other times the issue is quite narrow. A broad topic addresses several aspects of an issue, whereas a narrow topic focuses on one particular aspect.

For instance, a broad review about preventing falls in home-dwelling elders would have to include studies regarding the functional status of patients (e.g., balance and gait), the role of medications, orthostatic hypotension, environmental issues, and more. In contrast, a narrower review about environmental alterations to prevent falls in the home could focus on a smaller subset of studies having to do with floor surfaces, grab bars, lighting, steps, etc. Broad and narrow scope is not a good–bad issue; the scope depends on what clinicians in the area of practice need to know and what has already been summarized. However, broader topics require more resources to conduct the review, are more difficult to summarize, and require longer reports.

Types of Studies

Early on, the panel considers the types of studies they will include in the SR and how far back they will go in the search for studies and previous SRs. Sometimes changing technology or patterns of care signify that it does not make sense to go back beyond a certain date.

Reviewers can decide to include studies using the full range of designs or just those with certain design characteristics. For instance, a physician group interested in reviewing interventions for urinary incontinence in nursing home residents included only randomized trials (Fink, Taylor, Tacklind, Rutks, & Wilt, 2008). In contrast, a nurse reviewer interested in women's experiences of cardiac pain included only qualitative studies because she was interested in understanding the women's perspective (O'Keefe-McCarthy, 2008). The difference in the types of studies included in the two reviews was determined by the clinical issue of interest.

In the recent past, when conducting an SR about a clinical treatment or intervention, the interest was merely in treatment effectiveness, thus only randomized studies, i.e., experimental studies, were included. Increasingly, however, researchers are recognizing the need to go beyond summarizing studies about the treatment effect to address other issues related to the treatment such as: problems patients have following a particular treatment regimen and how the treatment affects their daily lives. Clearly, these are important considerations when evaluating the evidence in support of a treatment. They shed light on its actual use. In fact, real patient-world effectiveness of a treatment or intervention is most likely a combination of direct physiological or psychological effectiveness and patient response and use factors.

Studies about these real-world issues are conducted using qualitative and nonexperimental methods. Thus, increasingly, organizations producing SRs are working on how qualitative and nonexperimental quantitative studies can be used to inform and add to the information obtained from the randomized controlled studies (Cochrane Collaboration, 2015).

Early on, SR panels decide how they will handle studies that are of dubious or poor methodological quality. Some panels will include them but note their poor or modest quality, whereas other panels will eliminate them altogether. Still others will analyze the results of low-quality and high-quality studies together and then separately to determine if study quality affects the conclusions.

Search for Studies and Screen for Relevance

When the topic and scope have been clearly specified, the search for studies begins. Most review panels include a health science librarian who has expertise in locating research reports. The most common search-starting place is the computerized databases of the published healthcare literature (CINAHL, MEDLINE, PsycINFO, and others). Reviewers typically search several healthcare databases using a variety of search terms, combinations of search terms, and search options.

Usually, the panel's initial goal is to identify all potential studies on the issue; however, database indexing and retrieval may fail to identify some eligible studies, which can be a source of bias. Moreover, databases include only published studies, and some studies may have been done but not published. Thus, retrieval of eligible studies from databases is only a starting point. In an attempt to include findings from all relevant studies, panels often peruse reference lists, check research registries and conference presentations, contact colleagues, and even run searches using Web search engines.

At this point, hundreds of citations may be under consideration. Careful reading of abstracts can reduce the number considerably by eliminating those that are not research reports or are not on topic. Then, all potentially relevant research reports are retrieved. Using a prespecified set of inclusion–exclusion criteria, two or more persons decide which studies are eligible for the SR.

Appraise

All of the eligible studies should then be carefully appraised for quality; the goal of this appraisal is to eliminate studies that are biased or not credible because of the study methods. The number of studies that survive relevance screening and quality appraisal may be much smaller than the number initially identified during the search phase. It is not uncommon to have hundreds of citations identified by the search, but end up with 30, or even 8 studies, in the final review.

Extract and Analyze

The panel will then sort the final body of research reports into stacks by key questions or subtopics, such as those using similar forms of the intervention or those evaluating a particular clinical outcome. For instance, a study of the effectiveness of home palliative care looked separately at the outcomes of pain control, symptom burden for patients, caregiver grief, and cost (Gomes, Calanzani, Curiale, McCrone, & Higginson, 2013).

Basic information about design, sample, variables studied, and results are carefully extracted from the report and entered into evidence tables (see **Table 9-2**). Lists or coding may be used to help identify differences,

TABLE 9-2   Example of a Findings Table from an SRwNS Comparing Exercise Programs

Study	N Randomized/ Followed up*	Participants, Inclusion Criteria and Mean Age	Interventions	Primarily Aimed at†	Follow-up‡	Outcome measures§	Results⊘
Binder, 2002, USA	IG: 69/66 CG: 50/49	Two out of three criteria: Score 18–32 on modified PPT, peak oxygen uptake between 10–18 mL/kg/min, self-reported difficulty in max. 2 ADLs or 1 IADL (Mean age: 83)	IG: 9-month program provided by physiology exercise technicians consisting of three phases of each 36 sessions. Phase 1: Group format: 22 exercises on flexibility, balance, coordination, speed of reaction and strength. Phase 2: Progressive resistance training combined with shortened version of phase 1 exercises. Phase 3: Endurance training combined with shortened version of phase 1 and phase 2 exercises. CG: 9-month home exercise program including 9 of the 22 exercises from phase 1. Participants were asked to perform exercises 2–3 times a week and attended a monthly class.	Reduce or delay frailty	3, 6, and 9 months	Self-reported use of assistance or assistive technology (OARS ADL and IADL scale) Self-reported difficulty with ADL and IADL (Physical Function subscale of FSQ) Modified PPT items Knee extension/ flexion strength VO$_2$-peak Balance Body weight	No differences between groups (data not presented). Difference (SS) in favor of IG. Differences (SS) in favor of IG for modified PPT score knee strength, VO$_2$-peak and balance. No SS difference for body weight (data not shown).

Boshuizen, 2005, Netherlands	Experiencing difficulty in rising from chair and maximum knee extensor torque < 87.5 N-m (Mean age: ~79)	Increasing strength knee extensors	10–12 weeks	*IG:* High-guidance: 10-wk exercise program, each week two group sessions (60 min) by PT and one unsupervised home session. Focus on exercises with a variation in concentric, isometric, and eccentric knee-extensor activity.	Self-reported performance in activities of daily living (GARS)	No differences between groups.
IG: High guidance (HG) 24/16						
IG: Medium guidance (MG) 26/16				*IG:* Medium-guidance: Same program, though each week one supervised session and two unsupervised home sessions.	Knee extensor strength Walking function Balance Box stepping Timed Up and GO	Difference (SS) in knee strength and walking function for HG group compared to CG. Differences (NS) between HG and MG for walking function in favor of HG.
CG: 22/17				*CG:* No training or other encouragement		

(continued)

TABLE 9-2   Example of a Findings Table from an SRwNS Comparing Exercise Programs (*continued*)

Study	N Randomized/ Followed up*	Participants, Inclusion Criteria and Mean Age	Interventions	Primarily Aimed at†	Follow-up‡	Outcome measures§	Results[¶]
Chandler, 1998, USA	IG: 50/44 CG: 50/43	Inability to descend stairs step over step without holding the railing (Mean age: ~78)	IG: 10-wk exercise program, each week three individual in-home sessions by PT. Focus: Progressive resistive lower extremity exercises with Thera-Band. CG: No training or any encouragement.	Increasing lower extremity strength	10 weeks	Self-reported limitations in physical activities (MOS-36 physical functioning subscale) Lower extremity strength Physical performance	No significant differences between groups (data not presented). Greater lower extremity (SS) strength gain in favor of IG (data on physical performance not presented).

Adapted from Daniels, R., van Rossum, E., de Witte, L., Kempen, G. I., & van den Heuvel, W. (2008). Interventions to prevent disability in frail community-dwelling elderly: A systematic review. *BMC Health Services Research, 8,* 278. Retrieved from http://www.biomedcentral.com/content/pdf/1472-6963-8-278.pdf

*Randomized relates to the number of participants randomized to intervention guidance (IG) and control group (CG). Followed up relates to the numbers of participants taken into data analysis.

†Outcome that the authors primarily aimed to improve by conducting the intervention.

‡Follow-up measurement in weeks or months after randomization.

§Measured disability concept and instrument, followed by outcome measures for frailty components.

[¶]SS = Statistically significant difference if *p* < 0.05; NS = Not statistically significant.

commonalities, and patterns across the studies. Different research questions, contexts, ways of measuring a variable, or timing of the outcome measurement are noted. Similarities and differences in findings are identified and reasons for the variations explored.

Synthesize/Conclude

The goal of synthesis is to reach conclusions that represent the findings of the individual studies as elements of a body of findings, which is different from looking at each one in isolation from the others. This combining of findings from many studies in the form of integrated conclusions is referred to as *synthesis* because new knowledge claims are produced—claims that go beyond what any single study produced. The term *synthesis* makes the process of bringing research findings together sound quite exacting—which is not quite the reality. In the conduct of all three forms of SRs, even when the reviewers are conscientious, interpretation is inherent in the process; assumptions, decisions about inclusion and exclusion, and faulty reasoning can affect the conclusions—and even produce misleading ones. However, these sources of bias can be minimized by following the recognized ways of conducting SRwNSs.

Synthesis involves integrating the findings, with due consideration of differences, similarities, and relative methodological quality. In the case of SRwNS, the integration is achieved using inductive reasoning to produce conclusions, which are in essence new findings. In the case of SRs with meta-analysis, the data from the original studies are extracted and pooled for the statistical analysis that evaluates the overall direction and size of the effect. Often, the statistical estimate of treatment effect size (point estimate and 95% confidence interval) for each study in the SR is shown in a graph that makes clear how many studies found a benefit, how many found no benefit, and how large the benefit or lack of it was. For those readers interested in understanding the results of a meta-analysis, several references are provided on the text website; alternatively you can search online for "meta-analysis forest plots."

Report

SRwNS reports open by stating the issue they examine and why the reviewers think it is important. You should note if the review focused on a certain population or setting, and whether it is focused on one or several outcomes. For instance, a review about the effectiveness of relaxation techniques could focus just on the outcome of pain, or it could also include studies that examined relaxation techniques for anxiety, onset of panic attacks, or smoking cessation.

Next, the process that was used to search for study reports is described in detail, including databases searched, key terms used, and any inclusion or exclusion criteria used. The number of records identified, included and excluded, and the reasons for exclusions should be indicated, often using a flow diagram such as that in **Figure 9-1**. The process used to extract information from the reports and the methods used to evaluate the quality of the studies should also be described.

Typically, tables display much-abbreviated profiles of the studies and their findings. Table 9-2 is part of an evidence table from a review of exercise interventions to prevent disability in frail community-dwelling elderly (Daniels, van Rossum, de Witte, Kempen, & van den Heuvel, 2008). Note how this table provides a quick overview of the methods and the results of the studies.

In the text, findings that are consistent, conflicting, and equivocal, as well as gaps in the research base, are reported, and bottom-line conclusions are set forth. Finally, the panel or authors indicate whether and how their conclusions square with any prior work that has been done on the topic, summarize the limitations of the body of research, and offer opinions regarding the clinical implications of the conclusions.

Use of SRwNS

SRwNSs are being published in clinical journals with increasing frequency, which is very helpful to clinician teams designing nursing protocols. Locating a well-conducted, recent SRwNS saves a clinical project team all the work of identifying, retrieving, appraising, analyzing, and summarizing the research findings pertaining to the protocol they are designing.

At the same time, users of SRwNSs need to keep in mind that the conclusions are interpretations of findings. Two review groups examining the same body of research findings could arrive at different conclusions. From the search of studies to the appraisal of the quality of the individual studies and on through the conclusions, there are numerous points at which the opinion of two review groups could differ. One group may discount the findings of a study that another group thinks is important. One group

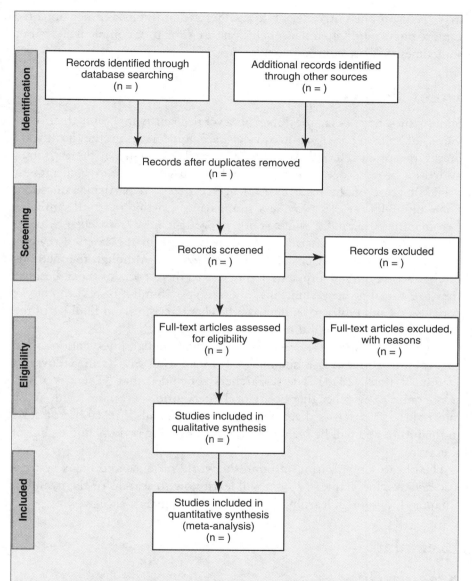

Reproduced from Moher, D., Liberati, A., Tetzlaff, J., Altman, D. G., The PRISMA Group. (2009). Preferred reporting items for systematic reviews and meta-analyses: The PRISMA statement. *PLOS Med 6*(6): e1000097. doi:10.1371/journal.pmed1000097

Figure 9-1   PRISMA 2009 Flow Diagram

may focus on one outcome, while another group thinks another outcome is more important. Often the conclusions are similar or complementary but sometimes they are contradictory.

Umbrella SRs

Some issues have been the topic of several, even many, SRs; thus overviews of existing systematic reviews are appearing in the healthcare literature—often referred to as *umbrella reviews*. Many of these reviews address a broad scope of issues related to a topic of interest and present a wide picture of the research evidence related to a particular question. Some umbrella reviews provide a summary of existing research syntheses (Aromataris et al., n.d.), whereas others produce new knowledge by combining information, patterns, and inconsistencies in the existing reviews into new conclusions (Conn & Coon Sells, 2015). Although the methods of conducting umbrella reviews are rigorous, the reports of them, because they are aimed at busy clinicians, often use a minimum of text to convey conclusions and tables to summarize the characteristics and findings of the individual SRs (Becker, n.d.).

An SR of existing SRs regarding behavior change interventions used to promote condom use summarized 13 existing SRs (von Sadovszky, Daudt, & Boch, 2014). The researchers concluded that "There is a preponderance of evidence that behavioral interventions promote condom use and reduce STIs across diverse groups of individuals" (p. 107). For sure, in the future you will be seeing more SRs of existing reviews in the clinical literature.

Healthcare organizations around the world produce and index systematic reviews. In Chapter 12, you will learn how to search for them, and in Chapter 15, you will learn how to appraise the quality of SRwNS.

Exemplar

Reading Tip

The additional files (supplementary material) mentioned in the report can be accessed from the electronic version in the "Additional File" box near the end of the article.

Graverholt, B., Forsetlund, L., & Jamtvedt, G. (2014). Reducing hospital admission from nursing home: A systematic review. *BMC Health Services Research, 14*,36. Retrieved from http://www.biomedcentral.com/1472-6963/14/36. Creative Commons license available at http://creativecommons.org/licenses/by/2.0.

Research article: Reducing hospital admissions from nursing homes: A systematic review

BIRGITTE GRAVERHOLT[1,2*], LOUISE FORSETLUND[3], AND GRO JAMTVEDT[1,3]

[1]Centre for Evidence-Based Practice, Bergen University College, Bergen PB 7030, 5020, Norway. [2]Department of Global Public Health and Primary Care, University of Bergen, Bergen, Norway. [3]The Norwegian Knowledge Centre for the Health Services, Oslo, Norway.

Abstract

Background: The geriatric nursing home population is vulnerable to acute and deteriorating illness due to advanced age, multiple chronic illnesses and high levels of dependency. Although the detriments of hospitalising the frail and old are widely recognised, hospital admissions from nursing homes remain common. Little is known about what alternatives exist to prevent and reduce hospital admissions from this setting. The objective of this study, therefore, is to summarise the effects of interventions to reduce acute hospitalisations from nursing homes.

Methods: A systematic literature search was performed in Cochrane Library, PubMed, MEDLINE, EMBASE and ISI Web of Science in April 2013. Studies were eligible if they had a geriatric nursing home study population and were evaluating any type of intervention aiming at reducing acute hospital admission. Systematic reviews, randomised controlled trials, quasi randomised controlled trials, controlled before-after studies and interrupted time series were eligible study designs. The process of selecting studies, assessing them, extracting data and grading the total evidence was done by two researchers individually, with any disagreement solved by a third. We made use of meta-analyses from included systematic reviews, the remaining synthesis is descriptive. Based on the type of intervention, the included studies were categorised in: 1) Interventions to structure and standardise clinical practice, 2) Geriatric specialist services and 3) Influenza vaccination.

Results: Five systematic reviews and five primary studies were included, evaluating a total of 11 different interventions. Fewer hospital admissions were found in four out of seven evaluations of structuring and standardising clinical practice; in both evaluations of geriatric specialist services, and in influenza vaccination of residents. The quality of the evidence for all comparisons was of low or very low quality, using the GRADE approach.

Conclusions: Overall, eleven interventions to reduce hospital admissions from nursing homes were identified. None of them were tested more than once and the quality of the evidence was low for every comparison. Still, several interventions had effects on reducing hospital admissions and may represent important aspects of nursing home care to reduce hospital admissions.

Keywords: Nursing home, Homes for the aged, Hospitalization, Hospitalisation, Acute care, Hospital admission

Background

Longevity, chronic illness, frailty and deficits in activities of daily living are common characteristics of the geriatric nursing home population. These features are predispositions to a trajectory of health with acute incidences which raises the question about acute care hospitalisation. Acute flares in nursing home residents' health may call for services not necessarily available in the nursing homes, such as diagnostic procedures, particular interventions or a shift towards end-of-life care. Indeed, studies from a range of different countries with well-developed nursing home sectors have demonstrated that acute hospital admissions occur commonly, with annual rates from 9% up to 60% [1–7]. Noteworthy, large variations in hospital admission rates from nursing homes are not only observed between countries, but also within countries and in small geographic areas [1,8,9].

Adding to this picture, a number of studies have pointed to the detrimental impacts that hospitalisations may have on elderly people, including iatrogenic illnesses, like infections to functional and cognitive decline [10–16]. Additionally, the nursing home population is appointed to account for many potentially unnecessary hospitalisations, with estimates between 19–67% [17–20]. As such, a reduction of hospital admissions among nursing home residents may potentially serve a dual benefit of improving care for residents, as well as reducing use and monetary cost of specialist health care.

Although it is strongly communicated that nursing home residents represent an overuse of specialist services [17–20], it is not clear what strategies can best substitute hospitalisations. Thus, enforced by healthcare reforms that warrant for a shift in the provision of health care from specialist to primary care settings, there is an increasing interest for care models that can replace frequent and perhaps unnecessary use of hospital admissions from nursing homes [21,22]. Still, it is not clear what strategies can best substitute hospitalisations, to achieve the twofold aim of providing high quality services and reducing cost in specialist health care.

The objective of this systematic review is therefore to summarise the effects of interventions to reduce acute hospitalisations from nursing homes.

Methods

This is an update of a systematic review published in Norwegian by the Norwegian Knowledge Centre for the Health Services [23]. A protocol for the first version, including eligibility criteria, search strategy and methods of analysis, was developed in advance and made available in PROSPERO [24].

Eligibility criteria

We considered studies with a geriatric nursing home study population, evaluating any type of intervention aiming at reducing hospitalisation, compared to care as usual or a different intervention. The primary outcome measure of interest was acute hospital admission. The secondary outcomes, listed in the protocol, are only reported in the supplementary summary of findings tables (Additional file 1: Tables S4–S12). Study designs eligible for this review were systematic reviews, randomized controlled trials (RCT), quasi-randomized controlled trials, controlled before-after studies and interrupted time series. We imposed no restriction on language or publication year in the search. We decided to deal with languages as they emerged and to draw on language proficiency levels in the review group, among colleagues or to translate studies if necessary. The two studies in Spanish and Austrian was managed in the review team and no studies were excluded due to language.

Literature search

The updated literature searches were carried out from the inception and until April 2013 in the following databases: The Cochrane Library, PubMed, MEDLINE Ovid 1946, EMBASE Ovid 1974, ISI Web of Science and CINAHL Ebsco. The search strategy was developed using keywords and standardised key words, where appropriate. The search terms derived from the population/setting (nursing home) and the primary outcome (hospitalisation). The complete search strategy is available in the (Additional file 1: Table S1) and in the protocol [24].

Study selection and assessment

Titles and abstracts that the literature search brought fourth were screened independently by two researchers (LF, BG). Any potentially relevant publication was ordered in full-text and assessed for inclusion and exclusion according to eligibility criteria, following the same procedure. Any disagreement in the process of selecting, assessing and collecting data was solved by a third researcher (GJ).

Reviews that fulfilled criteria for inclusion were assessed for methodological quality using a check list based on international criteria for assessing reviews [25]. Only reviews of high quality were included. From the included SRs, we only used data from included primary studies that were relevant to our eligibility criteria. We used the review authors' own assessment of risk of bias. For primary studies we used the risk of bias tool from Cochrane Handbook [26]. We used GRADE (Grading of Recommendations, Assessment, Development and Evaluation) to assess and grade the quality of the overall documentation for each outcome as high, middle, low or very low quality [27].

Data extraction process

For each included study, we extracted the following information: Full reference, the number of study participants, type of intervention, type of control intervention, the setting and outcomes. If the outcome was measured several times in a study, we used the last observation.

Synthesis of results

Where possible, we reported the overall effect estimate from meta-analyses in included systematic reviews (Additional file 1: Tables S11–S12) [28,29]. For the remaining included studies, analyses were descriptive, due to differences in interventions. We used RevMan 5 to recalculate estimates if we considered that this would improve the reporting of the effect estimates, the preferred presentation being relative risks (RR) with 95% confidence intervals (CI).

Results

Study selection

The literature search identified a total of 6 250 unique references. Of these, 54 studies were retrieved in full text and assessed according to eligibility criteria. A total of four systematic reviews and five primary studies met the inclusion criteria and were included. **Figure 1** holds the details of the selection process. A table of excluded studies and reason for exclusion is available as an (Additional file 1: Table S2).

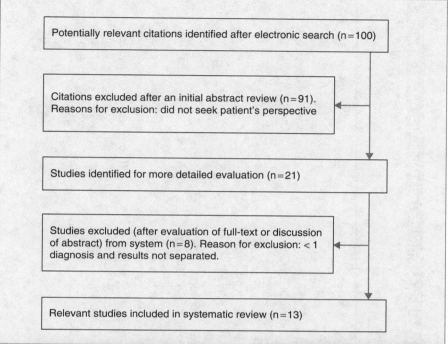

Potentially relevant citations identified after electronic search (n=100)

Citations excluded after an initial abstract review (n=91). Reasons for exclusion: did not seek patient's perspective

Studies identified for more detailed evaluation (n=21)

Studies excluded (after evaluation of full-text or discussion of abstract) from system (n=8). Reason for exclusion: < 1 diagnosis and results not separated.

Relevant studies included in systematic review (n=13)

Figure 1   Flow chart of the selection process

Characteristics of included studies

Four systematic reviews and five primary studies, evaluating a total of 11 different interventions were included. All but two of the included studies were in English; these two were Austrian and Spanish [30,31]. Follow-up periods varied between 30 days up to 3 years. The interventions varied fundamentally and made it unfeasible to do meta analyses; the exception being two included Cochrane reviews on the effect of influenza vaccination [28,29].

We classified the type of interventions into three categories; Interventions to structure or standardise clinical practice, geriatric specialist services and influenza vaccination. The categories were decided after the inclusion of studies, to cluster studies according to type of intervention. The results are presented according to these categories: Tables 1, 2, 3 hold descriptions of included studies and Additional file 1: Tables S4–S12 are summary of findings.

Only the results for the primary outcome (hospitalisation) are reported in the manuscript. The results for other outcomes are included in the summary of finding tables (Additional file 1: Tables S4–S12).

Table 1 Table of included studies in the category interventions to structure and standardise clinical practice

Study, design, included studies if SR*	Population	Intervention	Control	The setting and nationality
Robinson 2012 [32], Systematic review, 3/4 studies were relevant for inclusion	People with cognitive impairment	Defined as 'Any kind of advance care planning' by review authors.	Usual care	Any care environment, including nursing homes
Caplan 2006, Controlled before-after design		A structured educational programme (Let Me Decide) for health personnel, residents and their families		Nursing homes in Canada, Australia and USA
Molloy 2000, Randomised controlled trial		The Let Me Decide programme in addition to hospital-to-the-nursing-home		
Morrison 2005, Non-randomised controlled trial		Half-day course for social workers in guiding residents and families in ACP. Feedback to physicians was given in intervention group to initiate referral to palliative care.		
Hall 2011 [33], Systematic review	Residents of care homes for older people	Defined as 'All types of palliative care service delivery interventions' by review authors.	Not specified	Setting defined as 'collective institutional settings where care is provided' Nursing homes in USA

1/3 studies was relevant for inclusion: Casarett 2005, Randomised controlled trial

Study	Population	Intervention	Comparison	Setting
Hutt 2011 [34], Controlled before-after study	Nursing home residents with symptoms of systemic lower respiratory tract infection	Multifaceted implementation of a national guideline for management of nursing-home-acquired pneumonia	Usual care	16 nursing homes in Colorado, USA (8 intervention homes and 8 control homes)
Loeb 2006 [35], Cluster randomised controlled trial	Nursing home residents with pneumonia	On-site treatment of pneumonia according to pathway	Usual care	22 nursing homes Ontario, Canada
Lee 2002 [36], Cluster randomised controlled trial	Nursing home residents with chronic obstructive pulmonary disease	Community nurses followed up residents for 6 months post-hospitalisation according to a care protocol	Usual care	45 nursing homes in Hong Kong, China

*See included systematic review for full reference of included primary studies.

Methodological quality

Overall, using GRADE, we judged the quality of the evidence as being low or very low for all outcomes. All but one comparison was downgraded because of a high or unclear risk of bias. Imprecision was the second most frequent reason to downgrade and indirectness was a problem in several studies. The evidence from one of the systematic reviews was additionally downgraded due to inconsistency of results between studies. In the supplemental file, all judgements for assessing methodological quality are made explicit (Additional file 1: Tables S4–S12).

Effects of interventions

Interventions to structure and standardise clinical practice

Seven different interventions in this category had been evaluated in two systematic reviews and three single studies **(Table 1)**. One systematic review summarised the effect of advance care planning in people with cognitive impairment, and included three studies relevant for this review [32]. Two of the studies, a cluster randomised controlled trial and a controlled before after study, both investigated a structured program aimed at residents, families and health personnel in the intervention homes, but the latter additionally provided hospital-to-nursing-home services. Both studies found that intervention homes reported fewer hospitalisations than the control homes (mean 0.27 hospitalisations vs. 0.48, $p = 0.001$, and RR 0.89, 95% CI: 0.85–0.93, respectively). In the third study, a cluster-RCT, social workers in intervention wards received a course in how to do structured interviews with residents to identify needs for advance directives.

Table 2   Table of included studies in the category geriatric specialist services

Study, design	Population	Intervention	Control	The setting and nationality
Díaz-Genúndez 2011 [30], Controlled before-after study	Nursing home residents	Ambulatory geriatric team doing comprehensive geriatric assessments of residents and revision of their medication, in addition to providing educational sessions and support to staff	Usual care	14 nursing homes in Spain (10 voluntary intervention homes, 14 control homes)
Shippinger 2012 [31], Controlled before-after study	Nursing home residents	Mobile GEriatric Consultant geriatric service (GECO) in addition to usual care	Usual care	Two nursing homes in Austria (one intervention home and one control home)

Table 3 Table of included studies in the category influenza vaccination

Study, design, Included studies if SR*	Population	Intervention	Control	The setting and nationality
Thomas 2010 [29], Systematic review	Healthcare workers caring for elderly residents in institutions	Promotion of vaccination of healthcare workers with any influenza vaccine given alone or with other vaccines	Usual care	Any type of institution for elderly, including nursing homes
2/5 studies were relevant for inclusion: Hayward 2006, Lemaitre 2009, Cluster-randomised controlled trials				Nursing homes in England and France
Jefferson 2010 [28], Systematic review	Elderly people	Vaccination with any influenza vaccine	Usual care	Irrespective of setting, including nursing homes
One to 27 out of 75 studies were relevant: Feery 1976, Saah 1986b, Horman 1986, Fyson 1983a, Patriarca 1985a, Goodman 1982, Straburg 1986, Fyson 1983b, Meiklejohn 1987, Cartter 1990c, Cartter 1990a, Cartter 1990, Aylor 1992, Morens 1995, Monto 2001, Murayama 1999, Ruben 1974, Saah 1986a, Arroyo 1984, Coles 1992, Patriarca 1985b, Caminiti 1994, Deguchi 2001, Howells 1975a, Howells 1975b, Howells 1975c, Saah 1986c, Strassburg 1986, Arden 1988, Cartter 1990b, Taylor 1992, Mukerjee 1994, Isaacs 1997, Leung 2007, D'Alessio 1969, Currier 1988, Saito 2002a, Saito 2002b, Gross 1988, Cuneo Crovari 1980, Howarth 1987a, Howarth 1987b				Nursing homes in USA, Australia, Canada, Japan, Italy, China, UK

*See included systematic review for full reference of included primary studies.

The effect of this intervention on number of hospitalisations was unclear (RR 0.60, 95% CI 0.28–1.28) (Additional file 1: Table S4).

The other review evaluated the effectiveness of palliative care service delivery interventions in nursing homes, and one of three included studies met our eligibility criteria [33]. This was an RCT aimed at increasing the use of hospice services by supporting physicians in identifying residents in need for this. The intervention group reported lower hospitalisation rate (mean annual admissions 0.28 per bed (SD ± 0.70) vs. 0.49 (SD ± 0.89), $p = 0.004$) (Additional file 1: Table S5).

Hutt and colleagues [34] tested the effect of a multifaceted implementation strategy of a national guideline for management of nursing home acquired pneumonia in a cluster-RCT [34]. The risk difference between intervention and control group was a statistically non-significant reduction in hospitalisation for the intervention group (Additional file 1: Table S6). Loeb and colleagues [35] compared the use of a clinical care pathway to usual care for nursing home residents developing symptoms of lower respiratory infections, also using a cluster-RCT design (Additional file 1: Table S7) [35]. Among the intervention homes there was a statistically significant lower hospital admission rate (weighted mean difference of 12% [95% CI:5–18%, $p = 0.001$]). In the last of the three primary studies, Lee and colleagues [36] compared a care protocol with usual care for residents recently hospitalised with chronic obstructive pulmonary disease (COPD) (Additional file 1: Table S8) [36]. There was not a statistical significant difference in re-hospitalisation rates between the groups in number of COPD-related readmissions (p-value = 0.67).

The quality of the evidence for the results for this category was graded low or very low quality (Additional file 1: Tables S4–S8).

Geriatric specialist services

The use of geriatric specialist services in nursing homes was evaluated in two single studies [30,31]. Both of these tested the effectiveness of providing ambulant specialist services, in addition to usual care, but in different facets. Schippinger [31] evaluated a service where a physician did regular and on-call visits intended to provide services otherwise associated with hospitalisation (Additional file 1: Table S10) [31]. The intervention home had fewer cases of hospitalisation than the control home (6.1 cases vs. 11.7 cases per 100 residents, $p < 0.01$). Dìaz-Gegùndez [30] evaluated an ambulant team with a nurse and a physician, doing comprehensive geriatric assessments of residents as well as reviewing medications and providing support to staff (Additional file 1: Table S9) [30]. Also in this study, the intervention group reported fewer hospitalisations than the control group (56 cases vs. 32 cases per 100) (RR 0.58, 95% CI: 0.52–0.65) (calculated by us, based on numbers given in the study).

The quality of the evidence for the results for this category was graded very low (Additional file 1: Tables S9–S10).

Influenza vaccination

Two Cochrane reviews concerning influenza vaccination were relevant for this review; one reviewing studies where health personnel were encouraged to vaccinate and another where effects of influenza vaccination among residents were reviewed [28,29]. In the first review by Thomas [29], two out of five included studies were relevant to us, but the effect of influenza vaccination in health personnel on hospitalisation of residents was unclear (RR 0.89, 95% CI: 0.75–1.06) (Additional file 1: Table S11) [29]. In the review by Jefferson [28], the meta-analysis showed a favourable effect on hospitalisation for the residents that were vaccinated (RR 0.51, 95% CI: 0.33–0.66) (1.1% in intervention group vs. 1.7% in control group) (Additional file 1: Table S11) [28].

The quality of the evidence for the effect of vaccinating health personnel or nursing home residents was graded low and very low, respectively (Additional file 1: Tables S11–S12).

Discussion

We set out to systematically review the effects of interventions to reduce acute hospital admissions from nursing homes. Four systematic reviews and five primary studies were included, evaluating a total of eleven different interventions. Overall, using GRADE, the quality of the evidence for all outcomes was low or very low. In systematic reviews, the quality of evidence reflects the extent of confidence that an estimate of effect is correct [37]. As such, our confidence in the findings is weak. Still, we believe that this review is an important contribution as the first truly systematic and transparent approach to the topic. Further, several of the included studies showed promising effects on hospital admission, but were downgraded, in many cases because of the relatively few included patients. Among the seven interventions to structure or standardise treatment, a reduction in hospital admissions was found for four of them. This was the case for two out of three advance care planning interventions, one intervention to enhance the use of palliative care services and one where a care pathway for lower respiratory tract infections was tested. For the three remaining interventions in this category; an ACP-intervention involving social workers, one multifaceted implementation of a national guideline for the treatment of pneumonia and a care protocol for residents with COPD, a statistical significant difference in hospitalisation between the intervention and control group was not found. Two single studies tested geriatric specialist services, both involving flexible and add-on special competence and human resources to the care in nursing homes. Both of these reported fewer hospitalisations in favour of the intervention. Two Cochrane reviews respectively tested influenza vaccination among residents and health personnel. The case of vaccinating residents, although many studies were identified, only observational design studies were found, making it infeasible to draw conclusive inferences from the findings. Also, noteworthy, all of the studies failed to show an effect on laboratory-confirmed influenza, raising serious doubt in the inherent conceptual mechanism of the intervention. Further, it is not clear whether promoting influenza vaccination among health personnel makes a difference on hospitalisations of nursing home residents.

Limitations

Although the literature searches were conducted by a research librarian using well-developed search filters and strategies, there is always a possibility of missing relevant studies due to the structural complexity of the literature databases, lack of use of pregnant text words in abstracts and also, in some instances, inconsistent indexing of articles. In our search we required that the references should be either indexed with terms for hospitalisations or having used 'hospitalisation' or a synonym in the abstract.

The screening process introduced predicament for a few studies, where hospitalisation was an outcome measure but where the intervention was not aimed at reducing hospitalisations. In these cases hospitalisation was measured as a possible adverse effect of an intervention that, in turn, was not aimed at reducing hospitalisations. When in doubt, we used the aim of the study to determine whether the intervention could coherently impact on acute hospitalisation admissions. This may have led to different decisions in the hands of other reviewers.

Most often, the comparison of the intervention was against usual care, however, this can obviously have different meanings in various settings and usually the descriptions leave it somewhat unclear what the comparison really was. Caution must be shown when judging the transferability of findings and circumstances from one nursing home setting to another, particularly across nationalities.

Implications and future research

The clinical usefulness of this review is weakened by the low quality of the evidence of the included studies, as well as the limited numbers of evaluations for each comparison. Unfortunately, this is not a stand-alone example in the sphere of research in nursing homes, as the body of evidence with robust designs to inform decisions is generally small, with few interventions evaluated more than once [38]. Several intervention studies were excluded because of a weak before-after study design, such as the INTERACT studies [39,40]. The fact that the quality of evidence for every comparison in this review was downgraded is not equivalent to claiming the interventions do not impact on hospitalisation, though. Rather, this renders the need for further studies, to increase the confidence of the findings.

As healthcare policies around the globe are seeking ways to increase efficacy and reduce strain on specialist services, reducing emergency admissions is often accentuated as the key to achieve this. However, it is currently debated whether the frail and old really represent much of a potential in this case [41–43]. Although remaining a target population in the health-policy discourse, it appears that much of the rhetoric is based on anecdotal arguments. This review brings together what is available evidence to inform the case for acutely ill nursing home residents. The fact that we found few studies fulfilling our eligibility criteria, even as accepting less rigorous designs for evaluating effectiveness of interventions, confirms that little research effort is placed on this matter. This is an evidence-policy gap with an urgent need to better inform current policies and reforms in the case of nursing home residents. A larger and better body of evidence is required before recommendations and incitements come in place. Moreover, research policies should request trials in the intersection between primary and secondary care for frail and old residents, emphasising which methodological demands are necessary for the research to have impact.

Most of the studies referred to introductorily, to underpin the argument for reducing hospitalisations, are based on observational studies [10–16], without control groups. Intuitively, reducing hospitalisations for this very frail group of elderly is favourable, but prospective studies with control groups are required to provide more solid evidence for the well-used arguments. Secondly, the studies where many hospitalisations are claimed to be ambulatory care sensitive, and thus potentially unnecessary, are mostly based on secondary analysis of administrative data [17–20]. These judgments are thus made in retrospect, where contextual information is lost.

For future studies evaluating interventions to reduce hospitalisations, adherence to the framework of complex interventions is recommended, where barriers and facilitators for treating the residents on-site, and process evaluations are addressed

[44,45]. Clearly, the potential for interdisciplinary innovations across levels of health care is present, and necessary. It goes without saying, but interventions reducing hospitalisations must hold proof of being a more gentle option for the frail and old, in addition to being equally safe and effective.

Conclusions

Few evaluations are conducted on the effects of interventions to reduce hospital admissions from nursing homes. Eleven evaluated interventions were identified, but none were tested more than once with a rigorous study design. Although the quality of evidence was low for all comparisons in this review, some of the interventions had effects on reducing hospital admissions. These interventions, such as advance care planning, palliative care, care pathways and geriatric specialist services, may represent important aspects of nursing home care to reduce hospital admissions and should be studied further. Our findings suggest an evidence-policy gap, where current policies and practices are lacking evidence-based management strategies to underpin them.

Additional file

Additional file 1: An additional file is available (Supplementary File), containing the complete search strategy (Table S1), table of excluded studies with reason for exclusion (Table S2), risk of bias assessments of primary studies (Table S3) and GRADE summary of findings tables (Table S4–S12).

Competing interests

All authors declare they have no competing interests.

Authors' contributions

BG, LF, and GJ made substantial contributions to conception of the study and to the development of the protocol of this review, the acquisition of data and interpretation of the data. BG drafted the manuscript and LF and GJ has been involved in revising it critically before submission. Approval of the final version has been given from all authors.

Acknowledgements

Research librarian Mariann Mathiesen, The Norwegian Knowledge Centre for the Health Services, made a substantial contribution to setting up and carrying out the literature search for the studies.

Received: 1 August 2013; Accepted: 21 January 2014
Published: 24 January 2014

References

1. Grabowski DC, Stewart KA, Broderick SM, Coots LA: Predictors of nursing home hospitalization a review of the literature. *Med Care Res Rev* 2008, 65(1):3–39.

2. Graverholt B, Riise T, Jamtvedt G, Ranhoff AH, Kruger K, Nortvedt MW: Acute hospital admissions among nursing home residents: a population-based observational study. *BMC Health Serv Res* 2011, 11:126.

3. Condelius A, Hallberg IR, Jakobsson U: Medical healthcare utilization as related to long-term care at home or in special accommodation. *Arch Gerontol Geriatr* 2010, 51(3):250–256.

4. Godden S, Pollock AM: The use of acute hospital services by elderly residents of nursing and residential care homes. *Health Soc Care Community* 2001, 6(9): 367–374.

5. Ronald LA, McGregor MJ, McGrail KM, Tate RB, Broemling A-M: Hospitalization rates of nursing home residents and community-dwelling seniors in British Columbia. *Can J Aging* 2008, 27(1):109–116.

6. Gruneir A, Bell CM, Bronskill SE, Schull M, Anderson GM, Rochon PA: Frequency and pattern of emergency department visits by long-term care residents—a population-based study. *J Am Geriatr Soc* 2010, 58(3):510–517.

7. Jensen PM, Fraser F, Shankardass K, Epstein R, Khera J: Are long-term care residents referred appropriately to hospital emergency departments? *Can Fam Physician* 2009, 55(5):500–505.

8. Carter MW, Porell FW: Variations in hospitalization rates among nursing home residents: the role of facility and market attributes. *Gerontologist* 2003, 43(2):175–191.

9. Graverholt B, Riise T, Jamtvedt G, Husebo BS, Nortvedt MW: Acute hospital admissions from nursing homes: predictors of unwarranted variation? *Scand J Public Health* 2013, 41(4):359–365.

10. Creditor MC: Hazards of hospitalization of the elderly. *Ann Intern Med* 1993, 118(3):219–223.

11. Hirsch CH, Sommers L, Olsen A, Mullen L, Winograd CH: The natural history of functional morbidity in hospitalized older patients. *J Am Geriatr Soc* 1990, 38(12):1296–1303.

12. Covinsky KE, Palmer RM, Fortinsky RH, Counsell SR, Stewart AL, Kresevic D, Burant CJ, Landefeld CS: Loss of independence in activities of daily living in older adults hospitalized with medical illnesses: increased vulnerability with age. *J Am Geriatr Soc* 2003, 51(4):451–458.

13. Lefevre F, Feinglass J, Potts S, Soglin L, Yarnold P, Martin GJ, Webster JR: Iatrogenic complications in high-risk, elderly patients. *Arch Intern Med* 1992, 152(10):2074.

14. Wilson RS, Hebert LE, Scherr PA, Dong X, Leurgens SE, Evans DA: Cognitive decline after hospitalization in a community population of older persons. *Neurology* 2012, 78(13):950–956.

15. Ehlenbach WJ, Hough CL, Crane PK, Haneuse SJ, Carson SS, Curtis JR, Larson EB: Association between acute care and critical illness hospitalization and cognitive function in older adults. *JAMA* 2010, 303(8):763–770.

16. Boyd CM, Landefeld CS, Counsell SR, Palmer RM, Fortinsky RH, Kresevic D, Burant C, Covinsky KE: Recovery of activities of daily living in older adults after hospitalization for acute medical illness. *J Am Geriatr Soc* 2008, 56(12):2171–2179.

17. Saliba D, Kington R, Buchanan J, Bell R, Wang M, Lee M, Herbst M, Lee D, Sur D, Rubenstein L: Appropriateness of the decision to transfer nursing facility residents to the hospital. *J Am Geriatr Soc* 2000, 48(2):154–163.

18. Ouslander JG, Lamb G, Perloe M, Givens JH, Kluge L, Rutland T, Atherly A, Saliba D: Potentially avoidable hospitalizations of nursing home residents: frequency, causes, and costs: [see editorial comments by Drs. Jean F. Wyman and William R. Hazzard, pp 760–761]. *J Am Geriatr Soc* 2010, 58(4):627–635.

19. Walker JD, Teare GF, Hogan DB, Lewis S, Maxwell CJ: Identifying potentially avoidable hospital admissions from Canadian long-term care facilities. *Med Care* 2009, 47(2):250–254.

20. Grabowski DC, O'Malley AJ, Barhydt NR: The costs and potential savings associated with nursing home hospitalizations. *Health Aff (Millwood)* 2007, 26(6): 1753–1761.

21. Blumenthal D, Dixon J: Health-care reforms in the USA and England: areas for useful learning. *Lancet* 2012, 380(9850):1352–1357.

22. The Norwegian Ministry of Health and Care Service: *The coordination reform. Proper treatment—at the right place and right time. Summary in English: report No. 47 (2008–2009) To the storting.* Oslo: Norwegian Ministry of Health and Care Services; 2009.

23. Forsetlund L, Graverholt B, Mathisen M: Effekter av tiltak for å redusere akutte sykehusinnleggelser fra sykehjem. In *The Norwegian Knowledge Centre for the Health Services.* Oslo; 2013. (Rapport fra Kunnskapssenteret nr 7-13, ISBN 978-82-8121-530-6).

24. Effectiveness of interventions to reduce acute hospitalisations of nursing home residents. A systematic review. PROSPERO 2012:CRD42012002473..

25. The Norwegian Knowledge Centre for the Health Services: *Slik oppsummerer vi forskning. Håndbok for Nasjonalt kunnskapssenter for helsetjenesten [English title: Handbook for summarising research].* 32nd edition. The Norwegian Knowledge Centre; 2013. ISBN: 978-82-8121-427-9.

26. Higgins JPT, Green S (Eds): Cochrane handbook for systematic reviews of interventions, Version 5.0.2. The Cochrane Collaboration 2009. [http://www.cochrane-handbook.org]

27. GRADE working group. http://www.gradeworkinggroup.org/.

28. Jefferson T, Di Pietrantonj C, Al-Ansary LA, Ferroni E, Thorning S, Thomas RE: Vaccines for preventing influenza in the elderly. *Cochrane Database of Systematic Reviews* 2010(2). Art. No.: CD004876. DOI:10.1002/14651858. CD004876.pub3.

29. Thomas RE, Jefferson T, Lasserson TJ: Influenza vaccination for healthcare workers who work with the elderly. *Cochrane Database of Systematic Reviews* 2010, (2). Art. No.: CD005187. doi:10.1002/14651858.CD005187.pub3.

30. Díaz-Gegúndez M, Paluzie G, Sanz-Ballester C, Boada-Mejorana M, Terré-Ohme S, Ruiz-Poza D: Evaluación de un programa de intervención en residencias geriátricas para reducir la frecuentación hospitalaria. *Rev Esp Geriatr Gerontol* 2011, 46(5):261–264. doi:10.1016/j.regg.2011.03.001.

31. Schippinger W, Hartinger G, Hierzer A, Osprian I, Bohnstingl M, Pilgram E: Mobiler geriatrischer konsiliardienst für pflegeheime: untersuchung der effektivität eines internistisch-fachärztlichen konsiliardienstes zur medizinischen versorgung von pflegeheimbewohnern (originalien). *Z Gerontol Geriatr* 2012, 45(8):735–741.

32. Robinson L, Dickinson C, Rousseau N, Beyer F, Clark A, Hughes J, Howel D, Exley C: A systematic review of the effectiveness of advance care planning interventions for people with cognitive impairment and dementia. *Age ageing* 2012, 41(2):263–269.

33. Hall S, Kolliakou A, Petkova H, Froggatt K, Higginson IJ: Interventions for improving palliative care for older people living in nursing care homes. *Cochrane Database of Syst Rev* 2011, (3). Art. No.: CD007132. doi:10.1002/14651858.CD007132.pub2.

34. Hutt E, Ruscin JM, Linnebur SA, Fish DN, Oman KS, Fink RM, Radcliff TA, Van Dorsten B, Liebrecht D, Fish R: A multifaceted intervention to implement guidelines Did Not affect hospitalization rates for nursing home–acquired pneumonia. *J Am Med Dir Assoc* 2011, 12(7):499–507.

35. Loeb M, Carusone SC, Goeree R, Walter SD, Brazil K, Krueger P, Simor A, Moss L, Marrie T: Effect of a clinical pathway to reduce hospitalizations in nursing home residents with pneumonia. *JAMA* 2006, 295(21):2503–2510.

36. Lee DT, Lee IF, Mackenzie AE, Ho RN: Effects of a care protocol on care outcomes in older nursing home patients with chronic obstructive pulmonary disease. *J Am Geriatr Soc* 2002, 50(5):870–876.

37. Guyatt GH, Oxman AD, Kunz R, Vist GE, Falck-Ytter Y, Schünemann HJ: Rating quality of evidence and strength of recommendations: what is "quality of evidence" and why is it important to clinicians? *BMJ* 2008, 336(7651):995.

38. Gordon A, Logan P, Jones R, Forrester-Paton C, Mamo J, Gladman J: A systematic mapping review of Randomized Controlled Trials (RCTs) in care homes. *BMC Geriatr* 2012, 12(1):31.

39. Ouslander JG, Lamb G, Tappen R, Herndon L, Diaz S, Roos BA, Grabowski DC, Bonner A: Interventions to reduce hospitalizations from nursing homes: evaluation of the INTERACT II collaborative quality improvement project. *J Am Geriatr Soc* 2011, 59(4):745–753.

40. Tena-Nelson R, Santos K, Weingast E, Amrhein S, Ouslander J, Boockvar K: Reducing potentially preventable hospital transfers: results from a thirty nursing home collaborativ. *J Am Med Dir Assoc* 2012, 13(7):651–656.

41. Roland M, Abel G: Reducing emergency admissions: are we on the right track? *BMJ* 2012, 345.

42. Hawkes N: Alternatives to hospital for older people must be found, says NHS chief. *BMJ* 2013, 346:f453.

43. D'Souza S, Guptha S: Preventing admission of older people to hospital. *BMJ* 2013, 346:f3186.

44. Craig P, Dieppe P, Macintyre S, Michie S, Nazareth I, Petticrew M: Developing and evaluating complex interventions: the new Medical Research Council guidance. *BMJ* 2008, 337:a1655.

45. Oakley A, Strange V, Bonell C, Allen E, Stephenson J: Health services research: process evaluation in randomised controlled trials of complex interventions. *BMJ* 2006, 332(7538):413.

Profile & Commentary

STUDY PURPOSE

The authors are quite clear in the *Background* section regarding why they thought this SR needed to be done. The great variation in the percentage of nursing home residents admitted to acute hospitals across countries is interesting. I had to wonder where the rate was only 9%—that seems quite low given the frailty and conditions one would expect to find in nursing home residents; on the other hand, 60% is quite high. The authors cogently point out that hospitalization is usually detrimental to the frail elderly in that it often results in loss of physical function, infection, and cognitive decline. The objective of the SR was to examine the effects of interventions aimed at reducing acute hospital admissions from nursing homes.

METHODS

The review methods used are in line with widely recognized recommendations and with the steps set forth earlier in this chapter. Of interest in the eligibility criteria is that they could and did consider studies published in any language. Not all review panels have those language resources. The search used the usual databases and focused on the nursing home setting and on the outcome of hospitalizations. Per recommendations of PRISMA, a flow chart of the selection process is provided. Supplementary to the flow chart is an additional file that lists the studies excluded and the reason for doing so

(Table S2, which you can access from the online version of this SR which is available at http://www.biomedcentral.com/content/pdf/1472-6963-14-36. pdf); the link is in the "Additional File" box near the end of the article.) The most common reason for excluding studies was that they used retrospective chart data. Importantly, all studies included in the review were appraised in detail for methodological quality using GRADE standards (an internationally recognized grading system for quality of evidence). Four SRs and five primary studies passed relevance screening and met methodological quality standards. However, even though they qualified, several places in the report the authors point out that overall the quality of the SRs and primary studies was low or very low. The sources of bias in each study and findings tables are provided (via the *Additional File* link) in supplementary tables 3 and 4; the findings tables for each intervention type provide a fine-grained sense of the populations, methods, and results of the studies included in this SRR. Ultimately the low quality of the studies led the authors to lack confidence in their findings and to be tentative in their conclusions.

 CONCLUSIONS

WHAT

Once the reviewers were familiar with the studies, they divided them into three groups based on the type of intervention used to prevent hospital admissions. These groups were:

1. Interventions that structured or standardized clinical practice processes
2. Interventions that used geriatric specialists
3. Interventions that promoted influenza vaccination

Interestingly, none of the studies examined whether pneumonia vaccine given to patients is effective in reducing hospitalizations.

Within each of these categories the studies were compared; the details are provided in the tables and in the text. Looking at Table 1, studies pertaining to standardization of clinical care, you can see that the interventions tried were diverse: several addressed pneumonia management (Hutt et al., 2011; Loeb et al., 2006); three addressed advanced care directives (Robinson, 2012; Caplan, 2006; Molloy, 2000); and three others addressed services for person with particular illnesses (Morrison, 2005; Hall, Kolliakou, Petkova, Froggatt, & Higginson, 2011; Lee et al., 2002). Information about the individual studies is provided in detail, and in the *Discussion* section, the reviewers summarize and point out patterns across studies. For example, "Among the seven interventions to structure or standardize treatment, a reduction in hospital admissions was found for four of them" (p. 6). The same reporting format was used for the other two intervention groupings.

The reviewers' lack of confidence in their SR's findings is acknowledged in the *Implications* section. The observation that small and weak studies are common in the areas of research in nursing homes is interesting—and regretful, as is the relatively few studies being conducted on this population in general. In the end, the reviewers conclude "Eleven evaluated interventions were identified, but none were tested more than once by rigorous study design" (p. 7). So, several interventions were found to reduce hospital admissions, but the research evidence in support of their effectiveness is not strong.

REFERENCES

Aromataris, E., Fernandez, R., Godfrey, C., Holly, C., Khalil, H., & Tungpunkom, P. (n.d.). *Methodology for JBI Umbrella Review.* Retrieved from http://joannabriggs.org/assets/docs/sumari/ReviewersManual-Methodology-JBI_Umbrella%20Reviews-2014.pdf

Becker, L. (n.d.). *Umbrella reviews: What are they and do we need them?* Retrieved from http://www.slideshare.net/Cochrane.Collaboration

Chan, P. S., Jain, R., Nallmothu, B. K., Berg, R. A., & Sasson, C. (2010). Rapid response teams: A systematic review and meta-analysis. *Archives of Internal Medicine, 170*(1), 18–26.

Cleveland, L. M. (2008). Parenting in the neonatal intensive care unit. *Journal of Obstetric, Gynecologic, and Neonatal Nursing, 37,* 666–691.

Cochrane Collaboration. (2015). Cochrane Qualitative & Implementation Methods Group. Retrieved from http://methods.cochrane.org/qi/

Conn, V. S., & Coon Sells, T. G. (2015). WJNR welcomes umbrella reviews. *Western Journal of Nursing Research, 36*(2), 147–151.

Daniels, R., van Rossum, E., de Witte, L., Kempen, G. I., & van den Heuvel, W. (2008). Interventions to prevent disability in frail community-dwelling elderly: A systematic review. *BMC Health Services Research, 8,* 278. Retrieved from http://www.biomedcentral.com/

Fink, H. A., Taylor, B. C., Tacklind, J. W., Rutks, I. R., & Wilt, T. J. (2008). Treatment intervention in nursing home residents with urinary incontinence: A systematic review of randomized trials. *Mayo Clinic Proceedings, 83*(12), 1332–1343.

Gomes, B., Calanzani, N., Curiale, V., McCrone, P., & Higginson, I. J. (2013). Effectiveness and cost-effectiveness of home palliative care services for adults with advanced illness and their caregivers. *Cochrane Database of Systematic Reviews,* 6:CD007760. doi: 10.1002/14651858. CD007760.pub2.

Graverholt, B., Forsetlund, L., & Jamtvedt, G. (2014). Reducing hospital admission from nursing home: A systematic review. *BMC Health Services Research, 14,36.* Retrieved from http://www.biomedcentral.com/. doi:10.1186/1472-6963-14-36 36

Higgins, J. P. T., & Green, S. (Eds.). (2011). *Cochrane handbook for systematic reviews of interventions* (Version 5.1.0). The Cochrane Collaboration. Retrieved from http://www.mri.gov.lk/assets/Uploads/Research/Cochrane-Hand-booktext.pdf

Institute of Medicine. (2011). *Finding what works in health care: Standards for systematic reviews.* Retrieved from http://www.iom.edu

Joanna Briggs Institute. (2014). *Reviewers' manual.* Adelaide, South Australia: Author. Retrieved from http://joannabriggs.org/assets/docs/sumari/reviewers manual-2014.pdf

Maharai, R., Raffaele, I., & Wendon, J. (2015). Rapid response systems: A systematic review and meta-analysis. *Critical Care, 19,* 254–269. doi 10.1186/s13054-015-0973-y

O'Keefe-McCarthy, S. (2008). Women's experiences of cardiac pain: A review of the literature. *Canadian Journal of Cardiovascular Nursing, 18*(3), 18–25.

PRISMA Group. (2009). Preferred reporting items for systematic reviews and meta-analyses: The PRISMA statement. *British Medical Journal, BMJ, 338*,b2535. doi: http://dx.doi.org/10.1136/bmj.b2535

Von Sadovszky, V., Draudt, B., & Boch, S. (2014). A systematic review of reviews of behavioral interventions to promote condom use. *Worldviews on Evidence-Based Nursing, 11*(2), 107–117.

Whittemore, R., Chao, A., Jang, M., Minges, K. E., & Park, C. (2014). Methods for knowledge synthesis: An overview. *Heart & Lung, 43,* 453–461.

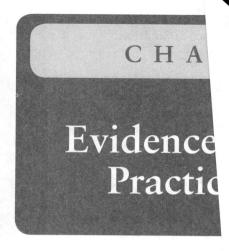

C H A

Evidence
Practic

212 CHAPTER 10 Evidence-Based C

Although EbCPGs are techni
the real world, if they are
evidence. So, when the
mendations of EbC
vidual studies.
In this cha
guidelines
plement
ers
is

Professional associations _____, long time produced position papers and care guidelines for clinical conditions in their specialty. However, only within the last 10 years has the standard of basing clinical guidelines on research evidence become widespread. Prior to this, guideline recommendations were based on one or several studies combined with a good amount of expert opinion. Now, the increased number of research studies and systematic reviews about clinical topics has made it possible to base guideline recommendations to a much greater extent on research evidence.

In brief, an evidence-based clinical practice guideline (EbCPG) is a set of recommendations for care that is informed by systematic reviews of evidence (IOM, 2011). Here's a short list of nursing-relevant EbCPGs, just to give you a sense of what is being produced:

- *Engaging Clients Who Use Substances* (Registered Nurses' Association of Ontario, 2015)
- *Care of the Patient with Mild Traumatic Brain Injury* (Association of Rehabilitation Nurses and American Association of Neuroscience Nurses, 2011)
- *Chemotherapy-Induced Nausea and Vomiting in Adults* (Oncology Nursing Society, 2012)
- *Clinical Practice Guideline for Carotid Artery Stenting* (Society for Vascular Nursing, 2013)
- *End-of-Life Care During the Last Days and Hours* (Registered Nurses' Association of Ontario, 2011)

cally a translation of research evidence, in
well produced, they are considered research
term *research evidence* is used, it refers to recom-
Gs, conclusions of SRs, and findings of original indi-

pter, the abbreviation *EbCPG* is used to make clear that the
being described are based on available research evidence com-
ed by expert opinion when necessary. Most guideline develop-
ecognize expert opinion as evidence—albeit at a low level because it
subjective. It is much like the testimony of a reliable eyewitness of an
event—better than no witness but not as strong as physical evidence. The
fact that expert opinion is the opinion of the whole guideline development
panel, not just one individual, adds to its credibility.

Forerunners to Care Protocols

EbCPGs are generic in that they are not designed for a particular organization or agency; rather, they are offered as guidelines for care in a variety of
settings. Although EbCPGs certainly can be used by individual clinicians,
often they are adapted by clinical project teams into care protocols specific
to their setting, patients, and staff. These care protocols serve as standards
of care in that they provide evidence-based guidance for care providers.
Importantly, standardizing the processes of care based on research evidence
has the potential to:

1. Increase the use of clinical actions that are effective.
2. Reduce the use of actions that are of minimal value or put patients
   at risk.
3. Reduce undesirable variation in care.

These kinds of process of care improvements have been found to improve
patient safety, quality of care, and patient outcomes (Graham, Harrison, &
Godfrey, 2014; Lavin, Harper, & Barr, 2015). Care protocols take many
forms, including standardized care plans, care maps, decision algorithms,
care bundles, standard order sets, clinical procedures, and clinical pathways. Increasingly, they are being incorporated into the electronic decision
support and communication systems of healthcare organizations.

Lest you be concerned that *standardized plan of care* sounds like
cookie-cutter care whereby every patient with a particular problem auto-
matically gets the same care regardless of their unique characteristics and

wishes, be assured that patient-centered care and standardized plans of care *are* compatible. However, the nurse must be observant and sensitive to patients' responses to care given in accordance with standardized plans. If the care recommended by the standardize plan is not acceptable to the patient or the patient is not responding well to it, the nurse must seek consultation with clinical leaders about how to proceed. Also, it should be said that most caregiving organizations expect professional caregivers to exert judgment and take into account the individual patient's condition, preferences, life situation, and personal goals when planning and giving care. Standardized plans of care benefit most but not necessarily all patients.

> **Patient-centered care and standardized plans of care are compatible.**

EbCPGs are an intermediate step on the rather long road from individual studies to evidence-based practice (see Figure 10-1). To a project team developing a care protocol, the advantages of working with an EbCPG rather than systematic reviews are that an EbCPG saves time in that a group with expertise has made the translation from research evidence to recommended care actions. Of course, the team still has to develop a plan for incorporating the recommendation or recommendations into the organization's care processes.

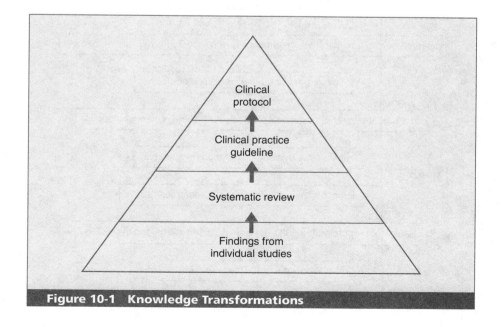

Figure 10-1   Knowledge Transformations

EbCPG Production

As part of the evidence-based practice movement, the process for producing EbCPGs has been widely agreed upon, and quality standards for them have been formulated. Multidisciplinary groups and professional associations in many countries provide manuals regarding the production of clinical practice guidelines (Australian Government National Health and Medical Research Council, 2011; Guidelines International Network, n.d.; Institute of Medicine, 2011; Registered Nurses' Association of Ontario, 2006; Scottish Intercollegiate Guidelines Network, 2014). Although there are some differences of opinion and emphasis, the production process is generally agreed upon as described in the sections that follow. The point in making you aware of the process is that in Part II of the text, knowing this process will help you to appraise guidelines as the production process used is an important criterion for judging whether a guideline is trustworthy.

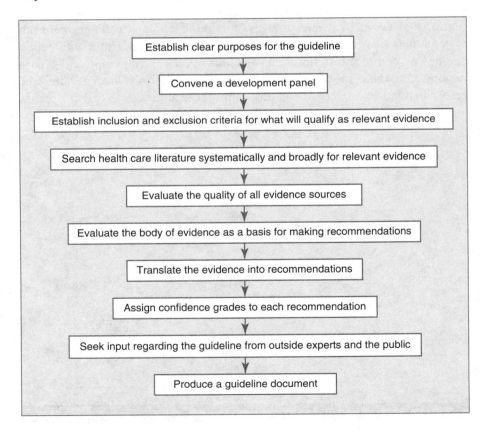

Clearly, this is a lengthy and rigorous process and the integrity of each step depends on the integrity of those that precede it.

Purposes

The organization or association commissioning the development of a guideline typically sets specific goals for the project. A clear purpose statement assures that the development panel proceeds in sync and on mission. Later, it conveys to potential users of the guideline what they can expect from it. The purpose statement may include a health condition that requires management or prevention, a patient population with a certain condition, or a specific care action or healthcare delivery process that requires procedural clarification.

Panel Composition and Expertise

Members are chosen to ensure that all affected healthcare stakeholders and the needed expertise are present at the table. That would include the following:

- Representation of all key professionals who will be influenced by the guideline
- Clinical expertise in the various issues the guideline will address
- Research expertise to help appraise study quality and interpret the study results
- Evidence-based practice expertise to ensure sound transfer of knowledge from science to clinical recommendations
- Information search and retrieval expertise to help locate research evidence
- Group process expertise to facilitate the development process, group dynamics, and consensus decision making
- For some guideline topics, a member of the public

Inclusion and Exclusion Criteria

The inclusion-exclusion criteria are to a large extent determined by the guideline's purpose, which may specify target population, outcomes of interest, or setting characteristics, but it may also include criteria regarding the types of study designs that will be included. It is not uncommon for guidelines aimed at making recommendations regarding treatment or intervention effectiveness to include only randomized controlled studies. However, to make recommendation regarding treatment issues other than effectiveness, such as helping patients adjust to the intervention, other study designs are included.

Search for Evidence

The search for relevant evidence should be systematic and wide. This undoubtedly requires the services provided by an information specialist or healthcare librarian skilled in searching the health-related databases. Ideally, the search would identify systematic research reviews relevant to the guideline's issues. However, if relevant SRs are not found or the ones found are not of acceptable quality or don't fully address the guideline's issues, reports of individual studies will have to be retrieved and the development team will have to perform its own SRs. These should be performed in accordance with recognized SR conduct standards as set forth in Chapter 9.

Evaluate Quality of all Evidence Sources

If working from existing SRs, the panel should appraise their quality and use only those of acceptable quality. Note that appraisal of the quality of the individual studies in the SRs is not required because good SRs will already have done this. However, if the panel has to conduct its own SR, it would appraise the quality of the individual studies in the process of producing it. Quality appraisal and elimination of poor quality evidence is a critical step in assuring trustworthy guidelines.

Evaluate the Body of Evidence

The panel then summarizes and evaluates the strength of *the body of evidence* pertaining to each issue about which it is considering making a recommendation. In so doing, the members should take into account a wide range of characteristics of the body of evidence, which are listed in **Box 10-1**. (Berkman et al., 2013; GRADE, n.d.).

In the guideline document the panel conveys its appraisal of the strength of the body of evidence by a combination of evidence tables, textual summarization of the evidence, or using an evidence-grading system that takes into account several characteristics of the body of evidence. Clearly, it is difficult to capture all the characteristics listed in Box 10-1 with a simple grading system, so the grading systems in use either focus on several characteristics of the body of evidence or use grades that convey the quality and strength of the evidence in general terms. The strength-of-evidence rating systems in **Box 10-2** and **Box 10-3**, grade evidence related to interventions; note that they are quite different.

BOX 10-1   Strength of a Body of Evidence

To evaluate the strength of evidence of a body of evidence, the panel takes into consideration:

- Whether the studies done were of the best design type for the issue being considered
- The methodological quality of the SRs and/or the individual studies
- The number of studies and/or SRs
- The consistency of the findings across studies
- Whether enough patients were studied to confer confidence on the findings
- If the estimated benefit of an intervention in the population is clinically significant
- Whether population/s studied in the body of evidence are the same as the target population for the guideline
- Whether the studies directly addressed important health outcomes

BOX 10-2 Rating Scheme for Strength of Evidence

Scheme for grading the strength and consistency of evidence in the guideline

A1 = Evidence from well-designed meta-analysis or well-done systematic review with results that consistently support a specific action (e.g., assessment, intervention, or treatment)

A2 = Evidence from one or more randomized controlled trials with consistent results

B1 = Evidence from high-quality evidence-based practice guideline

B2 = Evidence from one or more quasi-experimental studies with consistent results

C1 = Evidence from observational studies with consistent results (e.g., correlational, descriptive studies)

C2 = Evidence from observational studies or controlled trials with inconsistent results

D = Evidence from expert opinion, multiple case reports, or national consensus reports

Reproduced from Mentes J. C, & Kang S. (2011). Hydration management. University of Iowa College of Nursing and John A. Hartford Foundation Center of Geriatric Nursing Excellence. http://www.guideline.gov/content.aspx?id=34272

> **BOX 10-3   Strength of a Body of Evidence Scale**
>
> **HIGH** We are very confident that the estimate of effect lies close to the true effect for this outcome. The body of evidence has few or no deficiencies. We believe that the findings are stable, i.e., another study would not change the conclusions.
>
> **MODERATE** We are moderately confident that the estimate of effect lies close to the true effect for this outcome. The body of evidence has some deficiencies. We believe that the findings are likely to be stable, but some doubt remains.
>
> **LOW** We have limited confidence that the estimate of effect lies close to the true effect for this outcome. The body of evidence has major or numerous deficiencies (or both). We believe that additional evidence is needed before concluding either that the findings are stable or that the estimate of effect is close to the true effect.
>
> **INSUFFICIENT** We have no evidence, we are unable to estimate an effect, or we have no confidence in the estimate of effect for this outcome. No evidence is available or the body of evidence has unacceptable deficiencies, precluding reaching a conclusion.
>
> Reproduced from Owens, D. K., Lohr, K. N., Atkins, D., Treadwell J. R, Reston J. T., Bass, E. B., et al. (2009). Grading the strength of a body of evidence when comparing medical interventions. In Agency for Healthcare Research and Quality, Methods guide for comparative effectiveness reviews. Rockville, MD: Agency for Healthcare Research and Quality. Available at http://www.effectivehealthcare.ahrq.gov/index.cfm/search-for-guides-reviews-and-reports/?pageaction=displayproduct&productid=318

While the issue of whether the studies comprising the evidence were done using "the best design type" is important, it is just one aspect of the strength of evidence. Until recently, evidence pyramids ranking evidence relied almost exclusively on the design of the studies. In these pyramids, which were designed mainly for evidence about interventions and treatments, systematic review of randomized controlled trials, i.e., experimental studies, were ranked at the highest level followed by one or a few randomized controlled trials of good quality; nonexperimental and observational studies were ranked at a lower level. Now, evidence grading systems, even those for interventions and treatments, take more than the design of the studies into consideration.

In addition, randomized controlled trials are not the best type of design for every guideline issue. In recognition of this fact, the Joanna Briggs Institute uses a levels-of-evidence approach that is composed of different levels of evidence ranking systems for: (1) intervention effectiveness; (2) diagnosis; (3) prognosis); (4) economic evaluations; and (5) meaning of human experience, interaction, and culture. The highest form of evidence is different for each of the five issues (Joanna Briggs Institute, 2013).

To summarize the issue of how the panel conveys the overall strength of the evidence about an issue: panels developing guideline documents should in some way grade the overall strength of evidence about each issue or question. If the evidence about an issue is moderate or high quality, the panel usually will make a recommendation about it.

Translate Evidence into Recommendations

To some extent the details of how the panel moves from evidence to a recommendation is a bit of a black box—typically described as "informal consensus." Understandably, many of the conversations required involve a tangle of evidence that lacks consistency of populations studied, methods used, and results obtained, particularly certainty about the magnitude of benefit. Some developers are better than others at conveying what the panel discussed and took into account when making this translation. In the interests of transparency, the IOM standards (2011) require that development panels describe how decisions were made regarding whether or not to include a recommendation, how differences of opinion were resolved, and the part played by values, theory, and clinical experience.

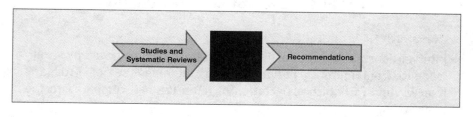

Assign a Certainty Level to Each Recommendation

Most guideline developers indicate the level of certainty they have in each recommendation. "When CPG developers are confident that the beneficial effects of a recommendation outweigh the harms, a strong recommendation can be made" (IOM, 2011, p. 113). The strength of evidence in support of a recommendation is certainly a major consideration in determining how confident the panel is in a recommendation. However, other factors are considered as well so that they can have certainty that the recommendation will produce desired patient outcomes without undue risk of harm and that the recommendations are feasible to use in practice (Guyatt et al., 2006). Some of the factors that enter into assigning a level of certainty to a recommendation are listed in **Box 10-4**.

Some guideline developers use just two grades for their confidence in the recommendation, e.g., *Strong* and *Weak* (GRADE, n.d.), while others use several levels. The recommendation grading system shown in **Box 10-5** is used by the Oncology Nursing Society for interventions in its *Putting Evidence Into Practice* guidelines (2012). It takes into account the amount of evidence, its quality and consistency, and a comparison of benefit and harm.

BOX 10-4   Certainty Considerations

Issues considered in assigning a level of certainty to a recommendation:

- The strength or quality of the supporting evidence
- Whether the populations and subpopulations to whom the recommendation would apply are clear
- The size of the benefit likely to be achieved by the recommendation, i.e., it is clinically significant
- The balance of benefits to risk of harm
- Whether patients value the outcomes likely to be achieved
- The cost and feasibility of implementing the recommendation

---

BOX 10-5   Levels of Recommendation

RECOMMENDED FOR PRACTICE

Interventions for which effectiveness has been demonstrated by strong evidence from rigorously designed studies, meta-analyses, or systematic reviews, and for which expectation of harm is small compared to the benefits.

LIKELY TO BE EFFECTIVE

Interventions for which effectiveness has been demonstrated from a single, rigorously conducted controlled trial, consistent supportive evidence from well-designed controlled trials using small samples or guidelines developed from evidence and supported by expert opinion.

BENEFITS BALANCED WITH HARM

Interventions for which clinicians and patients should weigh the beneficial and harmful effects according to individual circumstances and priorities.

EFFECTIVENESS NOT ESTABLISHED

Interventions for which insufficient or conflicting data or data of inadequate quality currently exist, with no clear indication of harm.

EFFECTIVENESS UNLIKELY

Interventions for which lack of effectiveness has been demonstrated by negative evidence from a single rigorously conducted controlled trial, consistent negative evidence from well-designed controlled trials using small samples, or guidelines developed from evidence and supported by expert opinion.

NOT RECOMMENDED FOR PRACTICE

Interventions for which lack of effectiveness or harmfulness has been demonstrated by strong evidence from rigorously conducted studies, meta-analyses, or systematic reviews, or interventions where the costs, burden, or harm associated with the intervention exceed the anticipated benefit.

EXPERT OPINION

Low-risk interventions that are consistent with sound clinical practice, suggested by an expert in a peer reviewed publication, and for which limited evidence exists. (An expert is an individual who has published peer reviewed material in the domain of interest.)

Reproduced from Oncology Nursing Society. (2012). ONS PEP(r)—Putting evidence into practice. Retrieved from http://www.ons.org/Research/PEP

Ideally, guideline producers provide both a strength-of-evidence grade and a certainty, or confidence, grade for each recommendation. However, other developers provide only a recommendation grade that incorporates consideration of the strength of the supporting evidence. I realize this is a bit confusing but that's the way it is.

Input

Once the guideline document is in near-final form, input should be sought from outside experts and the public. This review can identify lack of clarity, omission of key issues, and questions about feasibility of implementation. Some guideline developers put their guideline through a field test; this helps determine whether the recommendations are implementable and what the barriers to implementation might be. Ideas from outside reviews and field testing can lead to modification of the guideline document or to adding suggestions that will help users put the recommendations in place.

Guideline Formats

Many guidelines are quite long. There are several reasons for this, including the following:

1. The broad nature of a guideline's purpose.
2. The inclusion in the guideline of details about the research evidence.
3. Inclusion of a description of the guideline production process.
4. Recommendations for practice, education, and organizations.

Although there is no standardized format for EbCPGs, the one that follows is typical:

I. Title
II. Producing agency (date) and panel members
III. Table of contents
IV. Copyright statement
V. Background context
VI. Purpose and scope
VII. Practice recommendations
VIII. Levels of evidence
IX. Definitions
X. Discussion of evidence
XI. Evidence tables
XII. Production process
XIII. Plans for updating
XIV. Implementation strategies
XV. References

To make guidelines more usable for clinicians, often several of the elements just listed are not included in the main document; rather, they are available in associated documents, often via online links. Even more convenient, EbCPG producers issue quick-reference guides separate from the full version of the guidelines. Quick-reference guides typically list the recommendations and indicate an evidence grade or a certainty level for each recommendation. The Joanna Briggs Institute produces two- to six-page best practice sheets, which are designed for clinicians; some are free to nonsubscribers (http://www.joannabriggslibrary.org/index.php/JBIBPTR). The Registered Nurses' Association of Ontario (2016) makes abbreviated versions of its guidelines available via its BPG app (http://rnao.ca/bpg/pda/app).

An example of a well-produced and very useful, but long, guideline is *Prevention and Treatment of Pressure Ulcers: Clinical Practice Guideline,* which was produced by the National Pressure Ulcer Advisory Panel, European Pressure Ulcer Advisory Panel, and Pan Pacific Pressure Injury Alliance (2014a). Its recommendations for prevention and treatment are explicit, and there are sections devoted to the unique issues of special populations such as bariatric/obese individuals, older adults, individuals in the operating room, and individuals with spinal cord injury, to name a few. A strength of evidence and a certainty/confidence of recommendation level is provided for each recommendation; support documents describing production methodology, evidence appraisals, and evidence tables are provided, as are translations. Alas, the *Quick Reference Guide* (NPUAP, 2014b) is 75 pages long, but easy to navigate. I suggest you look at it.

In light of the fact that organizations and associations around the world are producing EbCPGs, it is becoming more common for several guidelines to exist about the same topic. In responses to this, several organizations have begun to produce syntheses of several guidelines. These syntheses lay out areas of agreement and difference and compare the recommendations. One of these syntheses, about prevention of pressure ulcers, is available at the National Guideline Clearinghouse website (Agency for Healthcare Research and Quality, n.d.).

Comorbidity

Recently, attention has been given to the reality that most guidelines address a single condition whereas real-world patients often have several conditions (Boyd & Fortin, 2010). Few guidelines take into account that many patients have several conditions (comorbidity) that could limit the applicability of a particular guideline to their care. An attempt to apply several guidelines to the care of a person with several conditions could result in the clinician being confronted by conflicting recommendations (IOM, 2011). Ultimately, addressing this dilemma will require changes in how research is conducted, how guidelines are developed, and the ability of the healthcare systems to support patient-centered care.

Guideline Producers

If you are interested in guidelines on a specific topic, five starting points for guidelines relevant to nursing would be:

- ▪ The Registered Nurses' Association of Ontario: http://rnao.ca/bpg
- ▪ The United States Preventive Services Task Force: http://www.ahrq.gov/professionals/clinicians-providers/guidelines-recommendations/guide/index.html

- The National Guidelines Clearinghouse: http://www.guideline.gov/browse/by-topic.aspx
- The University of Iowa College of Nursing Evidence-Based Practice Guidelines for Geriatric Care: http://www.iowanursingguidelines.com/category-s/125.htm
- The website of the professional association for your area of clinical interest; typically under the Practice tab

U.S. Preventive Services Task Force. (2015). *Final Recommendation Statement: Vitamin Supplementation to Prevent Cancer and CVD: Counseling.* Retrieved from http://www.uspreventiveservicestaskforce.org/Page/Document/RecommendationStatementFinal/vitamin-supplementation-to-prevent-cancer-and-cvd-counseling

Final Recommendation Statement

Vitamin Supplementation to Prevent Cancer and CVD: Counseling, February 2014

Recommendations made by the USPSTF are independent of the U.S. government. They should not be construed as an official position of the Agency for Healthcare Research and Quality or the U.S. Department of Health and Human Services.

Table 1 Summary of Recommendations and Evidence		
Population	**Recommendation**	**Grade***
Use of Multivitamins to Prevent Cardiovascular Disease or Cancer	The USPSTF concludes that the current evidence is insufficient to assess the balance of benefits and harms of the use of multivitamins for the prevention of cardiovascular disease or cancer.	I†

Population	Recommendation	Grade*
Single- or Paired-Nutrient Supplements for Prevention of Cardiovascular Disease or Cancer	The USPSTF concludes that the current evidence is insufficient to assess the balance of benefits and harms of the use of single- or paired-nutrient supplements (except β-carotene and vitamin E) for the prevention of cardiovascular disease or cancer.	I
Use of β-carotene or Vitamin E for Prevention of Cardiovascular Disease or Cancer	The USPSTF recommends against the use of β-carotene or vitamin E supplements for the prevention of cardiovascular disease or cancer.	D

*For an explanation of what the grades mean and suggestions for practice, see Appendix Table 1. For information on levels of certainty regarding net benefit, see Appendix Table 2.

† See the *Clinical Considerations* section for suggestions for practice regarding the I statements.

Source: U.S. Preventive Services Task Force.

Preface

The U.S. Preventive Services Task Force (USPSTF) makes recommendations about the effectiveness of specific clinical preventive services for patients without related signs or symptoms.

It bases its recommendations on the evidence of both the benefits and harms of the service and an assessment of the balance. The USPSTF does not consider the costs of providing a service in this assessment.

The USPSTF recognizes that clinical decisions involve more considerations than evidence alone. Clinicians should understand the evidence but individualize decision making to the specific patient or situation. Similarly, the USPSTF notes that policy and coverage decisions involve considerations in addition to the evidence of clinical benefits and harms.

This article was first published in Annals of Internal Medicine on 25 February, 2014.

Rationale

Importance

Use of dietary supplements is common in the U.S. adult population. Forty-nine percent of adults used at least 1 dietary supplement between 2007 and 2010, and 32%

reported using a multivitamin–multimineral supplement.[1] Supplement use is more common among women and older adults than men and younger adults.[2] Most dietary supplements are used to improve or maintain overall health.[1] The substantial effect of cardiovascular disease and cancer on health status and mortality in the United States has been well-described,[3] and many supplements are promoted to prevent these conditions.[4]

Benefits of Vitamin Supplementation

The USPSTF found inadequate evidence on the benefits of supplementation with multivitamins to reduce the risk for cardiovascular disease or cancer. The USPSTF found inadequate evidence on the benefits of supplementation with individual vitamins or minerals or functional pairs in healthy populations without known nutritional deficiencies to reduce the risk for cardiovascular disease or cancer. The USPSTF found adequate evidence that supplementation with β-carotene or vitamin E in healthy populations without known nutritional deficiencies does not reduce the risk for cardiovascular disease or cancer.

Harms of Vitamin Supplementation

The USPSTF found inadequate evidence on the harms of supplementation with multivitamins and most single vitamins or minerals or functional pairs. The USPSTF found adequate evidence that supplementation with β-carotene increases the risk for lung cancer in persons who are at increased risk for this condition. The USPSTF found adequate evidence that supplementation with vitamin E has few or no substantial harms.

USPSTF Assessment

The USPSTF concludes that the evidence is insufficient to determine the balance of benefits and harms of supplementation with multivitamins for the prevention of cardiovascular disease or cancer. The USPSTF concludes that the evidence is insufficient to determine the balance of benefits and harms of supplementation with single or paired nutrients (except β-carotene or vitamin E) for the prevention of cardiovascular disease or cancer. The USPSTF concludes with moderate certainty that there is no net benefit of supplementation with vitamin E or β-carotene for the prevention of cardiovascular disease or cancer.

Clinical Considerations

Patient Population Under Consideration

The focus of this recommendation is healthy adults without special nutritional needs. Populations studied were typically aged 50 years or older. This recommendation does not apply to children, women who are pregnant or may become pregnant, or persons who are chronically ill or hospitalized or have a known nutritional deficiency.

Suggestions for Practice Regarding the I Statement

Potential Preventable Burden

Evidence from in vitro and animal research and population-based epidemiologic studies supports the hypothesis that oxidative stress may play a fundamental role in the initiation and progression of cancer and common cardiovascular diseases.[3] If this hypothesis is correct, then some combination of specific supplements, a specific dose, a vulnerable host, and specific timing may be found to be useful.

Potential Harms

Important harms have been shown with the use of β-carotene in persons who smoke tobacco or have an occupational exposure to asbestos. There are several known adverse effects caused by excessive doses of vitamins; for example, moderate doses of vitamin A supplements may reduce bone mineral density, but high doses may be hepatotoxic or teratogenic. Otherwise, the vitamins reviewed by the USPSTF had few known risks. Because many of these vitamins are fat soluble, the lifetime effect of high doses should be taken into consideration.

The USPSTF did not address doses higher than the tolerable upper intake level, as determined by the U.S. Food and Nutrition Board. Vitamins A and D have known harms at doses exceeding the tolerable upper intake levels,[5] and the potential for harm from other supplements at high doses should be carefully considered.

The U.S. Pharmacopeia has developed reference standards to aid in quality control of dietary supplement production; however, the content and concentration of ingredients in commercially available formulations probably vary considerably. This variability in the composition of dietary supplements makes extrapolating results obtained from controlled clinical trials challenging.

Costs

Although dietary supplements themselves are not particularly costly, the cumulative effect of this class of agent on spending is substantial. In 2010, $28.1 billion was spent on dietary supplements in the United States.[6]

Current Practice

Surveys conducted by the dietary supplement industry suggest that many physicians and nurses have recommended dietary supplements to their patients for health and wellness.[7]

Additional Approaches to Prevention

Appropriate intake of vitamin and mineral nutrients is essential to overall health.[5] Despite the uncertain benefit of vitamin supplementation, the 2010 Dietary Guidelines for Americans[8] suggest that nutrients should come primarily from foods and provide guidance on how to consume a nutrient-rich diet. Adequate nutrition by eating a diet rich in fruits, vegetables, whole grains, fat-free and low-fat dairy products, and seafood has been associated with a reduced risk for cardiovascular disease and cancer.[9,10]

Specific groups of patients with well-defined conditions may benefit from specific nutrients. For example, women planning or capable of pregnancy should receive a daily supplement containing folic acid to help prevent neural tube defects. The USPSTF also recommends vitamin D supplements for older persons at risk for falling.

Useful Resources

The USPSTF has a large portfolio of recommendations for prevention of cardiovascular disease and cancer, including recommendations for smoking cessation; screening for lipid disorders, hypertension, diabetes, and cancer; obesity screening and counseling; and aspirin use (available at www.uspreventiveservicestaskforce .org).

Other Considerations

Research Needs and Gaps

A critical gap in the evidence is the lack of studies of multivitamin combinations in groups generalizable to the U.S. population. Two randomized, controlled trials (RCTs) of multivitamin supplements suggest a potential cancer prevention benefit in men but not women. Future trials should be more representative of the general population, including women and minority groups, and should have enough power to show whether there are true subgroup differences. Targeting research toward persons who can be identified as high-risk for nutrient deficiency rather than the general population may be more productive.

There are substantial challenges to studying nutrient supplementation by using methods similar to those used in studying pharmaceutical interventions. New and innovative research methods for examining effects of nutrients that account for the unique complexities of nutritional research but maintain rigorous designs should be explored.

The paucity of studies and general lack of effect of any single nutrient or nutrient pair makes it difficult to draw meaningful conclusions on the balance of benefits and harms without a coordinated research effort and focus. A general lack of standardized methods to determine relevant serum nutrient levels, agreement on thresholds for sufficiency and insufficiency, or predictive validity of current mechanistic models further hinders progress in understanding potential benefits of dietary supplements.

Discussion

Burden of Disease

Cardiovascular disease and cancer are the largest contributors to the burden of chronic disease in the developed world. In 2011, these diseases accounted for 23.7% and 22.8% of all deaths in the United States, respectively.[11]

Scope of Review

In order to update its 2003 recommendation, the USPSTF reviewed evidence of the efficacy of the use of multivitamin or mineral supplements in the general adult population for the prevention of cardiovascular disease and cancer.[3,12] The value of vitamins that naturally occur in food and the use of vitamin supplements for the prevention of other conditions (for example, neural tube defects) and for the secondary prevention of complications in patients with existing disease are outside the scope of this review.

Effectiveness of Preventive Medication

Multivitamin and Antioxidant Combinations

The USPSTF reviewed 4 RCTs and 1 cohort study assessing health outcomes of a multivitamin supplement.[3] The studies varied in the nutrients and doses used. No effect on all-cause mortality was found in the three trials that assessed this outcome. Two trials assessed cardiovascular disease outcomes. Overall, there was no effect on incidence of cardiovascular disease events. One trial reported a borderline significant decrease in fatal myocardial infarctions.

Two large trials, the Physicians' Health Study II[13] and the SU.VI.MAX (Supplementation in Vitamins and Mineral Antioxidants) study,[14] showed a decrease in overall cancer incidence in men (pooled unadjusted relative risk, 0.93 [95% CI, 0.87 to 0.99]).[3] The Physicians' Health Study II included 14,641 male U.S. physicians with an average age of 64.3 years. The intervention used a commercially available multivitamin that contained 30 ingredients. The unadjusted relative risk for total cancer incidence was 0.94 (95% CI, 0.87 to 1.00) after 11.2 years of follow-up. The homogeneity of this study population (primarily older white male physicians) limits its generalizability.

The SU.VI.MAX study was conducted in France in 13,017 men and women with an average age of 49 years. The intervention supplement included nutritional doses of vitamins C and E plus β-carotene, selenium, and zinc. Outcomes were reported for the end of the intervention phase at 7.5 years and again at 12.5 years after randomization. During the supplementation period, overall cancer incidence was not affected in women but decreased by 31% in men (adjusted relative risk, 0.69 [95% CI, 0.53 to 0.91]). The lack of effect in women and the use of different supplement formulations in the two trials make extrapolating these findings to the general population difficult.

Single and Paired Vitamins and Minerals

The USPSTF reviewed 24 studies of individual vitamins or minerals or functional nutrient pairs.[3] Across all of the supplements studied, there was no evidence of beneficial effect on cardiovascular disease, cancer, or all-cause mortality. However, there are only a limited number of studies for most individual nutrients and differences in study designs make pooling effects across supplements difficult. Therefore, the USPSTF is not able to conclude with certainty that there is no effect. The evidence for each individual nutrient is discussed here.

Vitamin A: The USPSTF reviewed three RCTs and two cohort studies of vitamin A.[3] None of the studies reported cardiovascular disease incidence. One good-quality trial showed an increased risk for lung cancer and related death. The baseline population (smokers and workers who had been exposed to asbestos) was at high risk for lung cancer, so the increased mortality may be attributable to the β-carotene component. Two trials reported all-cause mortality, but no significant difference was observed between intervention and control groups at the longest follow-up. Increased risk for hip fractures was observed in one large prospective cohort study of postmenopausal women.

Vitamin C: Two RCTs studied the effects of vitamin C, either alone or in combination with other supplements, and found no statistically significant effect on cardiovascular disease, cancer, or all-cause mortality.[3]

Vitamin D With or Without Calcium: Three trials studied the effects of vitamin D on cardiovascular disease and cancer.[3] Two trials found no effect on cardiovascular disease incidence or mortality. One trial reported cancer incidence and death and found no difference between intervention and control groups. Two trials reporting all-cause mortality found no statistically significant difference.

Two trials studied vitamin D and calcium combined. One small, fair-quality study found a statistically significant decreased risk for cancer with supplement use.[15] The WHI (Women's Health Initiative) trial, a larger, good-quality trial using lower doses of vitamin D and calcium supplements, found no effect on cancer incidence or mortality.[16] A post hoc subgroup analysis of women who were not receiving supplements at baseline showed an association between use of vitamin D and calcium supplements and lower total cancer and breast cancer incidence.[17]

Only the WHI trial reported cardiovascular disease incidence and mortality and all-cause mortality, and it found no effect after 7 years of follow-up. Four trials of calcium supplementation found no effect on overall cardiovascular disease, cancer, or all-cause mortality.[3]

Vitamin E: Six RCTs assessed vitamin E supplementation.[3] Three trials reported cardiovascular disease incidence and mortality. One trial in women reported a lower cardiovascular disease mortality rate in the intervention group, but mortality rates for myocardial infarction and stroke did not differ statistically. One trial found an increased risk for hemorrhagic stroke in the intervention group.

Four RCTs reported cancer incidence. Overall, there was no significant effect on incidence of all types of cancer or on cancer mortality rates. No effect on all-cause mortality was observed in the five trials reporting this outcome.

Vitamin E was not found to have any effect on site-specific cancer incidence, although the results for prostate cancer were mixed. The ATBC (Alpha-Tocopherol, Beta Carotene Cancer Prevention) study[18] reported a decreased incidence of prostate cancer, but the effect did not persist with longer follow-up. Conversely, SELECT (Selenium and Vitamin E Cancer Prevention Trial)[19] reported an increased risk for prostate cancer after extended follow-up.

β-Carotene: A consistent body of evidence from six clinical trials suggests that β-carotene supplementation does not decrease the risk for cardiovascular disease events, overall cancer incidence, or cancer mortality.[3] Two trials, the ATBC study[18] and CARET (Carotene and Retinol Efficacy Trial),[20] showed an increased risk for lung cancer incidence and mortality and all-cause mortality in participants with a high baseline risk for lung cancer. A meta-analysis of β-carotene trials reported an increased risk for lung cancer (pooled odds ratio, 1.24 [95% CI, 1.10 to 1.39]) in current smokers.[21]

Selenium: Two trials studied selenium alone or in combination with other nutrients and found no effect on cardiovascular disease or all-cause mortality.[3] The effect on cancer was mixed. One trial found a decrease in risk for cancer incidence and mortality; the other found no significant difference. Additional analyses showed a decrease in cancer incidence only in men with the lowest levels of selenium, suggesting a potential effect resulting from treatment of selenium deficiency. No differences in all-cause mortality were found in either trial.

Folic Acid: Only one trial studied folic acid.[3] It found no effect on cardiovascular disease incidence or all-cause mortality. There was an increased incidence of cancer, attributed to an excess number of deaths from prostate cancer in the intervention group.

Potential Harms of Preventive Medication

Overall, few significant harms were reported from these interventions except for β-carotene. As described previously, two trials reported increased risk for lung cancer and lung cancer mortality in smokers, especially heavy smokers. No trials observed an increased risk for cancer in nonsmokers.

The literature contains reports of less serious harms, such as hypercarotenemia or yellowing of the skin (multivitamins and β-carotene), rashes (multivitamins), minor bleeding events (multivitamins), and gastrointestinal symptoms (calcium and selenium). Rare but more serious harms were associated with some nutrient trials, including hip fractures (vitamin A), prostate cancer (folic acid), and kidney stones (vitamin D and calcium).

Estimate of Magnitude of Net Benefit

The USPSTF found inadequate evidence on the effectiveness of multivitamin supplements to prevent cardiovascular disease or cancer. Therefore, the USPSTF concludes that the evidence is lacking and the balance of benefits and harms cannot be determined. The USPSTF also found inadequate evidence on the effectiveness of supplementation with most single or paired vitamins or minerals and is therefore unable to determine the balance of benefits and harms of their use to prevent cardiovascular disease or cancer.

Only two vitamin supplements have sufficient data to estimate net benefit. β-Carotene has been associated with a statistically significant increased risk for lung cancer in smokers. The USPSTF concludes with moderate certainty that the net benefit of β-carotene supplementation is negative (that is, there is a net harm).

A large and consistent body of evidence has shown that vitamin E supplementation has no effect on cardiovascular disease, cancer, or all-cause mortality. The USPSTF concludes with moderate certainty that the net benefit of vitamin E supplementation is zero.

How Does Evidence Fit With Biological Understanding?

The risk factors for cardiovascular disease are well established. Risk factors for cancer are considerably more complex because of the heterogeneous nature of different types of cancer and environmental and genetic influences. Inflammation, oxidative stress, and methionine metabolism have been theorized as common pathologic mechanisms for cardiovascular disease and cancer.

The potential antioxidant and anti-inflammatory effects of many nutrient supplements are the basis their proposed use to prevent cardiovascular disease and cancer.[3] The oxidative properties of antioxidants are not fully understood; however, research has suggested that these properties may vary in relation to other factors, such as the concentration of the nutrient and presence of other oxidants or antioxidants. The harmful association between β-carotene and lung cancer suggests that other variables may influence whether β-carotene acts as an antioxidant versus a pro-oxidant.

Response to Public Comments

A draft version of this recommendation statement was posted for public comment on the USPSTF website from November 12 to December 9, 2013. In response to these comments, the USPSTF added language emphasizing that the harms of β-carotene were found in persons at increased risk for lung cancer. The discussion of vitamin E was revised to clarify the consistency of evidence showing a lack of benefit.

Update of Previous USPSTF Recommendation

This recommendation updates the 2003 USPSTF recommendation on vitamin supplementation to prevent cardiovascular disease or cancer. At that time, the USPSTF concluded that the evidence was insufficient to recommend for or against the use of supplements of vitamins A, C, or E; multivitamins with folic acid; or antioxidant combinations for the prevention of cardiovascular disease or cancer (I statement). The USPSTF also recommended against the use of β-carotene supplements, either alone or in combination with other supplements, for the prevention of cardiovascular disease or cancer (D recommendation).

In the current recommendation, the USPSTF considered evidence on additional nutrient supplements, including vitamin D, calcium, selenium, and folic acid, for the primary prevention of cardiovascular disease and cancer. New evidence on the use of vitamin E increased the USPSTF's certainty about its lack of effectiveness in preventing these conditions.

Recommendations of Others

An independent consensus panel sponsored by the National Institutes of Health concluded that the present evidence is insufficient to recommend for or against the use of multivitamins to prevent chronic disease.[22] The Academy of Nutrition and Dietetics (formerly the American Dietetic Association) noted in a 2009 position statement that, although multivitamin supplements may be useful in meeting the recommended levels of some nutrients, there is no evidence that they are effective in preventing chronic disease.[23]

The American Cancer Society found that current evidence does not support the use of dietary supplements for the prevention of cancer.[10] The American Institute for Cancer Research determined in 2007 that dietary supplements are not recommended for cancer prevention and recommended a balanced diet with a variety of foods rather than supplements.[24]

The American Heart Association recommends that healthy persons receive adequate nutrients by eating a variety of foods rather than supplementation.[25] The American Academy of Family Physicians' clinical recommendations are consistent with the USPSTF recommendations.[26]

Members of the U.S. Preventive Services Task Force

Members of the U.S. Preventive Services Task Force at the time this recommendation was finalized[†] are Virginia A. Moyer, MD, MPH, *Chair* (American Board of Pediatrics, Chapel Hill, North Carolina); Michael L. LeFevre, MD, MSPH, *Co-Vice Chair* (University of Missouri School of Medicine, Columbia, Missouri); Albert L. Siu, MD, MSPH, *Co-Vice Chair* (Mount Sinai School of Medicine, New York, and James J. Peters, Veterans Affairs Medical Center, Bronx, New York); Linda Ciofu Baumann, PhD, RN (University of Wisconsin, Madison, Wisconsin); Susan J. Curry, PhD (University of Iowa College of Public Health, Iowa City, Iowa); Mark Ebell, MD, MS (University of Georgia Athens, Georgia); Francisco A. R. García, MD, MPH (Pima County Department of Health, Tucson, Arizona); Jessica Herzstein, MD, MPH (Air Products, Allentown, Pennsylvania); Douglas K. Owens, MD, MS (Veterans Affairs Palo Alto Health Care System, Palo Alto, and Stanford University, Stanford, California); William R. Phillips, MD, MPH (University of Washington, Seattle, Washington); and Michael P. Pignone, MD, MPH (University of North Carolina, Chapel Hill, North Carolina). Previous Task Force member Wanda K. Nicholson, MD, MPH, MBA, also made significant contributions to this recommendation.

Appendix Table 1 What the USPSTF Grades Mean and Suggestions for Practice		
Grade	Definition	Suggestions for Practice
A	The USPSTF recommends the service. There is high certainty that the net benefit is substantial.	Offer or provide this service.

† For a list of current Task Force members, go to www.uspreventiveservicestaskforce.org/members.htm.

Grade	Definition	Suggestions for Practice
B	The USPSTF recommends the service. There is high certainty that the net benefit is moderate or there is moderate certainty that the net benefit is moderate to substantial.	Offer or provide this service.
C	The USPSTF recommends selectively offering or providing this service to individual patients based on professional judgment and patient preferences. There is at least moderate certainty that the net benefit is small.	Offer or provide this service for selected patients depending on individual circumstances.
D	The USPSTF recommends against the service. There is moderate or high certainty that the service has no net benefit or that the harms outweigh the benefits.	Discourage the use of this service.
I	The USPSTF concludes that the current evidence is insufficient to assess the balance of benefits and harms of the service. Evidence is lacking, of poor quality, or conflicting, and the balance of benefits and harms cannot be determined.	Read the clinical considerations section of USPSTF Recommendation Statement. If the service is offered, patients should understand the uncertainty about the balance of benefits and harms.

Source: U.S. Preventive Services Task Force.

Appendix Table 2 Levels of Certainty Regarding Net Benefit	
Level of Certainty*	**Description**
High	The available evidence usually includes consistent results from well-designed, well-conducted studies in representative primary care populations. These studies assess the effects of the preventive service on health outcomes. This conclusion is therefore unlikely to be strongly affected by the results of future studies.
Moderate	The available evidence is sufficient to determine the effects of the preventive service on health outcomes, but confidence in the estimate is constrained by such factors as: ■ The number, size, or quality of individual studies. ■ Inconsistency of findings across individual studies.

Level of Certainty*	Description
	■ Limited generalizability of findings to routine primary care practice.
	■ Lack of coherence in the chain of evidence.
	As more information becomes available, the magnitude or direction of the observed effect could change, and this change may be large enough to alter the conclusion.
Low	The available evidence is insufficient to assess effects on health outcomes. Evidence is insufficient because of:
	■ The limited number or size of studies.
	■ Important flaws in study design or methods.
	■ Inconsistency of findings across individual studies.
	■ Gaps in the chain of evidence.
	■ Findings not generalizable to routine primary care practice.
	■ Lack of information on important health outcomes.
	More information may allow estimation of effects on health outcomes.

*The USPSTF defines certainty as "likelihood that the USPSTF assessment of the net benefit of a preventive service is correct." The net benefit is defined as benefit minus harm of the preventive service as implemented in a general, primary care population. The USPSTF assigns a certainty level based on the nature of the overall evidence available to assess the net benefit of a preventive service.
Source: U.S. Preventive Services Task Force.

Copyright and Source Information

This document is in the public domain within the United States.

Source: This article was first published in *Annals of Internal Medicine* on 25 February, 2014.

Disclaimer: Recommendations made by the USPSTF are independent of the U.S. government. They should not be construed as an official position of the Agency for Healthcare Research and Quality or the U.S. Department of Health and Human Services.

Financial Support: The USPSTF is an independent, voluntary body. The U.S. Congress mandates that the Agency for Healthcare Research and Quality support the operations of the USPSTF.

Potential Conflicts of Interest: None disclosed. Disclosure forms from USPSTF members can be viewed at www.acponline.org/authors/icmje/ConflictOfInterestForms .do?msNum=M14-0198.

Requests for Single Reprints: Reprints are available from the USPSTF website (http://www.uspreventiveservicestaskforce.org).

References

1. Bailey RL, Gahche JJ, Lentino CV, Dwyer JT, Engel JS, Thomas PR, et al. Dietary supplement use in the United States, 2003–2006. *J Nutr*. 2011;141(2):261–6.

2. Gahche J, Bailey R, Burt V, Hughes J, Yetley E, Dwyer J, et al. Dietary supplement use among U.S. adults has increased since NHANES III (1988–1994). *NCHS Data Brief*. 2011;(61):1–8.

3. Fortmann SP, Burda BU, Senger CA, Lin J, Beil T, O'Connor E, Whitlock EP. *Vitamin, Mineral, and Multivitamin Supplements for the Primary Prevention of Cardiovascular Disease and Cancer: A Systematic Evidence Review for the U.S. Preventive Services Task Force*. Evidence Synthesis No. 108. AHRQ Publication No. 14-05199-EF-1. Rockville, MD: Agency for Healthcare Research and Quality; 2013.

4. Denham BE. Dietary supplements—regulatory issues and implications for public health. *JAMA*. 2011;306:428–9.

5. Otten JJ, Hellwig JP, Meyers LD (eds). *Dietary Reference Intakes: The Essential Guide to Nutrient Requirements*. Washington, DC: National Academies Press; 2006.

6. Nutrition Business Journal. *NBJ's Supplement Business Report: An Analysis of Markets, Trends, Competition and Strategy in the U.S. Dietary Supplement Industry*. New York: Penton Media; 2011.

7. Dickinson A, Boyon N, Shao A. Physicians and nurses use and recommend dietary supplements: report of a survey. *Nutr J*. 2009;8:29.

8. U.S. Department of Agriculture and U.S. Department of Health and Human Services. *Dietary Guidelines for Americans, 2010*. 7th ed. Washington, DC: U.S. Government Printing Office; 2010.

9. Lichtenstein AH, Appel LJ, Brands M, Carnethon M, Daniels S, Franch HA, et al; American Heart Association Nutrition Committee. Diet and lifestyle recommendations revision 2006: a scientific statement from the American Heart Association Nutrition Committee. *Circulation*. 2006;114:82–96.

10. Kushi LH, Doyle C, McCullough M, Rock CL, Demark-Wahnefried W, Bandera EV, et al; American Cancer Society 2010 Nutrition and Physical Activity Guidelines Advisory Committee. American Cancer Society guidelines on nutrition and physical activity for cancer prevention: reducing the risk of cancer with healthy food choices and physical activity. *CA Cancer J Clin*. 2012;62:30–67.

11. Hoyert DL, Xu J. Deaths: preliminary data for 2011. *Natl Vital Stat Rep*. 2012;61(6):1–52.

12. Fortmann SP, Burda BU, Senger CA, Lin JS, Whitlock EP. Vitamin and mineral supplements in the primary prevention of cardiovascular disease and cancer: an updated systematic evidence review for the U.S. Preventive Services Task Force. *Ann Intern Med*. 2013;159:824–34.

13. Gaziano JM, Sesso HD, Christen WG, Bubes V, Smith JP, MacFadyen J, et al. Multivitamins in the prevention of cancer in men: the Physician's Health Study II randomized controlled trial. *JAMA*. 2012;308(18):1871–80.

14. Hercberg S, Galan P, Preziosi P, Bertrais S, Mennen L, Malvy D, et al. The SU.VI.MAX Study: a randomized, placebo-controlled trial of the health effects of antioxidant vitamins and minerals. *Arch Intern Med.* 2004;164(21):2335–42.

15. Lappe JM, Travers-Gustafson D, Davies KM, Recker RR, Heaney RP. Vitamin D and calcium supplementation reduces cancer risk: results of a randomized trial. *Am J Clin Nutr.* 2007;85(6):1586–91.

16. Wactawski-Wende J, Kotchen JM, Anderson GL, Assaf AR, Brunner RL, O'Sullivan MJ, et al. Calcium plus vitamin D supplementation and the risk of colorectal cancer. *N Engl J Med.* 2006;354(7):684–96.

17. Bolland MJ, Grey A, Gamble GD, Reid IR. Calcium and vitamin D supplements and health outcomes: a reanalysis of the Women's Health Initiative (WHI) limited-access data set. *Am J Clin Nutr.* 2011;94(4):1144–9.

18. Alpha-Tocopherol Beta Carotene Cancer Prevention Study Group. The effect of vitamin E and beta carotene on the incidence of lung cancer and other cancers in male smokers. *N Engl J Med.* 1994;330(15):1029–35.

19. Lippman SM, Klein EA, Goodman PJ, Lucia MS, Thompson IM, Ford LG, et al. Effect of selenium and vitamin E on risk of prostate cancer and other cancers: the Selenium and Vitamin E Cancer Prevention Trial (SELECT). *JAMA.* 2009;301(1):39–51.

20. Omenn GS, Goodman GE, Thornquist MD, Balmes J, Cullen MR, Glass A, et al. Effects of a combination of beta carotene and vitamin A on lung cancer and cardiovascular disease. *N Engl J Med.* 1996;334(18):1150–5.

21. Tanvetyanon T, Bepler G. Beta-carotene in multivitamins and the possible risk of lung cancer among smokers versus former smokers: a meta-analysis and evaluation of national brands. *Cancer.* 2008;113(1):150–7.

22. National Institutes of Health State-of-the-Science Panel. National Institutes of Health State-of-the-Science Conference Statement: multivitamin/mineral supplements and chronic disease prevention. *Am J Clin Nutr.* 2007;85(1):257S–64S.

23. Marra MV, Boyar AP. Position of the American Dietetic Association: nutrient supplementation. *J Am Diet Assoc.* 2009;109(12):2073–85.

24. World Cancer Research Fund; American Institute for Cancer Research. *Food, Nutrition, Physical Activity, and the Prevention of Cancer: A Global Perspective.* Washington, DC: American Institute for Cancer Research; 2007.

25. American Heart Association. *Vitamin and Mineral Supplements.* Dallas: American Heart Association; 2013. Accessed at http://www.heart.org/HEARTORG/GettingHealthy/NutritionCenter/Vitamin-and-Mineral-Supplements_UCM_306033_Article.jsp on 22 January 2014.

26. American Academy of Family Physicians. *Clinical Recommendations: Vitamin Supplementation.* Leawood, KS: American Academy of Family Physicians; 2014. Accessed at www.aafp.org/patient-care/clinical-recommendations/all/vitamin.html on 22 January 2014.

Profile & Commentary

GUIDELINE PURPOSES

This clinical guideline, issued by the U.S. Preventive Services Task Force (USPSTF), addresses three specific questions that are not explicitly stated in the *Final Recommendation Statement* reprinted here but can easily be inferred from the recommendations. They are:

1. In healthy adults without special nutritional needs, do multivitamins prevent cardiovascular disease (CVD) or cancer?
2. In healthy adults without special nutritional needs, do single- or paired-supplements prevent CVD or cancer?
3. What is the balance of benefits and harms for multivitamins and vitamin supplements?

Importantly, only the preventive effects on these two disease categories were considered. Also, in the *Clinical Considerations* section, we learn that the studies examined and the recommendations made apply only to "healthy adults without special nutritional needs" and that different supplement formulations were used in the studies, which make generalization to the general population difficult.

METHODS

The USPSTF's methods for producing a clinical guideline are available from a link on its home page: http://www.uspreventiveservicestaskforce .org/Page/Name/recommendations. An 84-page USPSTF procedural manual describes the methods used to ensure that its recommendations are scientifically sound, reproducible, and well documented. Its production process is consistent with the ideal process set forth earlier in this chapter.

In the *Scope of Review* section, there is a statement alluding to a systematic review that was done to address the questions of interest; this systematic review is referenced with footnotes 3 and 12. The dimness of this statement in unfortunate as it is important to some clinicians to be able to easily access the evidence on which the recommendations are based. Nevertheless, tracking footnote 3 got me to a report of that systematic review at http://www .ncbi.nlm.nih.gov/books/NBK173987/. The *Summary of Evidence* section (particularly the evidence tables) of that report details the evidence for each supplement. Some clinicians will be interested in the details of the evidence whereas others will trust that the USPSTF followed its guideline production standards and accept the more general information about the evidence that is included in this *Final Recommendation Statement* document. The bottom line is: an extensive and rigorous systematic review was conducted and used as the evidence for the recommendations made.

The guideline starts out with the recommendations and general statements about the sufficiency of evidence on which each recommendation was based. Two of the recommendations are actually non-recommendations and one is a recommendation against two supplements. Do note that the five evidence grades used by USPSTF are defined in *Appendix Table 1* and the certainty levels for recommendations are defined in *Appendix Table 2*.

RECOMMENDATIONS AND EVIDENCE

The guideline document first conveys in general terms the strength of the evidence for three supplements: multivitamins, individual supplements, and for β-carotene and vitamin E. The latter breakout was necessary because there was sufficient evidence regarding them whereas the evidence for the other individual supplements was insufficient.

For the question about the preventive effect of multivitamins, the evidence was insufficient to make a recommendation one way or the other for either CVD or cancer; there were five large studies relevant to this question. In the systematic review cited earlier, I learned that these studies consisted of four good-quality RCTs (n = 28,607) and one good-quality cohort study (n = 72,337).

The evidence about individual vitamins was also insufficient to make recommendations except for β-carotene and vitamin E for which there was sufficient evidence. In the case of β-carotene, there was consistent evidence from six clinical trials indicating that it does not decrease the risk for CVD. Additionally, a meta-analysis of the β-carotene trials detected an increased risk for lung cancer in smokers and/or those with asbestos exposure. This is the meaning of the sentence "A meta-analysis of β-carotene trials reported an increased risk for lung cancer (pooled odds ratio, 1.24 [CI 1.10 to 1.39] in current smokers." (Since 1 is not in the confidence interval, the risk for smokers is 10–39% greater than for nonsmokers.) The evidence about this risk in combination with sufficient evidence that it does not reduce CVD or cancer risk in the larger population led to a general recommendation against taking it that was issued with moderate certainty.

In contrast, for vitamin E, the evidence was sufficient to conclude there is no CVD or cancer prevention benefit to taking it, although there is no indication of harm, which is different than β-carotene, which was associated with risk in the named groups. Still, in both cases the recommendation is graded as *D*, meaning the USPSTF recommends with moderate to high certainty not taking them.

In the section *Potential Harms*, the authors recognize the potential for harm from high doses of the fat-soluble vitamins A and D, although the evidence reviewed did not examine studies of high-dose vitamin supplementation.

In sum, this was a soundly produced clinical practice guideline that was able to issue just two recommendations (against β-carotene and vitamin E); the research evidence regarding the other supplements was insufficient to make recommendations about them.

REFERENCES

Agency for Healthcare Research and Quality. (n.d.). Retrieved from http://www.guideline.gov/syntheses/synthesis.aspx?id=47794

AGREE Collaboration. (2013). *Appraisal of guidelines for research and evaluation, AGREE II update.* Retrieved from http://www.agreetrust.org/about-the-agree-enterprise/agree-research-teams/agree-collaboration/

Australian Government National Health and Medical Research Council. (2011). *Information for guideline developers.* Retrieved from http://www.nhmrc.gov.au

Berkman, N. D., Lohr, K. N., Ansari, M., McDonagh, M., Balk, E., Whitlock, E. . . . Chang, S. (2013). Grading the strength of a body of evidence when assessing health care interventions for the effective health care program of the Agency for Healthcare Research and Quality: An update. Methods guide for comparative effectiveness review. *AHRQ Publication No. 13(14).* Rockville, MD: Agency for Healthcare Research and Quality. Retrieved from https://www.effectivehealthcare.ahrq.gov/ehc/products/457/1752/methods-guidance-grading-evidence-131118.pdf

Boyd, C. M., & Fortin, M. (2010). Future of multimorbidity research: How should understanding of multimorbidity inform health system design? *Public Health Review, 32*(2), 451–474. Retrieved from http://www.publichealthreviews.eu/upload/pdf_files/8/PHR_32_2_Boyd.pdf

GRADE (Grading of Recommendations Assessment, Development and Evaluation Working Group). (n.d.). *The GRADE approach.* Chapter 12, section 12.2.1. Retrieved from http://handbook.cochrane.org/

Graham, I., Harrison, M. B., & Godfrey, C. M. (2014). Guideline dissemination and implementation intervention for nursing: A systematic review. *International Journal of Evidence-Based Healthcare, 12*(3). doi: 10.1097/01.XEB.0000455125.82499.33

Guidelines International Network. (n.d). Retrieved from http://www.g-i-n.net/

Guyatt, G., Gutterman, D., Baumann, M. H., Addrizzo-Harris, D., Hylek, E. M., Phillips, B., . . . et al. (2006). Grading strength of recommendation and quality of evidence in clinical guidelines. *CHEST, 129*(1), 174–181.

Institute of Medicine (IOM). (2011). *Clinical practice guidelines we can trust.* Retrieved from http://www.iom.edu/Reports/

Joanna Briggs Institute. (2013). *New JBI levels of evidence.* Retrieved from http://joannabriggs.org/assets/docs/approach/JBI-Levels-of-evidence_2014.pdf

Lavin, M., Harper, E., & Barr, N. (April 14, 2015). Health information technology, patient safety, and professional nursing care documentation in acute care settings. *OJIN: The Online Journal of Issues in Nursing, 20*(2). doi: 10.3912/OJIN.Vol20No02PPT04

Mentes, J. C., & Kang, S. (2011). *Hydration management.* University of Iowa College of Nursing and John A. Hartford Foundation Center of Geriatric Nursing Excellence. Retrieved from http://www.guideline.gov

National Pressure Ulcer Advisory Panel, European Pressure Ulcer Advisory Panel, Pan Pacific Pressure Injury Alliance. (2014a). *Prevention and treatment of pressure ulcers: Clinical practice guideline.* Washington, DC: National Pressure Ulcer Advisory Panel.

National Pressure Ulcer Advisory Panel, European Pressure Ulcer Advisory Panel, Pan Pacific Pressure Injury Alliance. (2014b). *Quick reference guide.* Retrieved from http://www.npuap.org. Also see: http://www.internationalguideline.com/ or a modified form at https://www.guideline.gov/content.aspx?id=48867

Oncology Nursing Society. (2012). *ONS PEP*[(r)]*—Putting evidence into practice.* Retrieved from http://www.ons.org/Research/PEP

Oncology Nursing Society. (2016). *PEP rating system overview.* Retrieved from https://www.ons.org/practice-resources/pep

Registered Nurses' Association of Ontario. (2006). *BPG development methodology.* Retrieved from http://rnao.ca/bpg/guidelines/methodology

Registered Nurses' Association of Ontario. (2010). *Condensed guidelines for personal digital assistants (PDAs).* Retrieved from http://rnao.ca/bpg/pda

Registered Nurses' Association of Ontario. (2016). Nursing best practice guidelines app. Retrieved from http://rnao.ca/bpg/pda/app

Scottish Intercollegiate Guidelines Network. (2014). *SIGN 50: A guideline developer's handbook.* Retrieved from http://sign.ac.uk/pdf/qrg50.pdf

PART II

Evidence-Based Practice

From Part I, hopefully you have acquired an appreciation of and basic knowledge about the different kinds of research studies that are used to study nursing phenomena and the desirable features of each. You also have basic knowledge about how systematic reviews are done and how evidence-based clinical practice guidelines are produced. **Figure PII-1** graphically portrays the ground covered in the first part of the text. This knowledge is essential to using research evidence in your own nursing practice and to participating in evidence-based practice (EBP) projects in your work setting.

Going Forward

However, research knowledge is not enough; you also need to be able to find research evidence, appraise it, and strategically use it in practice—and that is what this part of the text addresses. To this point, the focus has been on research evidence, and that will continue to be the focus in the remaining chapters, albeit more from the consumer of research evidence perspective.

Do notice the order of Chapters 14, 15, and 16. These chapters on appraisal of evidence first consider evidence-base clinical practice guidelines (EbCPGs), then systematic reviews (SRs), then original, individual studies. This is the reverse of how you learned about them in Part I of the text. The reason for the reversal is that EbCPGs and SRs are more reliable and ready for translation into practice, whereas the order in Part I was based on the natural learning order.

In Chapter 17, the lens is opened up and you will learn how caregiving organizations use research evidence in combination with other types of evidence. Evidence-based practice's contribution to clinical care will be described in the real-world contexts in which it comes

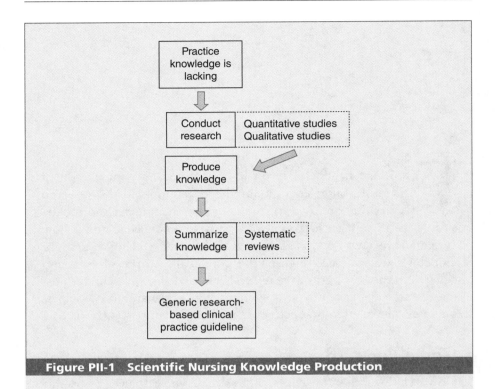

Figure PII-1   Scientific Nursing Knowledge Production

to life. In Chapter 19, the individual nurse's use of research evidence is described. The steps individual nurses use to incorporate research evidence into clinical decision making for individual patients and to refine their own methods of practice are similar to those used by organizations, albeit performed with less rigor (Eddy, 2005).

Not all writers differentiate between evidence-based practice as an organizational activity and the individual's use of research evidence, but I think a distinction is important. A distinction between the two ways of using research evidence retains high standards for translating research evidence into clinical protocols while recognizing the value of individual nurses seeking better information when organizational protocols are lacking or are not applicable to a particular patient situation. A distinction also recognizes EBP as an organizational activity, and point-of-care design as the individual professional nurse's responsibility. Maximally effective nursing care for patients requires translation of research into practice at both levels.

Figure PII-2   EBP Impact Model

The Evidence-Based Practice Impact Model

The evidence-based practice impact model shown in **Figure PII-2** depicts the major steps in achieving effective evidence-based practice in a healthcare organization. Importantly, each step should be thoughtfully and strategically carried out to ensure that the organizational protocol produced is truly evidence based and that the implementation of the protocol has the desired effect on provider behavior and on patient outcomes. To achieve this level of translation of research evidence into practice, EBP projects are conducted by units, service lines, or agency teams composed of members with clinical, managerial, and EBP knowledge.

The EBP impact model is similar to other, more detailed models that are used as working frameworks for implementation of evidence-based practice programs in healthcare organizations. The evidence-based practice impact model serves as a map for this part of the text.

REFERENCE

Eddy, D. M. (2005). Evidence-based medicine: A unified approach. Two approaches to using evidence to solve clinical problems and how to unify them. *Health Affairs, 24*(1), 9–17.

CHAPTER ELEVEN

Asking Clinical Questions

> Ask ▶

Ｔhe starting point for a clinical team embarking on a project to develop an evidence-based protocol is to formulate a clinical question in a way that will guide the search for research evidence and keep the project on mission. First, we need to consider how an issue might have risen to the level of the agency deciding to develop a care protocol regarding it. In the Iowa model of evidence-based practice, these initiators are referred to as *triggers* (Titler et al., 2001).

Triggers

Information pointing to a problem with care can come from various places in the caregiving system and trigger an initiative to find more effective approaches. Sources of triggers can be a staff member, quality management monitoring, risk management, financial reports, infection control monitoring, or a discharge planning coordinator. The trigger can also come from outside the agency in the form of new standards of care from a professional association, regulatory agency, or accrediting organization.

Clinical Practice

Care providers who are thoughtful and not robotic while giving care see what, in spite of good intentions, could be done better and ask questions such as the following:

■ What groups of people should we be screening in the emergency department for domestic violence?

- Should I recommend vitamin D supplements to my elderly patients?
- Should we be using bladder scans to determine urinary residual on all patients who have had an indwelling/Foley catheter removed?
- What nonpharmacologic measures can we use to prevent and treat muscle spasms in persons who have had cervical fusion surgery?
- Is acetaminophen or ibuprofen more effective and safer in treating fever in young children?
- Why do some adolescent girls in poor, urban neighborhoods aspire to good diet, exercise, good grades, and sexual abstinence?
- What factors determine whether middle-aged men working in an industrial plant follow recommendations regarding how to avoid back injury?

These kinds of questions can be answered in part by examining the knowledge produced by research.

Quality Data

All healthcare organizations collect a great deal of information to prove to third-party payers, accrediting agencies, and the public that important aspects of care are being given consistently and that their patients are attaining the appropriate outcomes. For example, a hospital might track the following information about people who have a discharge diagnosis of ischemic stroke:

- Readmission within 30 days
- Global disability status at discharge
- Discharge destination
- Special after-hospital services required
- Adverse events rates
- Complication rates

The hospital may also receive information from an accrediting agency, third-party payer, or a voluntary quality monitoring coalition about care and outcomes at other similar organizations. To be more specific: if a hospital's poststroke patients who were discharged on an anticoagulant medication had more emergency care visits for bleeding than similar patients discharged from other similar hospitals, the clinical staff would be obliged to reevaluate their teaching and discharge protocols for patients taking anticoagulants. If a current protocol was found to not represent current evidence-based standards of care, an EBP project to design a new protocol might be initiated.

Thus, quality monitoring data, whether internal or shared, may shed light on a deficiency in care and thereby serves as a trigger for an EBP project. Quality monitoring and its relationship to EBP are discussed more extensively in Chapter 17.

Professional Standards

When national professional associations issue evidence-based guidelines, caregiving organizations are obligated to take notice and decide if they should change the way they are giving care. Similarly, when licensing and accrediting agencies, such as the Centers for Medicare and Medicaid Services (CMS) or the Joint Commission set forth new standards of care, caregiving organizations have to decide how they will meet them, and this initiates a search for research evidence to help develop a new protocol. This was the case when the Joint Commission and the CMS required inpatient psychiatric settings to report data regarding their use of holding patients in seclusion rooms.

At a less formal level, a staff nurse might see an article or a research report in a clinical journal about a care approach that seems promising. Or he may learn about a new guideline in a session at a conference or workshop. After thinking about the matter, he may come to the conclusion that this aspect of care as it is being done in his setting is of dubious effectiveness. Taking the concern and idea to a nurse leader, clinical nurse specialist, or case manager might lead to a search for research evidence about the alternative approach to care.

Questions Not Answerable by Research Evidence

Before looking at how to formulate a focused clinical question for an evidence-based project, it might be helpful to address the issue of the kinds of questions that cannot be answered by research evidence.

One type of question that often cannot be answered with research evidence is a question involving very new technology. If studies are available about a new technology, they may have been conducted by the manufacturer and therefore should be appraised carefully. An example would be if scientists were able to produce an external device that senses seizures just minutes before they occur; the early users of such a device would most likely have very little research evidence to go on.

Another question for which research evidence may not be available is the application of an existing intervention to a new population. There may be considerable evidence regarding the intervention in the population for which it was developed but none in the population with whom the agency is considering using it. A digital device that monitors whether children use their asthma inhaler correctly may have been tested with children and found effective but may not have been tested in children with attention-deficit/hyperactivity disorder. Another example is that a body of research about the use of an intervention may have been conducted mainly with middle class women but there is no or very little research about the use of the intervention with poor, inner-city women. In these situations, the research available is informative, but clinical protocols for the new population cannot be truly based on the available evidence.

A third type of question that cannot be definitively answered with research evidence is a question pertaining to the care of an individual patient who does not want a standardized intervention. The ethical principle is that each competent patient has the right to determine what happens to his person and body, and this principle must be respected regardless of what research evidence shows. Questions about what care should be given to an individual must be decided by the patient and his care providers. Research evidence can provide useful information to consider in the discussion, but ultimately the decision is the patient's or that of his designated healthcare proxy.

In light of the ethical principle just described, research evidence is also of limited use in questions having to do with values or deciding what is a moral or ethical course of action. The question, "Should we treat pneumonia in nursing home residents older than 90 years of age who have severe cognitive deficits?" is essentially a moral question. Research may shed some light on the question by providing data regarding the percentage of this population that has an uncomplicated recovery and return to their former functional status when treated with antibiotics, but research cannot answer the question. In fact, the question cannot be answered in general. It must be answered on a case-by-case basis because the answer depends on how cognitively compromised the person was prior to the onset of the pneumonia, whether intubation is a likely possibility, and what the patient's end-of-life wishes were when last expressed—again, the ethical principle of self-determination. These ethical reminders are necessary to assure that research evidence is used for the purposes it inherently serves and not as a means of controlling individual lives.

Forming a Useful Project Question

To keep the project on target and to avoid spending a lot of time searching for and sifting through a large number of citations, it helps to formulate a focused project question—as opposed to a very broad or vague one. One of the previously listed questions asked about doing an ultrasound bladder scan on patients who have an indwelling catheter removed. This is a legitimate question, but it is vague and requires more focus. Let us assume that in the process of developing a postoperative order set for adults after abdominal surgery, a medical–surgical practice council decides to consider the research on this issue.

The council might use an approach that many healthcare providers have found useful in focusing their evidence-based clinical projects; it is referred to by the mnemonic PICOT (Sackett, Straus, Richardson, Rosenberg, & Haynes, 2000; Stillwell, 2010). The PICOT format helps clinicians zero in on specific elements of a question that are of interest.

P	Patient population
I	Intervention/Issue
C	Comparison intervention
O	Outcomes
T	Timing
S	Setting

[handwritten annotations: patient population / intervention / issue / comparison intervention / outcomes / timing / setting]

Generally, when using PICOT, the patient population can be characterized by attributes such as age, illness experience (e.g., shortness of breath), disease, or risk, to name a few. The intervention of interest can be specified by naming a clinical intervention, a particular approach, or a group of interventions (e.g., school-based programs regarding weight loss). For some questions, the *I* could stand for an issue rather than an intervention; this would be the case if the question was about mobility obstacles associated with foot drop. A comparison of the intervention to another intervention or to usual care may be of interest; alternatively, the effectiveness of just one intervention may be what is under consideration. Patient outcomes are almost always of interest, particularly outcomes that are important to patients, such as improved functional ability or fewer episodes of hypoglycemia. The timing, in terms of clinical status, duration, and frequency of treatment or length of follow-up, may be relevant. You may have noticed I added an **S** to the PICOT mnemonic. I did so because specifying the setting of care can often help focus the question and reduce the number of citations retrieved that are not relevant. Case in point: Managing urinary incontinence in home care is quite different than managing it in hospital.

Getting back to the issue of bladder scanning after removal of an indwelling urinary catheter, a hospital practice council could develop a project question specific to postoperative patients using **PICOTS** as follows:

> **In patients who have an indwelling bladder catheter removed after surgery (P) (implies acute care setting S), does bladder scanning (I) after the first voiding (T) identify persons who have a large urine residual (O) and require further monitoring of their urination (O)?**

If you were to state this question specifying the population as patients who have had repair of a hip fracture, you probably would not find studies pertaining to it. So, it is possible to get too specific; sometimes some trial and error is required to get the question just right.

Another example: Nurses on an obstetrical unit are concerned about the discomfort and distress newborns experience during and immediately after having blood drawn. To look into the intervention options they formulated the following question:

> **What nonpharmacologic measures should nurses use (I) to reduce pain, discomfort, and agitation (Os) with full-term newborn infants (P) before, during, and after venipuncture and insertion of intravenous lines (T)?**

The intervention (nonpharmacologic measures) in this question is somewhat open ended—and that's okay as it could identify measures of which the nurses were not aware. Alternatively, they may just be interested in comparing two methods, in which the question might be:

> **Is oral sucrose pacifier or swaddling more effective (I and C) in controlling pain (O) during and after venipuncture (T) in full-term newborns (P)?**

Note that the population specified in both questions is newborns, so the team looking into this issue would not retrieve or review guidelines, systematic reviews, and studies done on premature infants or infants older than 28 days.

Although not every clinical question about an intervention will have every PICOTS element, it is useful to at least consider each one. Generally, PICOTS works best for questions about intervention effectiveness. Questions regarding patients' experiences, the meaning of illness, relationships among clinical variables, and risk require modification of the PICOTS format. Nonintervention questions typically seek background evidence useful in developing assessment guides, teaching protocols, plans of care, or even whole programs. The *I* then represents *Issue* or *Issues,* instead of *Intervention.*

A project team at a stateside military hospital opening a department to treat soldiers with traumatic brain injury could formulate their question in several ways:

> **In soldiers returning from combat with traumatic brain injury (P), what stateside, rehabilitation setting characteristics (Issue and S) promote partner support and renewal of family relationships (Os)?**
>
> **What issues and problems reconnecting with partner and families (Issue) are experienced by soldiers returning from combat with traumatic brain injury (P) to rehab units stateside (S)?**

The first question targets what the project team wants to know but research about it may not be available. The second question should access studies about the reuniting experiences of these returning soldiers to help the team comprehensively and deeply understand the soldiers' experiences and then develop setting-specific facilities and services that address them.

Sometimes project teams seeking evidence about background issues find it better to have two closely related questions rather than cramming the issues of interest into one question. For instance, a protect team developing a support program for men with urinary incontinence might look at qualitative and descriptive studies about the experience of urinary incontinence and self-management strategies these men find helpful. The project questions could be:

> 1. What experiences and self-management issues (I) do men with urinary incontinence (P) find stressful or difficult to manage (Os)?
> 2. What self-management actions and strategies help (Issue) these men (P) adjust to and cope with urinary incontinence (Os)?

Together these questions could result in retrieval of research evidence that would be useful in developing a clinical program that is patient centered and evidence based. Both questions have population, issue, and outcome elements but no comparison or time element.

Another example would be a project group developing a care protocol to support chronically ill mothers of young children; the questions guiding the project would be as follows:

> 1. When mothers of young children develop a chronic illness that affects physical functioning (P), how is their ability to mother their children affected (O)?
> 2. When mothers of young children become chronically ill (P), how do they and their partners (or immediate family) adjust to the situation (O)?

Okay, hopefully you get the idea: Make the project question as focused as possible by using the PICOTS format. If it turns out to be too specific (i.e., you cannot find any studies about it), you can either broaden one of the elements or drop it altogether. Doing so may open it up just enough that relevant evidence can be identified. If a project team has difficulty focusing its question, it sometimes helps to have several members spend a half hour muddling around in a database looking at various abstracts and articles about the issue. This muddling may help formulate a more focused question and help identify the terminology that will result in a productive search for evidence.

Moving on, assuming the protocol development team has a focused question that is consistent with the agency's commitments and resources, the next step is to conduct a search for research evidence related to that question.

REFERENCES

Sackett, D. L., Straus, S. E., Richardson, W. S., Rosenberg, W., & Haynes, R. B. (2000). *Evidence-based medicine: How to practice and teach EBM* (2nd ed.). Edinburgh, Scotland: Churchill Livingstone.

Stillwell, S. (2010). Asking the clinical question: A key step in evidence-based practice. *American Journal of Nursing, 110(3),* 58–61.

Titler, M. G., Kleiber, C., Steelman, V. J., Rakel, B. A., Budreau, G., Everett, L. Q., Goode C. J. (2001). The Iowa model of evidence-based practice to promote quality care. *Critical Nursing Clinics of North America, 13*(4), 497–509.

CHAPTER TWELVE

Searching for Research Evidence

> Search

Τhis chapter is short because the best way to learn how to search for research evidence is by actually doing it. Therefore, the suggestions offered in this chapter are merely starting points.

So, where to start? The answer obviously depends on the topic, how much time you have to devote to the search, and whether you are doing it as an individual or as part of a group developing an e-b protocol. Search strategy also depends to a great extent on the type of evidence you are looking for. There are places to look specifically for evidence-based clinical practice guidelines (EbCPGs) or for systematic reviews (SRs), but there are also resources that can be used to identify all three types of research evidence, i.e., EbCPGs, SRs, and individual study reports.

Also, searching from the point of care on a handheld device will be different than an extensive search for an e-b project. This chapter describes what is available from a health center or academic library. Point-of-care searching on handhelds will be addressed in Chapter 19.

For reasons stated earlier, most often it is best to start by looking for EbCPGs and SRs. You can search for both in a health science citation database or by going to the databases of organizations that indexes just EbCPGs or SRs. Let's start with the health science databases.

Health Science Databases

First the basics: A database is a collection of a specified type of data that is organized for storage, accessibility, and retrieval. The specific type of data of interest to evidence-based nursing is bibliographic information about journal articles (and other resources) in the health sciences. Three of the most widely used by nurses are described below.

PubMed/MEDLINE

The most accessible database listing healthcare-related publications is PubMed. It is the online version of MEDLINE and is available at http://www.ncbi.nlm.nih.gov/pubmed/. Even simple searches using keywords are aided by pop-up suggestions. A PubMed search produces a list of relevant article citations, often with abstracts, and sometimes with links for accessing the article (see the screen shot that follows).

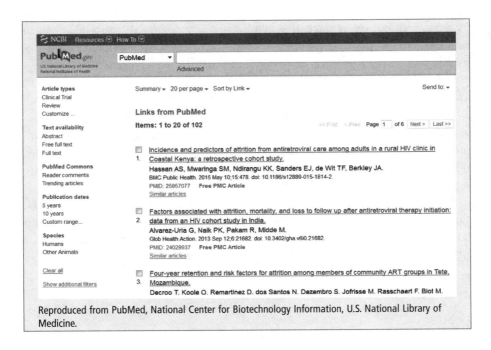

Reproduced from PubMed, National Center for Biotechnology Information, U.S. National Library of Medicine.

The PubMed search engine is quite powerful and has numerous features to help you get to the topic and evidence type of interest. Filters are available to help narrow your search by date, journal type, or language—to name just a few. Using the filter *Article type, Customize* you can limit your search to "practice guideline" and/or "systematic review." Beware, however, that not all the guidelines retrieved are evidence based and not all the systematic reviews meet the definition as set forth in Chapter 9.

Like with all the health science databases, it takes a bit of trial and error and practice to get good at using PubMed, but for those who rely on the Internet for doing their searching, the time would be well spent. To get you up to speed, the site provides a quick-start guide and tutorials.

For readers who have access to a health science library, you can access MEDLINE via the library's subscription. Most libraries have subscriptions to many journals, and often you can download the article right from the search engine the library uses. If a library doesn't have a subscription to a particular journal, it can usually obtain the article you are interested in via other means.

Cumulative Index to Nursing and Allied Health Literature

The Cumulative Index to Nursing and Allied Health Literature, better known as CINAHL, is an index of articles in nursing and allied health journals and other resources that are not included in MEDLINE, although there is considerable overlap between the two databases. CINAHL is available only by subscription, but all academic healthcare libraries and many hospital libraries have a subscription for use by students, their staff, and in many cases, by members of the public. Many articles are available in full text. Like PubMed, you can do a simple search using keywords and combine them with *AND* or *OR*. You can then limit your search by article type, date of publications, or age of the population of interest—to name a few of the limits possible. Again, tutorials are provided, and most librarians will assist you in learning to navigate it.

PsycINFO

This database is centered on the interdisciplinary literature in psychology and the behavioral and social sciences. Many health science libraries subscribe to it, and it is searchable in many of the same ways that CINAHL is. A fact sheet about it is available at http://www.apa.org/pubs/databases/psycinfo/psycinfo-printable-fact-sheet.pdf.

Nonprofit, International Organizations

There also are quite a few independent international organizations that produce or maintain databases of EbCPGs and SRs. The following is a sampling of these organizations.

Registered Nurses Association of Ontario

This organization produces high-quality guidelines on a wide variety of topics. It uses an explicit and transparent production process and has to date published and updated over 50 best practice guidelines, quite a few of which are available in languages other than English. Its guidelines are available free at its website, http://rnao.ca/bpg. It also offers condensed guidelines for mobile devices and implementation tool kits.

National Guideline Clearinghouse

The National Guideline Clearinghouse maintains an indexed database of clinical practice guidelines produced by a wide variety of organizations. The guidelines, which must meet inclusion criteria, are presented in a standardized format. Its index can be searched by disease/condition, by treatment/intervention, or by health service sector (e.g., profession, geographic area, or by the organization producing the guideline). National Guideline Clearinghouse guidelines are available free at http://www.guideline.gov/index.aspx.

U.S. National Preventive Services Task Force

This agency systematically reviews the evidence of effectiveness and develops recommendations for clinical preventive services. It offers an app to search for USPSTF recommendations by specific patient characteristics, including age, gender, and selected behavioral risk factors. Its website is http://epss.ahrq.gov/PDA/index.jsp.

Joanna Briggs Institute

The Joanna Briggs Institute is an international organization based in Australia with collaborating centers in over 40 countries. Its undertakings in the areas of developing and supporting the synthesis, transfer, and utilization of evidence is quite broad, but it does maintain a database of systematic reviews and implementation reports it and its international collaborating centers have produced. Most Joanna Briggs Institute resources are available only by subscription through a library; check to see if the library you use has a subscription. The Joanna Briggs Institute website is at http://joanna briggs.org/.

Cochrane Collaboration

Also an international organization, the Cochrane Collaboration promotes evidence-informed health decision making by producing high-quality systematic reviews. The Cochrane Database of Systematic Reviews includes reviews produced by the Cochrane Collaboration and its partner groups. As of this writing, its SRs become free for all readers 12 months after publication via open access; however, it is working to make them open access immediately. Its open access guidelines are available at http://www .cochrane.org/search/site.

Professional Specialty Organizations

Many professional specialty organizations produce and make available EbCPGs and SRs. Some organizations publish their guidelines in a book that can be purchased; others make them free to members, and others make their guidelines free online. The rigor of guideline development across the many producers varies. The list is long but here are a few that make guidelines available free online:

- American College of Physicians: https://www.acponline.org/
- Best Evidence Topics (BETs) Emergency Medicine: http://bestbets.org/ home/bets-introduction.php
- Emergency Nurses Association: https://www.ena.org/
- HIV Medicine Association: http://www.hivma.org/hiv_guidelines/
- Oncology Nursing Association: https://www.ons.org/practice- resources/pep

Wrap-Up

Obviously, many sources are available. The secret to locating research evidence relevant to your project is to become proficient in using at least one database and then identifying a few other sources that issue or index EbCPGs and SRs related to your clinical topic. Do poke around a bit to see what is applicable to your interests. And do consult with a librarian!

CHAPTER THIRTEEN

Appraising Research Evidence

>Appraise>

A ssuming that your database searches resulted in retrieval of at least one clinical practice guideline, systematic review, or report of an individual study, the next step is to appraise its quality to determine if you can have confidence in it. In this chapter, I will set forth the appraisal approach used in this text; in so doing when referring to all three forms of research evidence I will use the combination term *recommendations/conclusions/findings*, sometimes abbreviated as *r/c/f* (singular or plural).

Published guidelines, reviews, and individual study reports should not be accepted at face value, even when they are issued by professional associations or published in clinical and research journals. Reports of methodologically flawed evidence articles do get published. In addition to concerns about the trustworthiness of the r/c/f, the project team or individual considering using a piece of research evidence must also determine whether the r/c/f is likely to have significant clinical impact and whether it is feasible for their organization to base care on them. The term appraisal refers to an evaluation of the value of the evidence, both its inherent value and it value to a particular user.

Appraisal is a step beyond extracting the *why, how,* and *what* of the guideline, review, or study. It involves going beyond understanding how the r/c/f were produced to making a judgment about the soundness of the production methods. It involves moving beyond identifying the r/c/f to judging whether they are credible, clinically important, and applicable to a particular setting. However, appraisal as you will be doing it is not equivalent to a thesis or dissertation. Most of your time will be spent in reading the evidence report or guideline and marking it up for later reference. As a novice reader of research reports, however, reading for true understanding and extracting essential details can be a slow go. The time required for the actual appraisal is typically much less.

Appraisal Systems

Many appraisal systems for evaluating the quality of guidelines, systematic reviews, and studies exist. Six that are widely usesd are listed in Box 13-1; their websites are listed in the *Resources* section at the end of this chapter.

BOX 13-1 International Appraisal Systems

- The AGREE II instrument assesses the methodological rigor of how a clinical practice guideline was developed. It consists of 23 items organized within six domains, followed by two global rating items for an overall assessment.
- The GRADE system rates quality of evidence in systematic reviews and guidelines about the effects of health care using four explicitly defined levels (High to Very Low), and grades the strength of recommendations in guidelines (strong and weak).
- The Institute of Medicine issued a document called *Clinical Practice Guidelines We Can Trust* that sets standards for developing trustworthy clinical practice guidelines (CPGs). It sets forth eight standards with several more specific standards under each main standard.
- The *PRISMA Statement* is a guide for the reporting of systematic reviews and meta-analyses but also can be used for critical appraisal of systematic reviews. It consists of a 27-item checklist and several flow diagrams.
- *CONSORT 2010* focuses on the reporting of a randomized clinical trial—how the trial was designed, analyzed, and interpreted. It consists of a 25-item checklist and a flow diagram.
- *SRQR, Standards for reporting qualitative research* is a 21-item list of standards developed by 5 authors.

These appraisal tools—and others—require considerable research knowledge to complete. Therefore, the appraisal guides used in this text were developed specifically for students who are encountering evidence-based practice appraisal for the first time. Many of the questions that make up the premier guides were incorporated into the guides you will be using.

Appraisal in General

The goal of critical appraisal of any type of research evidence is to systematically and thoughtfully judge whether the research evidence is:

- Credible
- Clinically significant
- Applicable

In each of the appraisal tools, there are questions specific to each area of appraisal that will help you reach a bottom-line judgment for each area and ultimately make a decision that the r/c/f should be used as an evidence source. The bottom-line questions are:

Are the r/c/f credible?	☐ Yes	☐ No	☐ Some
Are the r/c/f clinically important?	☐ Yes	☐ No	☐ Some
Are the r/c/f applicable to our setting?	☐ Yes	☐ No	☐ Some
Should we proceed to design a protocol based on the r/c/f?	☐ Yes all	☐ Yes some	☐ No

The following sections are a brief introduction to each appraisal domain. In Chapters 14, 15, and 16, each appraisal domain will be discussed as it pertains to the three forms of research evidence.

Synopsis

The starting point for appraisal of all forms of research evidence is identifying why the guideline/systematic review/study was done, how it was produced, and what was found. Here you are on familiar ground; this is what you learned earlier in Part I of this text. Actually, you could write a useful synopsis using *why, how,* and *what* as a template. However, in the appraisal guides provided, you are asked more specific questions about each type of research evidence.

Writing a synopsis not only ensures that you have understanding of the evidence, but it also provides a brief to refer back to later. Importantly, a synopsis contains just the facts—no judgments or interpretations. Research articles typically are very dense, meaning that every sentence contains important information—there is little fluff. Consequently, you may find that to complete the synopsis you have to refer to the article quite a few times to answer the synopsis questions.

Credibility

The central issue in appraising the credibility of the evidence is to make a judgment about whether the r/c/f is to be trusted. The reason research evidence should not be trusted is if it is biased in a critical way. Bias in the evidence-based practice context is any tendency that influences the evidence produced in a way that is not truly objective or that distorts the truthfulness of the evidence. The source of this tendency can be in the researcher's inclinations and thinking or in the methods used. Bias is usually not intentional, rather unconscious or unrecognized by the researcher. Bias can occur during the conduct of a study, while conducting a systematic review, or during the production of a clinical practice guideline.

Sometimes bias is determined by the information reported about how the study was done, but other times it may be suspected by what was not reported or addressed. For instance, in a study comparing a posthospital, home-based exercise program to usual care without special follow-up, the authors concluded that those who received the program had higher exercise levels at 12 weeks after discharge than those who received usual care. The report showed that the control group had almost twice the loss to follow-up of the treatment group. However, the researchers did not analyze if or how the profiles of the groups were changed by the dropouts. This lapse makes it impossible to determine if the uneven dropout rates introduced bias.

One can envision several possible ways in which the results might have been affected. To consider just one: if the dropouts in the control group were younger than the stay-ins, the average age of the control group would have been raised, which would have disrupted the original age equality of the two groups created by randomization. Thus, age could have entered as an influence on scores by making the treatment group scores look better than they would have been had all the original control group contributed outcome data. This is an example of a potential source of bias not being acknowledged by the authors and thereby bringing the credibility of the findings of this study into serious doubt.

Unrecognized bias during the conduct of a study can be passed along to a systematic review, and bias at the review stage can be incorporated into the production of guidelines. Thus, it is important that appraisal be performed for each form of evidence in the credibility chain.

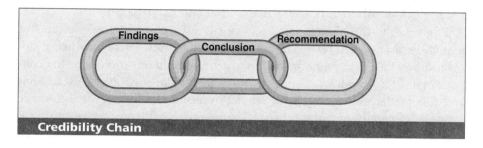

Questions to help you detect bias and to evaluate credibility chain issues are included in the appraisal guides you will be using.

Clinical Significance

In general terms, clinically significant findings are those that have enough impact or importance to make a difference in patients' health outcomes or life experiences should they be used as a basis for practice. Appraising clinical significance would lead you to ask questions such as the following:

- Is the average increase in patients' coping abilities found in the study sizeable enough to make practical differences in patients' everyday lives?
- Are the conclusions found in a systematic review about changes in women's attitudes regarding osteoporosis prevention after education about it likely to produce a change in their dietary, exercise, or smoking behaviors?
- Are the insights revealed by a systematic review with qualitative synthesis about the experience over several decades of living with a history of breast cancer after successful treatment informative enough to provide clinicians who see these women for follow-up with a fresh perspective on the care they give these women?

- Is the lower end of the 95% confidence interval around a difference in the means of an outcome variable enough of a difference that intervention A is likely to be more effective than intervention B in the population?
- Was panel producing the e-b clinical guideline made up of people with the necessary expertise?

In short, how robust is the evidence from a clinical perspective?

Regrettably, the clinical significance of research evidence is often not explicitly discussed in research reports and guidelines. There may be a clinical implications paragraph in the discussion section but too often this consists mainly of opinions about the ways the findings could be used. That is different than interpreting the results in terms of whether the difference found is clinically meaningful or, for qualitative evidence, an issue or social process uncovered is clinically informative. As a result, sometimes you will have to piece together your judgment about the clinical significance of recommendations, conclusions, and findings from what is reported in combination with your clinical knowledge. The fact that clinical significance is not always explicitly addressed is not a reason to gloss over it in appraisal—it is an important consideration.

Applicability

If an r/c/f is judged credible and clinically significant, you will then proceed to determine whether it is applicable to your setting, patients, and resources. If it is not credible and clinically significant, you need not proceed to appraising **applicability** because the r/c/f/ should not be used as a basis for practice. The applicability questions that should be asked will vary depending on the form of the evidence being translated into a care protocol and the nature of the change or changes being considered. Generally, the questions fall into four categories:

1. Fit of the evidence to the setting's patients
2. Safety
3. Expected benefit
4. Feasibility of incorporating the change

Fit of the Evidence   The fit question is, "Were the persons who made up the samples of the studies similar to those in our setting?" Making a judgment regarding this fit will require taking note of the profile of persons who participated in the studies and the characteristics of the settings in which the studies were conducted. Sometimes, a subgroup of patients studied will match the patients in your setting and you can pay particular attention to the evidence from that subgroup.

Safety and Expected Benefit   Safety and expected benefit are important considerations. Both safety and expected benefit must be thoughtfully considered prior to deciding to introduce a new care protocol or make a major change in practice. If a new approach to care is likely to produce meaningful benefits to patients and has few associated risks, the other hurdles can usually be overcome. The expected benefit and possible adverse events should actually be quantified. The quantification of the expected benefit is informed by what was found in the research studies. The agency then collects data to determine if its patients achieved the expected level of benefit.

Let's say a new care protocol for patient self-monitoring of blood glucose and administration of insulin is being introduced in a clinic. The goal is to have fewer patients whose blood glucose is not in optimal range. Based on findings from the research studies and on data indicating patients' current level of control, the expected benefit might be stated as, "We expect an absolute decrease of 5% in the percentage of patients whose hemoglobin HbA1c values are above 7." Such a specific target in combination with data about the percentage of patients not meeting the target would quantify the impact of e-b change in practice.

Feasibility   The ability of the setting to implement a clinical intervention in a way that is quite similar to the way it was delivered in the studies or guideline is another important consideration. If major changes have to be made because of limited resources or political forces, then the question could be raised as to whether the intervention being implemented will indeed be evidence based.

Feasibility also involves asking whether the change required could be implemented and maintained in the agency. Does it have the resources? Does it have the will? How much will it cost? The project team should consider whether their setting has the professional skills, support services, equipment, financial resources, and support of key persons to make the change and sustain it over time. A change that involves high cost or considerable effort on the part of direct care providers or support services faces an uphill road to successful implementation.

The applicability questions set forth in the guides are directed at making an organizational change in practice—that is, implementing a new approach to care. Making a change in individual practice would involve fewer issues; however, risk, resources needed, and people affected should still be considered.

The guides for individual studies do not include applicability questions. That is because changing clinical practice based on findings from any single study should always be undertaken with caution—particularly when the current approach to care is not causing major problems and is thought to be at least somewhat effective. The assumption is that before a change in practice is made, several studies will be considered and applicability will be appraised based on across-study conclusions, not on findings from just one original study. Analysis of findings across several studies is addressed in Chapter 16.

In summary, four domains (synopsis, credibility, clinical significance, and applicability) serve as a template for the appraisal criteria set forth in question form for the recommendations of clinical practice guidelines, for the conclusions of systematic reviews, and for the findings of original studies. The end point question of an appraisal is: Should we use the recommendation, conclusion, or finding to develop a unit, departmental, or agency clinical change in practice?

Practical Considerations

Even though appraisal of r/c/f is done using a set of objective criteria, appraisal inevitably involves a bit of judgment. Not infrequently, two appraisers using the same set of criteria will reach different judgments about the overall quality of a piece of evidence. The difference occurs for a variety of reasons, including the following:

- One appraiser may view a methodological weakness as minor whereas the other appraiser may view it as a critical flaw that undermines the credibility of the recommendations/conclusions/findings.
- One appraiser may consider bias or failure to control confounding influences in the way a study was done to be a major detractor from its credibility, but the other appraiser may view the same circumstances as inherent in the situation.
- One appraiser may conclude that the findings of several studies are similar, while the other appraiser may see an important difference in them.

For these reasons, appraisal of a body of research evidence is most often done by two or more appraisers so that consensus can be reached or arbitrated.

In a related issue, when appraising research evidence, you have to strike a balance between identifying critical flaws and being overly critical. There is no such thing as a perfect guideline/review/study. The goal is not to identify every weakness; rather, you want to detect methods that introduce the possibility of bias to the point that they put in doubt the credibility of the end products. Ultimately, this is a judgment. When researchers design guidelines, reviews, or studies, they often have to make trade-offs between the ideal and the possible or conduct their work with limited resources. Thus, you should reject only recommendations, conclusions, or findings that were produced in a seriously flawed way. Sometimes it is a fine line between being seriously flawed and of weak-but-acceptable quality. Appraisal guides can help you make that differentiation.

Importantly, these guides require a level of research knowledge appropriate to what a BSN nurse should possess. Therefore, you should be able to answer the questions in the appraisal guides with the knowledge you acquired in reading the first part of the book. Importantly, these appraisal guides will help you develop basic appraisal skills so that you can use more demanding appraisal guides in the future.

Appraisal guides specific to the three forms of research evidence are discussed in Chapters 14, 15, and 16; the guides themselves are in the appendices. The same template is used in all four guides (separate ones for qualitative and quantitative research), although the specific questions are different from one guide to another. The chapters are deceptively short because the real work of getting a handle on appraisal requires that you actually use the appraisal guides—and that will take considerable time. Just reading the chapters will not lead to true understanding of and skill in appraisal—you have to actually do several appraisals to begin to acquire appreciation for what is involved.

Already Appraised Evidence

Finally, in reading articles about evidence-based practice, you may see reference to "filtered evidence." Systematic reviews and evidence-based practice guideline are considered *filtered evidence* because, when well done, the studies and reviews incorporated in them have already been appraised for quality; the poor studies have been eliminated from analysis. However, the systematic review (SR) or evidence-based clinical practice guideline (EbCPG) itself should also be appraised to be sure that bias did not enter during its production. Do note that in the production of an EbCPG, if the studies in an SR were appraised for quality, they do not need to be appraised again.

Resources that summarize SRs and EbCPGs along with an appraisal of their strengths and weaknesses are increasingly becoming available. One such source is the journal *Evidence-Based Nursing*; high-quality reviews and original study articles are summarized in brief commentaries that address methods, findings, and clinical application of the findings. This type of resource will be discussed at length in Chapter 19 as it is particularly useful at the point of care.

RESOURCES

AGREE II. Retrieved from http://www.agreetrust.org/agree-ii/

CONSORT. Retrieved from http://www.consort-statement.org/

GRADE. Retrieved from http://www.gradeworkinggroup.org/FAQ/index.htm

Institute of Medicine. (2011). *Clinical practice guidelines we can trust*. Retrieved from http://iom.nationalacademies.org/Reports/2011/Clinical-Practice-Guidelines-We-Can-Trust.aspx

PRISMA. Retrieved from http://www.prisma-statement.org/

SRQR Standards for reporting qualitative research. (2014). Retrieved from http://www.mmcri.org/deptPages/core/downloads/QRIG/Standards_for_Reporting_Qualitative_Research___A_990451.pdf

CHAPTER FOURTEEN

Appraising Recommendations of Clinical Practice Guidelines

Appraise →

Even when a guideline carries a title indicating it is evidence based, a measure of skepticism is needed, because bias may have entered somewhere along the credibility chain and been ransmitted forward, or it may have entered into the production of the guideline itself. Several international organizations have set forth criteria for appraising the credibility of clinical practice guidelines: Australian Government National Health and Medical Research Council, 2011; Guidelines International Network, n.d.; GRADE Working Group, 2016; Institute of Medicine, 2011; Scottish Intercollegiate Guidelines Network (SIGN), 2014. Generally, the appraisal standards of these organizations require a somewhat advanced level of research knowledge and are quite detailed and lengthy. The appraisal guide provided in Appendix A includes the most important elements from these more in-depth guides and uses language appropriate to nurses with a basic Nursing degree.

The questions in the appraisal guide found in Appendix A will help you detect both transmitted and production sources of bias in guidelines as well as get a sense of how much clinical benefit might be expected and whether use of the guideline would be feasible in a particular setting. The guide is formatted using four domains: Synopsis, Credibility, Clinical Significance, and Applicability. In each domain, especially important questions are indicated by an asterisk (*), and depending on the guideline topic, you may have to enter *NA* for *Not Applicable* for some answers.

Synopsis

The first step in the appraisal of a clinical practice guideline is to get a grasp of the following:

■ The purpose of the guideline (health condition, intervention, population, and outcomes it addresses)
■ The production process that was used
■ Recommendations that were made
■ System used to grade the recommendations

At this point, I suggest you look at the synopsis questions in the *Appraisal Guide: Recommendations of a Clinical Practice Guideline* (Appendix A). You will see that the questions in the appraisal guide ask you to extract the information just listed.

Credibility

The major credibility issue is bias leading to recommendations that are not truly based on sound evidence and when implemented will not be likely to benefit patients. Sources of bias in the production of EbCPGs can take the following forms:

■ Search for relevant evidence was not systematic and comprehensive
■ Use of systematic reviews that did not eliminate studies of poor quality
■ Not recognizing differences in evidence for different populations and subpopulations
■ Not recognizing important differences in the interventions studied
■ Downplaying or not taking into account undesirable outcomes
■ Flawed judgments regarding the evidence for each recommendation

In broad terms, appraising the credibility of a guideline involves examining the following aspects of the guideline:

■ Whether the organization and persons that produced the guideline had the expertise to do so

- Whether the process used to produce the and free of bias
- Whether the recommendations are true to the evi
- The confidence the developers have in the recommen

Production Process

Ideally, the production process should be described in some detail (
2011); this allows potential adopters to determine if the guideline was pr
duced in accord with recognized standards. Do remember, however, that
the production standards may not be in the written document. Unfortunately, some guidelines make available no or very little information about
the production process. Omission of or sketchy information about the development process makes appraising the credibility of a guideline almost
impossible.

The *credibility* questions in the appraisal guide ask you to make judgments about the production process: the clarity of purpose, the search for
evidence, the sequence of steps, the quality of the systematic reviews used,
the link between evidence and recommendations, and whether the guideline is up to date. Perhaps the most frequently omitted steps by developers
are: (1) appraisal of the systematic reviews used to formulate the recommendations; and (2) a description or grading of the body of evidence in
support of each recommendation.

Recommendations Are True to the Evidence

The supporting evidence sources should be available either in the guideline
itself or in an accompanying document. Ideally, a table detailing each evidence source and a description of the body of the evidence in support of
each recommendation are the best ways of conveying the nature, strength,
and consistency of the evidence in support of a recommendation. Often
separate evidence tables are constructed for different issues; for example,
evidence pertaining to one type of intervention is in one table and evidence
pertaining to another intervention is in another table.

Based on the credentials of the developing organization, you can either
trust the rating of the evidence or you can look into the evidence tables
and description of supporting evidence to determine whether you agree
with their translation and rating. I obviously favor a bit of examination of
the linkage between the evidence and each recommendation. Most often I

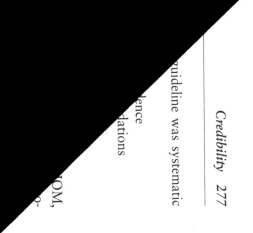

· go back to the original research

·ost guidelines rate the confidence
systems used are quite variable in
·ating levels. Often the confidence
·tion to rating the quality and/or
·lation rating systems combine the
·ing system along with other con-

> **FEATURES INDICATING SOUNDLY DEVELOPED RECOMMENDATIONS**
>
> - Clear guideline purposes
> - Production process that included all widely recognized steps
> - For each recommendation: A clear linkage between the evidence and the recommendation
> - Provision of the relevant sources of evidence and a discussion of the body of evidence
> - Grading of the confidence the panel has in each recommendation

Current Status If a guideline was produced 4 or more years ago, it would be advisable to search for more recent research evidence that might update the recommendations of the guideline. Many guideline developers require updates every 2–3 years (Vernooij, Sanabria, Sola, Alonso-Coello, & Garcia, 2014). Research on some clinical topics (such as management of the blood sugar levels of diabetics) is being done at a fairly fast rate; thus, a guideline or review done even 2 years earlier could be out of date. In contrast, other clinical topics receive much less research attention so that a guideline is stable for quite a few years.

Do look at the credibility questions in the appraisal guide.

Clinical Significance

Evaluating the clinical significance of guideline recommendations requires consideration of the following:

- Identification of essential elements of recommended action
- Magnitude of benefit associated with each recommendation
- Likelihood of benefit/outcome being realized
- Side effects and risks associated with the recommendation
- Acceptability and feasibility of the recommendation to patients
- Practicality of the recommendation in real world practice

Consideration of these issues determines whether the recommendation would be feasible to implement and make a difference in patients' state of wellness or well-being.

To truly have clinical impact, the set of recommendations that make up the guideline should address all the issues that are important to patients as well as all the important decisions care providers make while delivering care. Some guideline developers pilot test their guidelines prior to releasing them. If this is done, it addresses the clinical significance issue by providing future users with information about how patients and providers view the value and practicality of the recommendations and whether following the guidelines are likely to result in the presumed outcome.

Applicability

Assuming that the recommendations are credible and that the producers have reasonable level of confidence in the recommendations, the final appraisal task is to make a judgment regarding the fit between the recommendations and the setting in which you intend to implement them. As a student, if you are familiar with a caregiving setting, you should try to envision what would be involved in making the changes in practice that a new care protocol requires. The applicability questions will help you think through some of those requirements. At the very least, you should consider the applicability questions and appreciate what is involved in making an organizational change in care practice. The issue of implementation of a research-based change in practice receives more attention in Chapter 17.

A guideline can be soundly produced and make credible and clinically significant recommendations, but it may not be feasible for the setting in which a protocol project team intends to use it. Perhaps the population of patients or providers in the setting is not similar to those for whom the guideline was intended. Perhaps implementation of the protocol would require expenditure for training that is beyond what the setting can afford. Thus, one possible bottom line judgment resulting from appraisal of a guideline may be, "The guideline's recommendations are credible and clinically significant but are not applicable to our setting." Alternatively, some recommendations may be applicable but others may not be.

Appraisal Guide Format

The questions in the appraisal guide are stated so that a *Yes* answer indicates compliance with an appraisal criterion. Thus, a column of *Yes* answers in a domain indicates adequate quality and will undoubtedly lead you to a positive, bottom-line, decision for that appraisal domain. In contrast, a mix of *Yes* and *No* answers will cause you to debate the bottom-line decision for that domain. The four bottom-line decisions are in BOLD UPPERCASE font. Three pertain to decisions about quality in the domain, and the fourth asks for an overall decision about implementing the guideline's recommendations: **"SHOULD WE PROCEED TO DESIGN A PROTOCOL BASED ON THE RECOMMENDATIONS? YES ALL/ YES SOME/ NO".**

Generally, guideline recommendations are implemented as a whole, but this need not be the case. So, even though the questions ask about the guideline as a whole, there may be times when you should appraise the individual recommendations separately. The most common situation in which you would do this is when the strength of evidence or confidence rating is strong for one recommendation but is weak for another.

Your Turn

Now then, it's time to reread the clinical guideline about vitamins, *Vitamin, Mineral, and Multivitamin Supplements for the Primary Prevention of Cardiovascular Disease and Cancer: U.S. Preventive Services Task Force Recommendation Statement* (reprinted in Chapter 10), and complete an appraisal of its recommendations using the questions in the appraisal guide (it can be completed on paper or interactively on the text's companion website). Although most questions on the appraisal guide ask for a yes/no answer, for most purposes and particularly for student learning, a one- to three-sentence rationale for the yes/no answer should also be given. For the applicability questions, assume that you work in a multi-provider primary care practice and that you do intake interviews and meet briefly with returning patients before they see their primary care provider. The practice also runs a healthy aging workshop 4 times a year.

To get various perspectives, you might want to do the appraisal with one or several classmates. Afterwards, look at how a colleague and I appraised the guideline (Appendix B) and compare our judgments to yours.

REFERENCES

Australian Government National Health and Medical Research Council. (2011). Retrieved from http://www.nhmrc.gov.au/guidelines-publications/cp133-and-cp133a

GRADE Working Group. (2016). Criteria for applying or using GRADE. Retrieved from http://www.gradeworkinggroup.org/publications/Criteria_for_using_GRADE_2016-04-05.pdf

Guidelines International Network, Qaseem, A., Forland, F., Macbeth, F., Ollenschlager, G., Phillips, S., & van der Wees, P. (2012). Guidelines International Network: Toward International Standards for Clinical Practice Guidelines. *Annals of Internal Medicine, 156*(7), 525–531 Retrieved from http://annals.org/article.aspx?articleid=1103747

Institute of Medicine (IOM). (2011). *Clinical practice guidelines we can trust.* Retrieved from http://www.nationalacademies.org/hmd/

Vernooij, R. W. M, Sanabria, A. J., Sola, I., Alonso-Coello, P., & Garcia, L. M. (2014). Guidance for updating clinical practice guidelines: A systematic review of methodological handbooks. *Implementation Science, 9*, 3. Retrieved from http://www.implementationscience.com/content/9/1/3

CHAPTER FIFTEEN

Appraising Conclusions of Systematic Reviews with Narrative Synthesis

> Appraise

S ystematic reviews are important resources when designing evidence-based care innovations. The comprehensive synthesis they provide is essential to a complete understanding of clinical topics. However, research evidence in the form of the conclusions of systematic reviews, like the recommendations of clinical practice guidelines, must be critically appraised before using them as the basis for nursing care protocols or even for the care of an individual patient. Systematic review (SR) conclusions are a bit easier to appraise than are guideline recommendations because the translation of evidence into recommendations is not an issue. Still, there is much to consider because the move from individual findings to across-studies conclusions is susceptible to bias.

The appraisal framework discussed in this chapter uses the format introduced in Chapter 13: synopsis, credibility, clinical significance, applicability. The questions in the appraisal guide provided are specific to systematic reviews with narrative synthesis (SRwNS), the most common type of SRs seen in clinical nursing journals. The SRwNS from Chapter 9 about reducing hospital admissions from nursing homes is used to demonstrate appraisal of an SRwNS.

Several premier organizations have spelled out standards for conducting SRs (Cochrane Collaboration, 2010; Institute of Medicine, 2011; Joanna

Briggs Institute, 2014) and reporting SRs (PRISMA, 2015). The set of appraisal questions for SRwNSs presented in this chapter (see Appendix C) is representative of, albeit more basic than, the criteria of the premier producers and policy setters.

Synopsis

I have already made a case for completing a synopsis of the various forms of research evidence, so now I will just suggest looking at the synopsis questions specific to SRwNSs in the appraisal guide.

Credibility

SRwNS synthesis is prone to bias because it is all too easy for the reviewers to introduce their own predilections and beliefs into the review and synthesis process (Oxman & Guyatt, 1988). For this reason, the standards for SRwNSs include the requirements that the reviewers (1) set out the evidence from the individual studies, and (2) be explicit about how important steps in the review were done (IOM, 2011; Steinberg & Luce, 2005). This requires that SRwNS reports include the following elements:

- A clear objectives statement
- A description of how the search for relevant study reports was performed
- A description of the criteria for including or excluding studies
- A description of how the quality of individual studies was appraised and considered in the analysis
- A flow diagram giving number of studies, screened, assessed for eligibility, and included in the review with reasons for exclusions (PRISMA, 2009)
- Tables or narrative that describes the population, methods, and findings of the individual studies
- For each conclusion, a clear summary of the evidence that led to it, including the quality of studies, the quantity of studies, and the consistency of findings across the supporting studies (AHRQ, 2002; IOM, 2011)

When the research reviewers include these elements in their report, the reader is provided with information that can be used to decide if the conclusions are indeed derived from the across-studies synthesis of individual studies and are unbiased. If the reviewers do not provide this information, the reader is in the position of having to trust the reviewers' interpretation of the evidence, which is not in keeping with the explicit nature of scientific decision making.

The reviewers should be careful not to reach conclusions that are beyond what the evidence shows. This would be the case if the conclusions were applied to elders generally, but the studies had been done mainly with elders living in assisted living residences. Another example of going beyond the findings would be overstating the importance of the findings from several weak studies.

Importantly, when the evidence is inconclusive—that is, inconsistent across studies or from weak studies—the reviewers should not conclude that there is no effect, no difference, or no association. Rather, the conclusion should be that definitive evidence for or against an effect or association is lacking. A conclusion of *no effect* or *no association* assumes a clear finding of no effect based on consistent evidence, whereas a conclusion of *inconclusive evidence* or *insufficient evidence* recognizes that the evidence does not provide a clear and consistent answer regarding effect or association—two very different conclusions.

Recommendation	Evidence
Recommend	Sufficient, acceptable quality, and consistent
Recommend against	Sufficient, acceptable quality, and consistent
No Recommendation	Insufficient, low quality, and/or inconsistent

Clear connectivity between findings of the individual studies and the conclusions is established when the reviewers demonstrate a deep analysis of the data. The reviewers should convince you that they looked for patterns and similarities in findings and reasons for the differences. Reasons for different findings from one study to others would include differences in the samples studied, the form of an intervention, the outcomes studied, how the variables were measured, different measurement intervals, or length of follow-up. In short, conclusions based on a deep analysis give you, the consumer of the conclusions, confidence in their credibility.

Clinical Significance

To be clinically significant, the conclusions of a review should reflect issues that are important in everyday practice and that if incorporated into practice would make a difference in patient safety, comfort, or health outcomes. For reviews of interventions, this would include a conclusion that the treatment effect is large enough to be of benefit given costs and any burden to patients or staffs. This judgment is easier to make when measures of treatment effect such as absolute benefit improvement (ABI), numbers needed to treat (NNT) findings, and economic analysis are provided. Clinical significance is more difficult to appraise in SRwNSs of issues other than intervention effectiveness, although the consistency of the findings across the studies, the strength of the relationship between variables across the studies, and the informativeness of the conclusions can be considered.

Applicability

The judgment regarding whether the conclusions of a review are applicable to a particular setting is determined in part by the setting and patients that were included in the original studies reviewed. If they are similar, or the reporting is such that you can identify a subset of studies that were conducted in a setting similar to yours, then the results of that subset would be applicable to your setting. For instance, an emergency department in a rural hospital would have to consider whether the conclusions of a review about triage systems is applicable to its setting if all the studies included in the review were from inner-city or suburban emergency departments. The issues for the rural emergency department are very different—for instance, no option to close to admissions and divert ambulances elsewhere, and fewer clinical services available 24/7. Beyond the settings and patients studied, the feasibility of implementing, resources required, and costs of implementing should also be taken into account.

Your Turn

I suggest that you reread the Graverholt and colleagues' 2014 SRwNS about reducing hospital admissions from nursing homes that is reprinted in Chapter 9. For the purpose of answering the applicability questions, assume you are on a project team in a long-term care facility that is examining strategies for reducing hospital admissions. Then complete an appraisal of it using the *Appraisal Guide: Conclusions of a Systematic Review with Narrative Synthesis* (Appendix C or interactively on the text's website). Afterwards, look at the completed appraisal in Appendix D. You could further practice appraisal of SRwNSs by appraising one of the systematic reviews listed on the text's website. I suggest that readers new to appraisal not attempt appraisal of an SR with statistical analysis at this point.

REFERENCES

Agency for Healthcare Research and Quality (AHRQ). (2002). *Systems to rate the strength of scientific evidence: Summary*. Retrieved from http://www.ncbi.nlm.nih.gov/bookshelf/br.fcgi?book=erta47

Cochrane Collaboration. (2010). *For authors and MEs. Review production resources for Cochrane Review authors and managing editors*. Retrieved from http://www.cochrane.org/training/authors-mes

Graverholt, B., Forsetlund, L., & Jamtvedt, G. (2014). Reducing hospital admission from nursing home: A systematic review. *BMC Health Services Research, 14*, 36. Retrieved from http://www.biomedcentral.com/1472-6963/14/36. doi:10.1186/1472-6963-14-36

Institute of Medicine (IOM). (2011). *Finding what works in health care: Standards for systematic reviews*. Washington, DC: National Academy of Science.

Joanna Briggs Institute. (2014). *2014 JBI reviewers manual*. Retrieved from http://joannabriggs.org/assets/docs/sumari/reviewersmanual-2014.pdf

Oxman, A. D., & Guyatt, G. H. (1988). Guidelines for reading literature reviews. *Canadian Medical Association Journal, 138*, 697–703.

PRISMA. (2009). PRISMA Flow Diagram. Retrieved from http://prisma-statement.org/PRISMAStatement/FlowDiagram.aspx

PRISMA. (2015). *PRISMA Statement*. Retrieved from http://www.prisma-statement.org/PRISMAStatement/Default.aspx

Steinberg, E. P., & Luce, B. R. (2005). Evidence based? Caveat emptor. *Health Affairs, 24*(1), 80–92.

CHAPTER SIXTEEN

Appraising Findings of Original Studies

>Appraise>

I f your project group cannot find a sound and recent research-based clinical practice guideline or systematic review, you may decide to locate and appraise the findings of individual studies—first one study at a time and then as a group of findings from several studies (assuming more than one study was located). A finding of a single research study is like one block or stone in a wall—it is one piece contributing to knowledge about a topic. At some point there may be findings from only one or two studies about an issue, but gradually more studies are done and the knowledge about the topic becomes a more complete structure. Therefore, this chapter starts with a description of how to appraise the findings of individual studies and ends with a description of how to appraise findings across a group of studies.

Is This a Qualitative or Quantitative Study?

The differentiation between qualitative studies and quantitative studies requires that you be able to determine which type of study you are appraising. Often, the research report will inform you, but you should be able to make the determination on your own. Most often, determining if you are reading a qualitative study report or a quantitative one is quite straightforward. However, if you are not sure, the list in **Box 16-1** should help you decide what kind of study you are reading. Two appraisal guides are offered for the findings of individual studies: one for qualitative studies (Appendix E) and one for quantitative studies (Appendix F).

> ## BOX 16-1   Deciding What Type of Research Article You Are Reading
>
> **Is the study qualitative or quantitative, or was a mixed approach used?**
>
> - If the data consists of words, quotes, verbal descriptions, and/or themes, the study is a qualitative study.
> - If the data consists of scores, scales, numerical data, percentages, graphs, and/or statistics, the study is a quantitative study.
> - If both qualitative and quantitative data was presented, the study has a mixed design.

After you have determined the type of study you are reading, you will know which appraisal guide to use. If the study used a mixed design—a combination of qualitative and quantitative data collection methods, you should use a combination of both guides.

Broad Credibility Issues

Appropriateness of Design

The credibility of findings of both qualitative and quantitative studies depends on the researcher having used study methods that were appropriate to answer the research questions. So far, you have read about five different research designs but were not asked to challenge whether the researcher used the right design. Short of obtaining a doctoral degree, you may not be able to do this with 100% accuracy; however, there are a few things you should know. The study design used is determined by the question being asked—for some questions there is not a best design, but rather several that would be good although providing a slightly different perspective on the question.

If the question has to do with understanding the decision-making process used by parents of a child with moderate mental retardation when deciding whether to keep the child at home or place the child in residential care, a study using qualitative methods would get at the complexities of this very personal decision process and how that thinking evolves over time.

A related but different question, "What are the characteristics of families that keep a child with moderate mental retardation at home over at least a 5-year period?" could be studied using research methodology that quantifies characteristics such as number and ages of other children, ages of the parents, size of the extended family, social support, income, educational level, community services available, and housing situation. Such a study could produce a descriptive, quantitative profile of families who keep children with severe retardation at home.

If, instead of just quantifying family and community variables, the researcher also wanted to look for relationships among the variables, a correlation design could be used. This would be the case if the researcher looked for relationships between quantifiable family characteristics and the coping level of families who kept children with severe mental retardation at home. A more complex correlational design would examine a group of family and community variables to determine which ones are the best predictors of successfully keeping a child at home.

If the question was, "Does a day care service for children with mental retardation result in fewer children being placed in residential care than if families are paid to take care of their child 24 hours a day, 7 days a week with periodic paid respite?" A qualitative study, a descriptive study, or a correlational study would not get at the effectiveness of one intervention vis-à-vis the others. An experimental study would be best. Having said that, random assignment may not be possible, and a quasi-experimental design may have to be used.

Peer Review

You will note that the first question under credibility of both appraisal guides asks whether the research report was published in a journal requiring that all published articles be reviewed by peers. In asking this, the assumption is that research reports published in peer-reviewed journals are of higher quality than those published in journals that do not require review by peers prior to acceptance. In general, this is a good assumption because peer review assures the nonresearcher reader that the report has been reviewed by two or three knowledgeable persons in the field and was deemed worthy of publication.

Unfortunately, it is not always easy to determine if a journal requires peer review. Look for a statement regarding peer review on the journal's website or in the front material of an issue of the journal. In general, the absence of a statement on the website indicating that articles are peer reviewed should raise the possibility that they are not, which should cause you to be particularly careful in your appraisal of the study's credibility.

Appraisal of the Findings of a Qualitative Study

Credibility

When considering the credibility of the findings of a qualitative study, the main consideration is the rigor of the study's methods. Yet, criteria for rigor of qualitative studies are numerous, diverse, and not widely agreed upon (Dixon-Woods, Shaw, Agarwal, & Smith, 2004; Mackey, 2007). Given the many criteria of rigor, several frequently mentioned ones were incorporated into the qualitative appraisal guide in this chapter and in Appendix E. In general, the findings and interpretations of qualitative studies are considered credible if:

- The sampling of participants and observations served the purposes of the study (Fossey, Harvey, McDermott, & Davidson, 2002).
- Observation and/or interviewing were adequately prolonged and persistent (Lincoln & Guba, 1985).
- There was interaction between data collection and data analysis (Morse, Barrett, Mayan, Olson, & Spiers, 2002).
- The findings were rooted in the data (Dixon-Woods et al., 2004).

The findings of qualitative studies tend to be cohesive; that is, they hang together as a group rather than stand separately as findings of quantitative studies often do. Therefore, the findings of qualitative studies can be appraised as a group, although sometimes you might want to consider them separately.

Clinical Significance

Kearney (2001) made a strong case for evaluating the usefulness of findings from qualitative findings based on their richness and informativeness. Richness pertains to the demonstrated linking of findings into a web of connections and the creation of a truly new perspective on the phenomenon under study (Kearney, 2001, p. 146). Thus, the findings are informative to clinicians because they go beyond previous ways of thinking about the situation or experience. Vivid portrayal of the experience or situation and description of how context or events produce variations to the experience add to the usefulness of the findings to the clinician. As you read more qualitative studies you will see that some studies penetrate the experience or situation and produce new insights, whereas others fail to get much beyond what most clinicians in the field of practice already know. In brief, the clinical significance of qualitative findings pertains to their usefulness to clinicians. I suggest that now you look at the appraisal guide for findings of qualitative studies (Appendix E) and note how the issues just discussed were incorporated into the guide.

Applicability

As explained earlier, appraisal questions are not offered for applicability because generally an organization should not base care on the results of one study. However, the results of a single qualitative study may make a nurse more sensitive to patient experiences and preferences and may be used to fine tune her interpersonal approaches to assessment, patient teaching, and anticipatory guidance (Kearney, 2001; Zuzelo, 2007). The usefulness of the findings from single qualitative studies is derived from the fact that most qualitative researchers provide considerable detail about the study participants' thoughts and feelings, their experiences, and the contexts of their lives. Thus, it is often quite clear with whom or in what kind of situation the findings might add insight to care.

Appraisal of the Findings of a Quantitative Study

Credibility

In quantitative studies, the end products of the study typically are several, related findings, which are the researchers' data-based conclusions. Like all human conclusions, they can be right or wrong. In correlational and experimental studies, there are two possible correct conclusions and two possible erroneous conclusions.

The correct conclusions are the following:

1. Concluding that a relationship or difference exists in the population when in reality it actually does exist.
2. Concluding that no relationship or difference exists in the population when in reality it does not exist.

The two types of conclusion errors are the following:

1. Concluding that a relationship or difference exists in the population when in reality it does not exist (type 1 conclusion error).
2. Concluding that no relationship or difference exists in the population when in reality it does exist (type 2 conclusion error).

For a graphic of these possibilities, see Table 16-1.

TABLE 16-1   Reaching Correct Conclusion

		Does a real difference exist?	
		Yes	No
Researcher's conclusion	Real difference	Correct	Type 1 error
	No difference	Type 2 error	Correct

Avoiding Conclusion Error   The researcher is obviously aiming for correct conclusions and trying to avoid making conclusion errors. The ways in which she does this are as follows:

- Eliminate chance variation as an explanation.
- Avoid low statistical power.
- Control extraneous variables.
- Control bias.

Chance variation, which is always present to some degree when data is collected, can affect the statistical results of a study and lead to wrong conclusions. The researcher controls the role of chance variation by defining its limits. This is what is done when the researcher sets the maximal acceptable decision point p-level for significance at 0.05 or 0.01. In so doing, she is in essence saying, "I will accept only a low probability that my conclusion of a significant difference is due to chance variation." This in effect reduces the likelihood of a type 1 conclusion error.

Studies with small sample sizes can have statistical results indicating no relationship or effect when in fact the problem is that the sample size was not large enough (type 2 conclusion error). A too-small sample size results in insufficient statistical power to detect a significant difference; that is, the microscope was too weak. The problem is that there was insufficient data to allow the statistical analysis to detect a relationship or a difference amid the chance variation that is inevitably present. Using power analysis to determine sample size protects against type 2 conclusion errors. Remember power analysis from Chapter 7?

Other aspects of the study also determine whether a conclusion is right or wrong. As you learned earlier, researchers use inclusion/exclusion criteria, random assignment, adherence to study protocols, and awareness of what is going on in the research setting to eliminate or isolate the influence of the extraneous variables. However, it may not be possible to control all extraneous variables, or the researcher may not have thought to control a particular influence. Some extraneous variables enter a study without the researcher's awareness in the form of an event or change in the research setting, whereas still others are introduced by the research activities themselves.

Uncontrolled extraneous variables distort study results by mixing with the study variables and producing a statistical result that is an illusion. For example, a statistical result of a study may indicate that there is a significant difference in the outcomes of two treatment groups so the researcher would conclude that the experimental treatment was more effective than the control treatment. However, if the control group had considerably more persons with multiple comorbidities, that might be what caused the difference in outcomes, not the difference in treatments they received. The higher number of comorbidities in the one group was an extraneous variable that caused the difference in outcomes and led the researcher to make a type 1 conclusion error. Statistical analysis just works the numbers and does not shed any light on what caused the difference. Study design is what controls, eliminates, or identifies possible extraneous variables.

Extraneous variables can produce an illusion of a difference in effectiveness as in the example just given or an illusion of no difference in effectiveness when indeed there would have been one had the extraneous variable not been at work (i.e., type 2 conclusion error). In short, when evaluating the credibility of findings, you want to ask, "Was there anything else that could have produced the results obtained other than what the researcher concluded?" Said differently: "Is there any alternative explanation for the difference found or not found?"

Bias, which can enter a study at various points in the form of preconceived ideas about what the results will be or unconscious preference for one treatment over another, is also a potential source of erroneous conclusions. In quantitative studies, bias is controlled by research methods such as random sampling, random assignment, checks on adherence to research protocols, blinding of study observers and/or staff, and use of placebo treatments. Generally, researchers will not speak to bias in their reports; rather, you as the reader have to be alert to the possibility of it and decide whether adequate means were taken to prevent bias from affecting study results, findings, and conclusions.

Credible Versus Valid   The appraisal questions in the guide should assist you in identifying possible sources of wrong conclusions. When the researcher's conclusions are trusted as the best explanation for the results, not chance, extraneous variables, low statistical power, or bias, the findings are deemed credible (Stoddard & Ring, 1993). Although throughout this book the term *credible* has been used to convey that the researcher's conclusions are likely to be trustworthy, other appraisal guides ask, "Are the findings valid?" When used to characterize findings from a study, *valid* means that the findings are judged to be trustworthy reflections of reality and not the result of how the study was conducted or the result of an extraneous variable at work. Note that this usage of the word *valid* is a bit different from the way in which it was used to characterize measurement instruments. The term *valid* is more technical and more complex than the word *credible*. However, the word *credible* has more commonsense resonance and is an adequate substitute. I suggest that now you look at the credibility questions of the *Appraisal Guide: Findings of a Quantitative Study* (Appendix F) to see how the issues you just read about are incorporated into appraisal.

Clinical Significance

The clinical significance of the findings of a quantitative study is determined by the strength of the relationship between variables in correlational studies or the size of the difference in the outcomes of the two treatment groups in experimental or quasi-experimental studies. In a correlational study, one would consider the size of the r^2s, whereas in a study comparing interventions, one would consider (1) the difference in the means of the two groups, (2) the absolute benefit increase (ABI), (3) the numbers needed to treat (NNT), or (4) the relative risk (RR). Therefore, in intervention studies, the clinical significance question is: Is the treatment effect found in the study large enough to make a clinical difference in patient outcomes or well-being?

Applicability

Having stated the general principle that findings from a single study should not be used as the basis for a change in practice, an exception would be when a diligent search did not come up with another study and the basis for current practice is clearly not effective. Of course, the study should have been soundly conducted and the setting and sample should be similar to the patient group with whom the findings will be used. In the rare case when the findings of a single study will be used as the basis for practice, the applicability questions from the systematic review appraisal guide can be used.

Your Turn

At this point, I suggest you appraise the 2015 quantitative study by Canbulat, Ayhan, and Inal, reprinted in Chapter 7, using the appraisal guide for quantitative studies (Appendix F). Then read the appraisal of it that a colleague and I did, which is shown in Appendix G.

You should also consider completing an appraisal of the O'Lynn and Krautscheld (2011) qualitative study in Chapter 4 or one of the qualitative studies listed at the text's website to get some practice appraising qualitative studies. The more appraisals you do, the better you will get at using the questions to make a judgment regarding the credibility and clinical significance of study findings.

Across-Studies Analysis

Now that you have some skill in appraising individual studies, you need to at least be aware of what is involved in appraising several studies regarding a question or issue. This would have to be done when an agency team could not locate an evidence-based clinical practice guideline or systematic review, but did find several relevant studies. In addition to appraising each study separately, the several studies should be appraised as a body of studies; doing so is called across-studies analysis (Brown, 1999). In essence, the team has to do its own systematic review before translating the evidence into an agency protocol (Stetler et al., 1998). This will require identifying, retrieving, and appraising studies, then bringing together the findings from all relevant and sound studies.

Doing an across-studies review and summary is not something an individual should do. It is an advanced skill and is best done by a group in which the individual members' interpretations and thinking regarding the findings of the various studies can complement and correct one another. Generally, project teams who do across-studies analysis have a few members with master's or doctoral education. You may, however, be asked to be a member of an evidence-based practice (EBP) project team, in which case you will learn by direct observation how across-studies analysis is done. To prepare you for that, I offer a brief description of what across-studies analysis involves.

The goal in looking at a body of evidence is to answer the question, "What findings earn our confidence because they are well supported by one or more sound studies?" To answer this question, the protocol development team must determine the following:

- How many studies addressed the issue?
- Were the studies of good quality?
- Was the finding consistently produced by several well-conducted studies?
- If an intervention was studied, was the size of the treatment effect or the relationship of similar magnitude across the studies?
- Can inconsistencies regarding a finding be explained by study differences in patient populations or research methods?

Thus, the essential across-studies issues are the quality, quantity, and consistency of evidence across studies. If the project team is appraising two or more studies, they should work with a findings table (see **Table 16-2**). If the clinical issue has several subissues, such as prevention and management, the team might use separate findings tables for each subissue. And as mentioned earlier, the team may decide to weight studies with strong methodology or samples similar to their own population of patients more heavily than studies with weak methodology or samples that are very different.

Unlike the findings of single studies, for which the general recommendation was made that they not be used as the basis for clinical protocols, whenever clear conclusions are produced by across-studies analysis, the conclusions can be used as the basis for practice. The applicability questions in the SR appraisal guide will assist in planning implementation of across-studies conclusions.

Appraisal of findings from several or many studies involves decisions about the credibility, clinical significance, and applicability of the body of evidence. Ideally, these decisions should be reached in a deliberative way by the consensus of the EBP project team (Lomas, Culyer, McCutcheon, McAuley, & Law, 2005). A deliberative process requires the following:

- Clear objectives.
- Careful extraction of information from reports by at least two persons.
- Clear criteria for appraising the evidence.
- Clear rules regarding how to handle studies of poor quality.

TABLE 16-2   Findings Table

Author(s) and date	Questions, variables, objectives, hypotheses	Design, sample, setting	Findings	Notes

Topic _____   Date _____

- Good analytical thinking.
- Broad participatory dialogue.
- Formal polling to resolve differences of opinion.
- Skillful chairing.

Appendix H is a completed, partial findings table pertaining to fatigue in patients with congestive heart failure. Be advised that this findings table is not inclusive of all studies on this topic; rather illustrates the format typical of how a findings table on this topic might look.

Wrap-Up

Evaluating a body of finding from individual studies is definitely the long and labor intensive way of establishing the state of the science regarding an issue. However, sometimes a project group will have to do it; when necessary, it is important that the group include a person with knowledge of research methodology—be it an in-house person or a consultant.

REFERENCES

Brown, S. J. (1999). *Knowledge for health care practice: A guide to using research evidence*. Philadelphia, PA: Saunders.

Dixon-Woods, M., Shaw, R. I., Agarwal, S., & Smith, J. A. (2004). The problem of appraising qualitative research. *Quality & Safety in Health Care, 13,* 223–225.

Fossey, E., Harvey, C., McDermott, F., & Davidson, L. (2002). Understanding and evaluating qualitative research. *Australian and New Zealand Journal of Psychiatry, 36,* 717–732.

Kearney, M. H. (2001). Levels and application of qualitative research evidence. *Research in Nursing and Health, 24,* 145–153.

Lincoln, Y. S., & Guba, E. G. (1985). *Naturalistic inquiry*. Beverly Hills, CA: Sage.

Lomas, J., Culyer, T., McCutcheon, C., McAuley, L., & Law, S. (2005). *Conceptualizing and combining evidence for health system guidance*. Ottawa, Ontario, Canada: Canadian Health Services Research Foundation. Retrieved from http://www.chsrf.ca/migrated/pdf/insightAction/evidence_e.pdf

Mackey, M. C. (2007). Evaluation of qualitative research. In P. L. Munhall (Ed.), *Nursing research: A qualitative perspective* (4th ed., pp. 555–568). Sudbury, MA: Jones and Bartlett.

Morse, J. M., Barrett, M., Mayan, M., Olson, K., & Spiers, J. (2002). Verification strategies for establishing reliability and validity in qualitative research. *International Journal of Qualitative Methods 1*(2), article 2. Retrieved from http://www.ualberta.ca

Stetler, C. B., Morsi, D., Rucki, S., Broughton, S., Corrigan, B., Fitzgerald, J., . . . Sheridan E. A. (1998). Utilization-focused integrative reviews in a nursing service. *Applied Nursing Research, 11*(4), 196–206.

Stoddard, G. J., & Ring, W. H. (1993). How to evaluate study methodology in published clinical research. *Journal of Intravenous Nursing, 16*(2), 110–117.

Zuzelo, P. R. (2007). Evidence-based nursing and qualitative research: A partnership imperative for real-world practice. In P. L. Munhall (Ed.), *Nursing research: A qualitative perspective* (4th ed., pp. 481–499). Sudbury, MA: Jones and Bartlett.

CHAPTER SEVENTEEN

Evidence-Based Practice Strategies

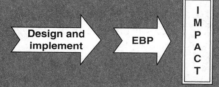

It is a long road from the conduct of research to patients actually receiving evidence-based care. You have learned that the findings of individual studies have to be appraised, and then the credible findings have to be summarized in the form of systematic reviews. Credible systematic reviews are then used to develop clinical practice guidelines. That brings the knowledge to caregiving settings in a practical form, but it still has to be integrated into practice. This final step, sometimes referred to as *planned change* or the *knowledge-to-action cycle* (Harrison et al., 2013), can be quite difficult because it involves changing organizational routines and human behavior.

The reality is that there can be very strong evidence showing the benefits of a clinical intervention, even a well-produced evidence-based clinical practice guideline from a respected organization, and yet the intervention won't get picked up by the majority of clinicians. Why is that so? It's because professional behavior is heavily influenced by work flow, the pace of work, one's peers, managers in the organization/agency/unit/ward, the culture of the workplace, and one's own comfort zone.

Research–Practice Lag

There is empirical data indicating that uptake of convincing evidence and e-b clinical practice guidelines is slow in the healthcare professions.

303

Sometimes clinicians are not aware of the recommendations from their professional association or a national agency (like the Centers for Disease Control and Prevention); other times they are aware of it but haven't changed how they do things.

In 2005, the American Association of Critical Care Nurses (AACN) issued an alert on verification of feeding tube placement (Bourgault et al., 2014); the alert included a warning that listening with a stethoscope (i.e., auscultation) for an air bolus over the stomach was not a reliable method of determining tube location. The alert was updated in 2009 and again in 2016 (AACN, 2016). Five recommendations related to verification of tube location and the evidence supporting them are set forth—it's definitely worth a look as it is a fine example of an evidence-based clinical practice guideline. Five years after the original alert, i.e., 2010, a survey of nearly 2,300 AACN members revealed that the auscultation method was still used by 79% of the respondents to verify placement prior to tube feeding (Metheny, Stewart, & Mills, 2012). A smaller 2011 survey of AACN members found that 55% were aware of the practice alert and 45% had adopted at least several of the recommendations, although only 23% avoided bolus auscultation per the recommendation (Bourgault et al., 2014). This situation reminds us that even strong evidence coupled with a persistent recommendation from a respected organization is not sufficient to protect patients from a potentially harmful practice. Even awareness of strong e-b best practice is often inadequate by itself.

And think about hand washing. The benefits to patients in terms of preventing hospital-, clinic-, or even home care-acquired infection have been well documented—the science is very strong (CDC, 2015). In addition, many clinicians see firsthand the distress to patients and the cost associated with infections acquired in care settings. Yet, many clinicians fail to wash their hands before and after a patient contact. Why? They forget; it isn't convenient; it's hard on the skin of their hands; it takes too much time; and so on. The reasons are numerous. The bottom line, however, is that it just isn't yet part of how they go about doing their daily job. The challenge for the organization is to make hand washing before and after a patient contact part of the culture, like saying *Hello* when meeting someone or seeing someone you know. There are a variety of strategies for getting there but it takes collaborative planning, feedback to clinicians about how they are doing, and persistence in delivering the message.

This chapter presents strategies healthcare organizations use to strategically introduce an evidence-based innovation into practice. Before examining strategies for unfreezing old habits and introducing the innovation, I want to place e-b innovation in an organizational context.

Embedding Evidence-Based Practice in Quality Improvement

All health service organizations are mandated by third-party payers, such as the Centers for Medicare and Medicaid Services (CMS), and by accreditors such as the Joint Commission, to provide documentation showing that the health services they provide are safe, effective, and cost-efficient. To achieve these goals, organizations collect data about their:

- Activities of care (what is being done)
- Processes of care (how it is done: when, where, by whom)
- Patient outcomes achieved
- Patient safety (low levels of adverse events in care environments)
- Patient satisfaction
- Cost

Analysis of this data and the performance improvement actions that accompany it most often go under the rubric *Quality Improvement*. Data collection is key to quality improvement (QI) at several points to identify problems, establish baseline performance, determine whether change made has led to improvements, and compare a health service system's outcomes to other organizations providing the same service. To evaluate systems of care, QI teams examine in detail processes such as patients' timely access to services, patient movement through a health service system, the patient experience of care, staff performance of key clinical actions, coordination of care, sequence of work, availability and functionality of equipment, and who does what when.

Sometimes QI and evidence-based practice (EBP) are viewed separately, but often EBP is viewed as part of QI (Health Resources and Services Administration, 2011). One could say that QI focuses on the processes and outcomes of care, whereas research evidence provides valuable knowledge about clinical practice actions that are likely to promote good care. Improvement can be achieved by addressing either component; however, the greatest impact is when both the systems of care and care actions are addressed at the same time because each adds value to the other (Levin et al., 2010; Seidl & Newhouse, 2012). Evidence-based protocols lose effectiveness if the delivery systems in which they are embedded are not safe, efficient, and patient centered. In reverse, it makes no sense to have safe, efficient, and patient-centered delivery systems if care protocols are not based on available and sound science.

> **QI** focuses on collecting data to evaluate and improve the systems, processes, and outcomes of care.
> **EBP** assembles scientific knowledge about clinical practice that is likely to achieve good patient outcomes and satisfaction and translates it into clinical protocols.

A Real-World Example

Nurses working on 32-bed general medical unit noted limited physical activity among patients on their unit and assembled an interdisciplinary team to implement an early mobility program (Wood et al., 2014). They reviewed the research literature on adverse effects of inactivity while in hospital, the barriers to mobility, and mobility interventions that have been tested. Drawing on this evidence, they (1) developed and implemented a two-level physical activity protocol (one level for ambulatory patients and another for nonambulatory patients), and (2) assigned a nurse's aide to assist patients in performing their exercises or ambulation; the mobility aide was trained and worked a regular 40-hour week. The outcomes of interest for their project were falls, patient lengths of stay, hospital readmission rates, and pressure ulcers. They collected baseline information and data on these outcomes at 3 months and 7 months after the change in practice was introduced. Although they fell short of their goal of patients' completing three activity sessions daily, a vast majority of patients completed at least two sessions per day. A slight reduction in falls and readmission within 30 days of discharge was realized, while pressure ulcer incidence and length of stay were essentially unchanged. The size of the reductions in falls and readmissions were small, but it must be acknowledged that these patient outcomes are influenced by many other factors, so even a small reduction suggests a promising impact from the intervention. Also, the unit was constrained to just one 5-day/week mobility aide position. One would assume that more consistent availability of a mobility aide would most likely increase the size of the impact on patient outcomes. Clearly, there were both QI and EBP components in this improvement project.

QI Models

The several QI models in use in health care go by various names, including total quality management and the continuous quality improvement model (HRSA, 2011; Seidl & Newhouse, 2012). A widely used one is PDCA cycle which has four stages:

Plan: Determine goals for a process and needed changes to achieve them.

Do: Implement the changes.

Check: Evaluate the results in terms of performance.

Act: Standardize and stabilize the change or begin the cycle again, depending on the results.

Source: http://www.lean.org/lexicon/plan-do-check-act

Other widely used quality improvement models in health care are *Six Sigma*, *Lean*, and *Root Cause Analysis*.

Organizational Structures

Organizational structure for QI and EBP responsibilities are quite variable. There may be a Best Practice Council at the departmental or division level whose mission includes supporting evidence-based practice and quality improvement. Alternatively, responsibility for EBP may reside at the operational level, i.e., unit, division or service line, while responsibility for quality improvement may reside in a department or with a QI coordinator. In sum, organizations use various ways to create synergy between QI and EBP and involve direct care providers in improvement activities. If you are currently employed in health care, you are undoubtedly aware of QI and EBP projects in your organization. If you are a basic nursing student, you may or may not have encountered either one of them during your clinical experience. But both of them are undoubtedly at work—although a bit behind the scenes.

Translating Evidence into Practice

Although QI and EBP are often part of the same project, there are times when a clinical practice group thinks it is important to introduce a clinical practice innovation apart from a larger QI purpose. Thus, there is a realm of study about the translation of research evidence into practice, and several models and theoretical frameworks for doing so (Rycroft-Malone & Bucknall, 2010). One of these is the iPARIHS framework, the acronym standing for integrated promoting action on research implementation in health services (Harvey & Kitson, 2015).

$$SI = Fac^n (I + R + C)$$

The model proposes that successful implementation of an innovation can be achieved when *fac*ilitation of the change takes into account the *i*nnovation being introduced, the *r*ecipients who will be affected by the change, and the various *c*ontexts that influence the care system. The superscript *n* recognizes that facilitation involves a range of activities to achieve the integration required for a successful implementation. This framework accommodates various theories of organizational behavior change, thus each element represents a complex domain of human activity with many interacting pieces. Still, the formula provides a useful overview of how to plan and implement a research-based change in practice.

Successful Implementation

Successful implementation occurs when (1) almost all providers and support services adopt the activities associated with the new intervention or way of doing things, (2) the performance goals and patient outcomes are achieved, and (3) the change is sustained over time (Rycroft-Malone et al., 2013).

Facilitation

Facilitation refers to activities that promote or enable the attainment of the project's goals. Facilitation in the iPARIHS model is considered the active ingredient that must integrate the three factors in the parenthesis. When the goal is implementation of an evidence-based change, facilitation involves working with the people who will be affected by the change to:

1. Make sense of the evidence leading to the change
2. See the benefits in making the innovation
3. Design the e-b innovation in a way that makes it as easy as possible for all those affected by it to incorporate it into their work routines
4. Support staff while making the change
5. Evaluate the impact of the change

These activities can be performed as an independent evidence-based practice project or within a quality improvement approach such as *Plan-Do-Check-Act*.

The facilitator can be an individual or a team in the system being changed. A dedicated lead facilitator with dedicated project time and prior experience in introducing e-b change in practice will undoubtedly increase the odds of successful implementation (Harrison et al., 2013). Importantly the team should represent all stakeholders in the proposed change and have a broad skill set including: operational knowledge of how the clinical processes and support systems of the setting work, sensitivity to the characteristics of the recipients and their current way of doing things, knowledge about how to appraise and translate research evidence into setting-specific protocols, and skill in working collaboratively with management and opinion leaders in the system into which the innovation will be introduced.

Innovation

Some innovations being introduced are relatively simple changes in how a nurse does an intervention but other innovations are quite complex and require organizational change in workflow, communications, and logistics (Stetler, Damschroder, Helfrich, & Hagedom, 2011). Research evidence should weigh heavily in considering how to design the innovation, but clinical experience, internal system and outcomes data, and the patient experience are also relevant forms of evidence.

Strong research evidence with a good fit to the implementation setting is obviously more persuasive than borderline evidence, but even strong research evidence by itself will not be sufficient by itself to change clinical behavior. Experts in the field of translations science express the view that translation of research evidence at the organization level should be done from systematic reviews and evidence-based clinical practice guidelines, not from individual studies—for reasons of basing the change on a more dependable body of findings and the advantages of a credible association having summarized and translated the evidence (GIN, 2010; Grimshaw et al., 2012). Importantly, in adapting high quality EbCPG to a particular care setting, the team must be vigilant to not weaken the evidence-based nature of the guideline recommendations.

Protocol Formats   E-b innovations often take the form of care protocols, which are set forth in diverse formats: standardized plans of care, standardized order sets, care bundles, decision algorithms, care maps, clinical pathways, policies, and procedures. References for each of these are listed on the text's website.

By way of definition, a care bundle is a group of e-b interventions related to a condition or treatment—generally three to five—that, when consistently performed together, result in improved patient outcomes (Institute for Healthcare Improvement, 2015). There are bundles for central line care, urinary catheter insertion and maintenance, reducing admissions for chronic obstructive pulmonary disease, and preventing sepsis, pressure ulcers, and falls, to name just a few. In ICUs the ABCDE bundle is being used to prevent and manage ICU-acquired delirium and weakness that result from prolonged mechanical ventilation and over-sedation (Balas et al., 2012). Based on the best available evidence, it involves coordinated awakening and breathing trials and early mobility. It is a complex clinical protocol to implement but one that produces considerable benefit to patients.

Decision algorithms are step-by-step instructions for reaching a decision or solving a problem; they are often formatted as a flow chart consisting of a series of yes/no questions leading to one of several possible decisions or actions. The use of an algorithm pertaining to the assessment and management of persistent pain in older adults is described in a quite readable and practical 2011 article (Jablonski, DuPen, & Ersek).

A clinical pathway, also called a care map, is a multidisciplinary specification of the actions to be implemented during the process of care for a well-defined group of patients over a specified period of time (DeBleser et al., 2006). A pathway explicitly sets forth key elements and sequences of care, time-specific goals and specification of performance and coordinating roles.

Although some decisions and actions in decision algorithms and clinical pathways will be based on high-quality, strong research evidence, others may be based on weaker evidence such as expert opinion. The ideal is that a companion document summarizing or grading the research evidence about the decision points and recommended actions is available to clinicians.

Recipients

To facilitate implementation of an innovation in care, the project team facilitating the implementation must identify the persons who will be affected by it, i.e., the stakeholders, and truly understand how they will be affected by the proposed change. Stakeholders should be viewed as both individuals and as a community of practice, i.e., all nurses working on the unit or in a department such as respiratory therapy. Developers of the iPARIHS framework emphasize that the implementation plan must be humanized (Harvey & Kitson, 2015). To do this they need to consider questions like:

- Who is going to be most affected and how can we ease their adoption of the change?
- Where is resistance likely to come from?
- Who will be the early adopters?
- Who will be a valuable source in identifying and working out the bugs in implementation?

Active involvement of the end users of an innovation in customizing a clinical practice guideline has been shown to lead to greater acceptance and adoption of the required actions (Harrison et al., 2013).

Making a change in practice typically encounters both enthusiasm and resistance. Cullen, Greiner, Greiner, Bombei, and Comried (2005) described the "tag-flag-nag" approach to supporting EBP innovation. Tagging involves identifying and visibly recognizing staff nurses who adopt the practice change. Flagging involves identifying less compliant staff and discussing with them how they can incorporate the change into their care. Nagging is the way of dealing with persistent noncompliers; it involves recruiting opinion leaders on the unit to talk with the noncompliers about their failure to adopt the new standard of care, and, if necessary, more firm ways of dealing with their resistance to change. Thus, leaders use a variety of carrot and stick strategies to convey that quality of care is the goal and that persons who detract from that goal will be held accountable for their failure to meet unit standards (Stetler, Ritchie, Rycroft-Malone, Schultz, & Charns, 2009).

Context

This is a broad category of considerations ranging from the routines of care delivery on a unit/ward or service line to the external forces that shape what direct care providers must do. In between are the variables of leadership support, identification of opinion leaders, the professional culture in the care system, resources available, and financial constraints.

For sure, change is and will continue to be the way of life in health care, but people can only absorb so much. Facilitators should pay attention to how many major changes the clinicians have had to make in the last several months and put off the change a while before hitting them with another major change. The reality is that in many hospitals patients' care is prescribed by as many as six care bundles, with patients in critical care units being on the most. In addition, nurses report difficulty giving care in complete accord with the bundles (Whelchel, Berg, Brown, Koepping, & Stroud, 2013). This is understandable as each bundle includes a set of 3–5 specific actions that must be incorporated into care. Keeping many standards in mind puts quite a cognitive strain on the nurse in that she not only has to be fully immersed in the immediate care situation, but also has to be keeping in mind the actions required by the bundles (Krichbaum et al., 2007). In response to this complexity, real-time clinical information systems are being developed to prompt clinical staff in delivering care in accord with the many standards.

In a sense, a care system is like an ocean liner in that quite a bit of energy has to be put forth to make even a small change in course. So, introducing a change in practice requires the strategic and coordinated efforts of quite a few people.

Evaluate the Impact

Even when an evidence-based protocol was carefully developed and introduced, checks on its uptake and ultimate impact are necessary. If the introduction of the e-b protocol or innovation was part of a large QI project, evaluation will naturally be undertaken. The measurements used to analyze the care system at baseline often can be repeated to determine if the protocol has been adopted and is having the desired impact.

Note that the appraisal guides for clinical practice guidelines and systematic reviews you learned about earlier include a question about how the protocol innovation will be evaluated. This question is included because the impact evaluation should be planned at the time the protocol is developed and introduced, not as an afterthought. Typically, measurement of performance and outcomes before, during, and after implementation of a change in practice is needed to be sure that the new protocol has resulted in the desired patient outcomes and that the change is being maintained over time. Too often improvements in performance and outcomes realized a few months after introducing an innovation are lost over time; thus monitoring of performance and outcomes should continue long term (Glasgow, 2011).

If Necessary, Revisit and Revise

If the anticipated results are not occurring, the protocol and the context in which it was embedded must be revisited to determine why it is not working, including the following questions:

- Was the evidence not interpreted correctly?
- Was the translation of the evidence into the agency protocol faulty?
- Was the implementation lacking in some way?
- Is the protocol unrealistic or in conflict with other job expectations?

The pursuit of quality care is indeed demanding and ongoing.

Information Technology[1]

Lest the preceding information about the complex process required to integrate research evidence into practice discourages you, you need to know that information technology offers promising assistance. Evidence-based protocols can be integrated into electronic health records (EHRs) to impact clinician decision making about individual patients at the point in time that decisions are made, i.e., in real time. When this is done it is referred to as clinical decision support (Berner & LaLande, 2007).

It works this way: A healthcare organization purchases a clinical decision support system from a vendor, e.g., Zynx Health, Elsevier Clinical Solutions, Lippincott ProVation Care Plans or Lippincott Solutions. (Check their websites for details about their products.) Organizations and vendor teams then adapt the decision support tools of the vendor and embed them in the organization's EHR so the care guidance is delivered when appropriate to providers during care planning and decision making for a patient. Decision support tools include e-b assessment forms, plans of care, order sets, and specifications of clinical procedures. When this content is embedded in the workflow of an electronic health record, it is described as "actionable" because it:

- Is relevant to the patient situation to which it has been linked.
- Fits into the workflow of clinical care.
- Is based on credible and current research evidence.
- Incorporates the quality and performance measures of regulatory and accrediting bodies (e.g., Centers for Medicare and Medicaid Services, 2012; Joint Commission).

---

[1]Thanks to Patricia S. Button, RN, EdD for consultation regarding this section.

Ideally the electronic health record supports the triggering of a care plan or order set from assessment data, interdisciplinary problem lists, and medical diagnosis at appropriate points across the care continuum. Importantly, the care plans and order sets, when used in the care of an individual patient, require the clinical judgment of the care provider to individualize the standard plan or order set to the unique needs of the specific patient. Decision support systems also provide hyperlinks to the evidence summaries or guidelines on which the vendor plan of care or standard order set is based and support links to relevant organizational policies, quality measures, and resources.

A caregiving organization purchasing a clinical decision support system can be saved a tremendous amount of effort and time investment in that it doesn't have to develop e-b standardized care protocols (i.e., plans of care, order sets, and procedures) from the ground up in that the vendor has done much of the early-stage work. Instead, the organization can focus on adapting the protocol to the organization, introducing it to staff, and monitoring the update of its actions. In other words, facilitation, recipients, and context (from the iPARIHS framework) must still be considered prior to the launch of each standardized plan of care or order set into the organization's EHR. Decision support vendors have resources to help organizations integrate their care planning tools into the EHR and to foster uptake of the care standards by clinicians.

An updated model of evidence for the future might recognize decision support tools as the highest form of evidence because the evidence has been translated into an integrated and usable form that is brought forward when a clinician needs it (**Figure 17-1**). Some health systems are already using evidence through decision support but others are just getting started.

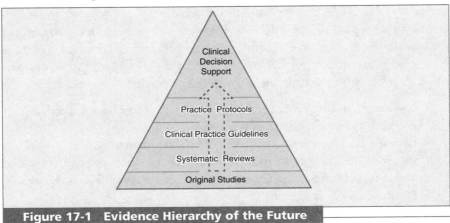

Figure 17-1   Evidence Hierarchy of the Future

Data from DiCenso, A., Bayley, L., & Haynes, R.B. (2009). Accessing pre-appraised evidence: Fine-tuning the 5S model into a 6S model. *Evidence-Based Nursing, 12*(4), 99–101.

Decision support can also be provided apart from the electronic health record. Vendors offer searchable libraries of summaries on clinical topics that are evidence based to the extent possible. The summaries include nursing care plans, recommendations from national guidelines, and quality core measures. Patient teaching handouts, procedure videos, and links to external sources are also part of these products. This type of decision support is considered *referential* information because the clinician must link out to it. It is also called *pull* guidance because it requires providers to interrupt their workflow and seek information. In contrast, clinical guidance embedded in an EHR is referred to as *push* guidance because it is provided to the clinician without any effort on her/his part. Generally, the availability of referential information is thought to have less impact on care planning and decision making than actionable information.

Present and Future

Most assuredly, access to research evidence and e-b best practice recommendations have greatly improved in recent years; the formats are more clinician friendly and professional associations are promoting awareness of e-b practices at conferences, on their websites, and in journals. Proprietary products are being upgraded; government and privately funded initiatives in many countries are promoting evidence-based practice and funding studies about how to translate research findings into practice. Thus, progress in moving research evidence into practice is well under way, but is still a work in progress (Moja et al., 2014).

Recap

At this point, I suggest you pause to consider all that has been presented to this point in this book. **Figure 17-2** portrays the really big picture beginning with recognition that knowledge for a particular issue of practice is lacking, proceeding through the steps of knowledge production and EBP and finally achieving best practice. It is a long path, but we owe it to our patients, to society, to our profession, and to ourselves as professional nurses to walk the EBP walk.

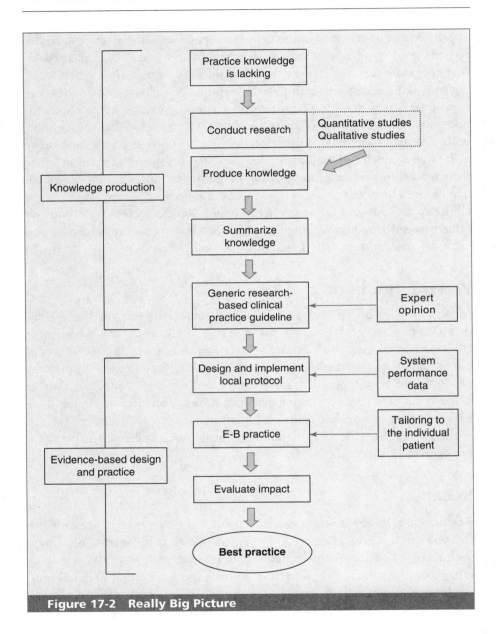

Figure 17-2 Really Big Picture

REFERENCES

AACN. (2016). AACN Practice Alert: Initial and Ongoing Verification of Feeding Tube Placement in Adult. *Critical Care Nurse Online*. Retrieved from http://www.aacn.org/wd/practice/docs/practicealerts/feeding-tube-pa.pdf

Balas, M. C., Vasilevskis, E. E., Burke, W. J., Boehm, L., Put, B. T., Olsen, K. M., . . . Ely, W. E. (2012). Critical care nurses' role in implementing the "ABCDE bundle" into practice. *Critical Care Nurse, 32*(2), 35–38, 40–48. Retrieved from http://www.aacn.org/wd/Cetests/media/C1223.pdf

Berner, E. S., & LaLande, T. (2007). Overview of clinical decision support systems. In E. S. Berner (Ed.), *Clinical decision support systems: Theory and practice* (2nd ed., pp. 3–22). New York, NY: Springer Science and Business Media.

Bourgault, A. M., Heath, J., Hooper, V., Sole, M. L., Waller, J. L., NeSmith, E. G. (2014). Factors influencing critical care nurses' adoption of the AACN practice alert on verification of feeding tube placement. *American Journal of Critical Care, 23*(2), 134–144). Retrieved from http://ajcc.aacnjournals.org

Centers for Medicare & Medicaid Services (CMS). (2012). *Hospital quality initiative.* Retrieved from http://www.cms.gov/Medicare/Quality-Initiatives-Patient-Assessment-Instruments/HospitalQualityInits/index.html?redirect=/HospitalQualityInits/

Centers for Disease Control and Prevention (CDC). (2015). *Handwashing: Clean hands save lives; Show me the science.* Retrieved from http://www.cdc.gov/

Cullen, L., Greiner, J., Greiner, J., Bombei, C., & Comried, L. (2005). Excellence in evidence-based practice: Organizational and unit exemplars. *Critical Care Nursing Clinics of North America, 17*, 127–142.

DeBleser, L., Depreitere, R., De Waele, K., VanHaecht, K., Vlayen, J., & Sermeus, W. (2006). Defining pathways. *Journal of Nursing Management, 14*(7), 553–563.

DiCenso, A., Bayley, L., & Haynes, R. B. (2009). Accessing pre-appraised evidence: Fine-tuning the 5S model into a 6S model. *Evidence-Based Nursing, 12*(4), 99–101.

Glasgow, J. (2011). *Introduction to Lean and Six Sigma approaches to quality improvement.* Retrieved from http://www.qualitymeasures.ahrq.gov

Grimshaw, J. M., Eccles, M. P., Lavis, J. N., Hill, S. J. & Squires, J. E. (2012). Knowledge translation of research findings. *Implementation Science, 7*, 50. Retrieved from http://implementationscience.biomedcentral.com/rticles/10.1186/1748-5908-7-50

Guidelines International Workgroup (GIN). (2010). *Guideline adaptation: A resource toolkit.* Retrieved from http://www.g-i-n.net/document-store/working-groups-documents/adaptation/adapte-resource-toolkit-guideline-adaptation-2-0.pdf

Harrison, M. B., Graham, I. D., van den Hoek, J., Dogherty, E. J., Carley, M. E., & Angus, V. (2013). Guideline adaptation and implementation planning: A prospective observational study. *Implementation Science, 8*, 49.

Harvey, G., & Kitson, A. (2015). *Implementing evidence-based practice in healthcare: A facilitation guide.* London, England: Rouldege.

Health Resources and Services Administration (HRSA). (2011). *Quality improvement.* Retrieved from http://www.hrsa.gov/quality/toolbox/508pdfs/quality improvement.pdf

Institute for Healthcare Improvement. (2015). *What is a bundle?* Retrieved from http://www.ihi.org/resources/Pages/ImprovementStories/WhatIsaBundle.aspx

Jablonski, A. M., DuPen, A. R., & Ersek, M. (2011). The use of algorithms in assessing and managing persistent pain in older adults. *AJN, American Journal of Nursing, 111*(3), 34–43.

Krichbaum, K., Diemart, C., Jacox, L., Jones, A., Koenig, P., Mueller, C., & Disch, J. (2007). Complexity compression: Nurses under fire. *Nursing Forum, 42*, 86–94.

Levin, R. F., Keefer, J. M., Marren, J., Vetter, M., Lauder, B., & Sobolewski, S. (2010). Evidence-based practice improvement: Merging 2 paradigms. *Journal of Nursing Care Quality, 25*, 117–126.

Metheny, N. A., Stewart, B. J., & Mills, A. C. (2012). Blind insertion of feeding tubes in intensive care units: A national survey. *American Journal of Critical Care, 21*(5), 352–360. Retrieved from http://ajcc.aacnjournals.org/

Moja, L., Kwag, K. H., Lytras, T., Bertizzolo, L., Brandt, L., Pecoraro, V., . . . Bonovas, S. (2014). Effectiveness of computerized decision support systems linked to electronic health records: A systematic review and meta-analysis. *American Journal of Public Health, 104*(12), 12–22. Retrieved from https://www.ncbi.nlm.nih.gov/. doi: 10.2105/AJPH.2014.302164

Rycroft-Malone, J., & Bucknall, T. (2010). Models and frameworks for implementing evidence-based practice: Linking evidence to action. Hoboken, NJ: Wiley-Blackwell.

Rycroft-Malone, J., Seers, K., Chandler, J., Hawkes, C. A., Chrichton, N., Allen, C., . . .Strunin, L. (2013). The role of evidence, context, and facilitation in an implementation trial: Implications for the development of the PARIHS framework. *Implementation Science, 8*, 28.

Seidl, K. L., & Newhouse, R. P. (2012). The intersection of evidence-based practice with 5 quality improvement methodologies. *Journal of Nursing Administration, 42*(6), 299–304.

Stetler, C. B., Damschroder, L. J., Helfrich, C., & Hagedom, H. J. (2011). A guide for applying a revised version of the PARIHS framework for implementation. *Implementation Science, 6*, 99.

Stetler, C. B., Ritchie, J., Rycroft-Malone, J., Schultz, A. A., & Charns, P. (2009). Institutionalizing evidence-based practice: An organizational case study using a model of strategic change. *Implementation Science, 4(1)*, 78.

Whelchel, C., Berg, L., Brown, A., Hurd, D., Koepping, D., & Stroud, S. (2013). What's the impact of quality bundles at the bedside? *Nursing, 43*(12), 18–21.

Wood, W., Tschannen, D., Trotsky, A., Grunawalt, J., Adams, D., Chang, R., . . . Diccion-MacDonald, S. (2014). CE: A mobility program for an inpatient acute care medical unit. *American Journal of Nursing, 114*(10), 34–40. Retrieved from http://journals.lww.com/ajnonline/Fulltext/2014/10000/CE_A_Mobility_Program_for_an_Inpatient_Acute.23.aspx

Evidence-Based Practice Participation

There are several scenarios in which you might get involved in an evidence-based practice (EBP) project. The first would be as a student; then other opportunities could arise in your work setting—present or future. I thought I could provide a bit of guidance in this regard. Six scenarios will be described, and suggestions will be made regarding each:

1. You decide to do your capstone project around some aspect of evidence-based practice.
2. As a participant in a patient care planning conference, you present research evidence relevant to the care of a patient with a complex issue.
3. As a member of a project team in your work setting, you could be asked to appraise one or several pieces of research evidence and give a short oral presentation about it.
4. You decide to submit an evidence-based poster to be displayed at a congress or conference.
5. You want to present an evidence-based clinical idea or concern to your nurse leader, clinical nurse specialist, or nurse manager.
6. Evidence-based practice really interests you, and you want to further develop your EBP knowledge and skills.

Capstone Project

A capstone project by definition requires you to use and connect what you have learned throughout your nursing program. A capstone project focused on evidence-based practice could require you to do some scholarly work but also some work in the clinical setting where you envision an e-b change in practice.

Your project could follow the process described in Part II of this text. That would include a sequence of steps as outlined in box below, but of course your proposal and submission would have to be adapted to the requirement of your program. The full proposal in the box is quite ambitious, but you could just do parts of it, e.g., steps, 1–9 or 4–7. Alternatively, if you are currently working in a setting and know of an issue and a credible e-b clinical practice guideline that you think should be implemented, your project could involve working with a nurse manager and others to develop an implementation and evaluation plan, and start the introduction process. Or you could take just one or two steps in the process and build an e-b project by pursuing those steps in depth from both a scholarly and a real world perspective.

Contribute to a Patient Care Conference

When a patient's care presents difficult problems or requires complex discharge arrangements, a patient care planning conference will often be called. The goal of such a conference is to bring together all the people involved in the patient's care to address a particular problem and come up with an approach to the problematic issue or issues.

These planning sessions design more effective strategies when someone is assigned to spend an hour looking for research evidence relative to a key issue or issues in the management of the patient's problems. Perhaps there is an evidence-based guideline that is relevant to the patient's sleeping problem. Maybe a systematic review (SR) that addresses the issue of whether a teenager can take a shower even though he has external skeletal pins in place can be identified. Increasingly, evidence-based information is being brought to the table at patient care planning conferences.

If a conference is called and you will be involved, you should give some thought to the problems or issues that may be, or should be, discussed. There may be one or two issues for which it would be helpful for all participants to understand effective approaches that are supported by research evidence. If the person who leads the conference does not assign anyone to look at the research evidence about the problem, you might lead the way by doing so.

At the conference, you could bring what you found in your brief search to the table—not in a lecturing way, but in a contributing way. In that

PROPOSAL FOR A CAPSTONE PROJECT AIMED AT DESIGNING AND INTRODUCING AN EVIDENCE-BASED CHANGE IN PRACTICE

1. Identify a nursing action or function or a patient problem/diagnosis that you think requires evaluation, improvement, standardization, or updating.
2. Identify a clinical mentor with whom you can discuss your perception; ask her/him to help you track down existing protocols and internal data pertaining to the issue to help understand the status of what you see as a weakness or deficiency in care. Consider talking with patients to obtain their perceptions about the issue.
3. Describe and summarize any process or outcome data or patients' perceptions about the issue.
4. Write a PICOTS question for a project.
5. Search databases and websites for research evidence relevant to your project. Search first for e-b clinical practice guidelines and systematic research reviews; if none are found or to supplement the EbCPG or SR found, search for original studies.
6. Appraise the evidence relevant to your PICOTS question.
7. Summarize the evidence related to your PICOTS.
8. Share with your mentor your evidence summary/summaries.
9. Compare and contrast current practice with the evidence found.
10. With at least one other person, preferably more, design your change in practice protocol. Consider: a plan of care; a care pathway; an algorithm; a new procedure; a new assessment guide; a patient education video.
11. Discuss with your mentor how you could go about introducing the change in practice/innovation in the setting (as if you were to actually do it).
12. List your strategies for introducing the change/innovation.
13. Identify how you would evaluate whether the change has been adopted and/or improved patient outcomes; be specific.

regard, I warn against the overused and vague phrase, "research shows." Instead, say something specific like, "I found one systematic review that looked at five studies about sleeping problems in hospitalized adolescents. The reviewers reached the conclusion that . . ." Have the article with you so anyone who chooses to can look at it. The inclusion of research-based information into the discussion will most likely be valued and will serve to take the exchange beyond opinions to more objective knowledge as the basis for care planning.

Join a Project Team

First, let's imagine a context for this scenario. You work as a staff nurse on an orthopedic unit. The unit is looking at its use of special beds and bed surfaces for patients at risk of skin breakdown. The work group is charged with developing a decision algorithm or decision tree regarding the use of special beds and surfaces. The unit already uses a risk assessment scale to quantify patients' risk for skin breakdown. In PICOTS terms, this question would be outlined as follows:

P. Patients with orthopedic injuries and/or recovering from orthopedic surgery who are at risk for skin breakdown
I. Special beds and mattress overlays
C. Effectiveness of each and when to use one rather than another
O. Prevention of skin breakdown
T. Before breakdown occurs
S. Inpatient orthopedics

The group decides to start by examining the effectiveness of various support surfaces aimed at preventing skin breakdown and then proceed to link risk assessment to the various surfaces. At the second meeting of this group, you are asked to appraise a systematic review regarding alternating air mattresses (Vanderwee, Grypdonck, & Defloor, 2008). The expectation is that you will extract information from the SR onto a findings table and at the next meeting give a less-than-5-minute summary and appraisal of the SR.

You could organize your talk in the following way:

- Give a summary of the SR along the same lines as the information in the synopsis part of the SR appraisal guide.
- State your overall impression of the credibility of the conclusions along with your reasons for confidence or concerns.
- State your opinion regarding the clinical significance of the conclusions.
- Address the applicability of the findings and conclusions to the patients seen on your unit and the resources that will be available.

Make a Poster

Professional conferences and congresses often issue calls for oral presentations or posters of research studies and EBP projects. A summary of evidence regarding a clinical question often makes a relevant and interesting poster. Posters are usually mounted on boards in specified areas at congresses, and people walk around and read them. Most congresses require that a person be present with the poster at specified times so people can ask questions.

So, let's say the bed surface-skin breakdown group's work is moving along well, and you notice a call from the National Association of Orthopaedic Nurses (NAON) for posters at its spring congress. Because your work group has not finished its work on the algorithm/protocol, you decide to submit a poster regarding just the evidence used to produce the algorithm. Most associations allow submission of work-in-progress posters. You would first submit to NAON an abstract of your poster's content. Then, if it is accepted, you would proceed to create the poster using PowerPoint or similar presentation software and produce it using a poster-making machine, which many agencies have on premises.

When making a poster, you have to be very selective about the information included. If it has too much information or if the information is presented in a disorganized way, people will avoid stopping to read it or will read part of it and walk away. The idea of a poster is to present the main ideas—it is like an abstract. If the person looking at the poster is interested in knowing more, she will ask you some questions. You (the person explaining the poster) are the real resource; the poster is mostly just a lure.

There are no ironclad rules for how to design a poster, but a few suggestions may help. In regard to design of the poster, information should be grouped in some logical way with a header for each block and three to five points under each header. You can use some abbreviations if you define them the first time you use them; of course this is not necessary if they are very common ones. You might want to have a list of the EbCPGs and SRs that are referenced in the poster for people who ask for them, or you could have interested persons write down their email address, and after the congress you can send a list of references to them.

The poster could look like the one in **Figure 18-1**. This is a low-budget poster, produced with only gray tones. Color would spruce it up considerably but would add to the cost. Note that the poster in the figure is fabricated—it does not represent an actual project or literature search.

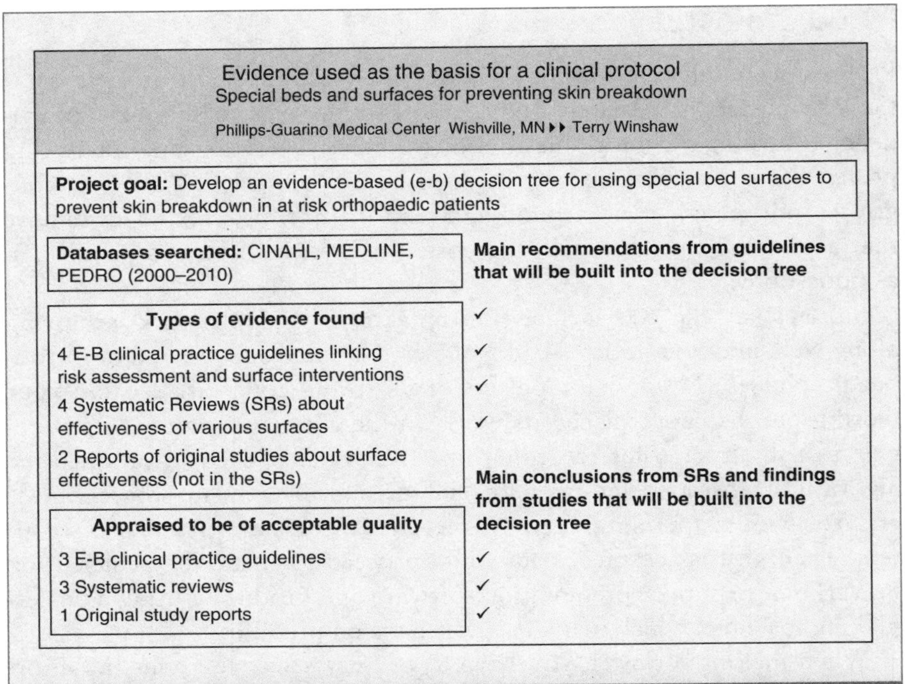

Figure 18-1   Poster

Having a poster at a congress is a fun and informative experience. A lot of people will talk with you, and you will learn a lot. It's definitely a recommended step in your professional growth and development.

Present an Idea or Concern

Let us say while you were at the congress, you went to a session about preventing and managing mental confusion in elderly patients with hip fractures. You went to the session because this issue has recently been a challenge in caring for several patients on your unit. You decide to see what research evidence is available on the topic and to talk with the clinical nurse specialist for your unit. A 15-minute search on CINAHL—using the terms *delirium, hip fracture,* and *interventions,* with the *research only* and *evidence-based practice* filters on—turns up two EbCPGs, an SR, and several research articles about preventing and managing delirium in patients with hip fracture; they indicate that pain relief is clearly important.

To talk to the clinical nurse specialist or nurse leader, it is best to make an appointment. Catch-as-catch-can in the hallway usually does not work; interruptions are bound to occur, or you may catch him when he has something else on his mind. Here are some suggestions for preparing for your appointment:

- Be able to give some recent examples of why you think delirium prevention and management is a problem on your unit. Specific patient examples would support your claim that delirium care is not as good as it could be.
- Briefly describe the research evidence you found on your quick search. It might be good to give him a copy of several of the research abstracts or URLs you found.
- If your unit already has a protocol about this topic, look at it before your appointment. If the protocol is evidence based and well written, maybe the appropriate action would be to bring it anew to the staff's attention along with any new research. If the protocol is not helpful, up to date, or consistent with newer research, point out its shortcomings.
- Ask his or her opinion about how to get things moving to make a change, but have an idea or two in mind beforehand.

There is no guarantee you will get a positive response and good follow-through, but the chances are good and the cause is a good one.

Build Your EBP Knowledge and Skills

If the transfer of scientific knowledge into practice really interests you, you should consider developing your EBP skills beyond what you have learned in the course you are now taking. You could take a graduate course or continuing education course about EBP. Some clinical congresses offer EBP precongress sessions or multiday EBP workshops. Alternatively, you might ask your nurse manager to give you paid time to attend an in-depth EBP workshop. The following list is a sampling of the opportunities available to advance your EBP knowledge and skills.*

- The Hirsh Institute of the Bolton School of Case Western Reserve University offers 2-day basic and intermediate EBP certificate programs. https://fpb.case.edu/Centers/Hirsh/basic_quikpay.shtm https://fpb.case.edu/Centers/Hirsh/intermediate.shtm

- The University of Iowa Hospitals and Clinics offers basic EBP internships and advanced workshops.
  https://www.uihealthcare.org/otherservices.aspx?id=22792
  https://www.uihealthcare.org/Nursing/Post.aspx?id=234195
- The Joanna Briggs Institute and collaborating centers around the world offer intensive training residencies.
  http://joannabriggs.org/jbi-education.html
  http://www.ebnp.org/fellows/fellowsresources.html
- The Institute for Johns Hopkins Nursing offers an EBP boot camp and online EBP course.
  http://www.hopkinsmedicine.org/evidence-based-practice/ebp_education.html
- Sigma Theta Tau International offers an annual grant to encourage nurses in clinical settings to apply evidence to practice and evaluate the effects on patient outcomes.
  http://www.nursingsociety.org/advance-elevate/research/research-grants/american-nurses-credentialing-center-evidence-based-practice-%28ebp%29-implementation-grant-program
- The Center for Transdisciplinary Evidence-based Practice in Columbus, Ohio, offers a 5-day EBP immersion program.
  https://ctep-ebp.com/5-day-clinical-ebp-immersion

* These links were live at the time this chapter was written, but as you know, links come and go.

The active learning that occurs in these kinds of programs will prepare you to fully participate in—even lead—EBP projects in your clinical unit or agency. Another option would be that when seeking employment at a large medical center, ask about in-house EBP training. Quite a few medical centers have them.

In summary, there are numerous ways to be involved in evidence-based practice and thereby contribute to good patient care and professional exchange.

REFERENCE

Vanderwee, K., Grypdonck, M., & Defloor, T. (2008). Alternating pressure air mattresses as prevention for pressure ulcers: A literature review. *International Journal of Nursing Studies, 45*(5), 784–801.

CHAPTER NINETEEN

Point-of-Care Adaptations

Evidence-based care protocols help incorporate scientifically supported care actions into care planning and promote consistency of care. However, as noted earlier, most scientific evidence is largely based on what works best *on average*. Thus, even when the research evidence is strong in support of a care approach for a specified patient group, we cannot expect everyone in that group to benefit from it. Additionally, even if it is clinically effective, the care approach may not be acceptable to all persons. For these reasons, nurses should enter into exchange with each patient during care planning and care delivery to determine if the care being given is accomplishing what it should and to learn what he wants from care.

When care is adapted or modified to individual responses and preferences, it is considered individualized, person-centered, or tailored to the individual. To achieve individualized care the nurse must:

- Truly be present to the patient when in his presence
- Be attuned to his problems, complaints, preferences, values, goals, and beliefs
- Share decision making about care

Individualized Care Story

A nurse saw a patient in a diabetes mellitus clinic. Listening to his chest, she heard mild wheezes so looked into his healthcare record to determine how his asthma was being managed. He was prescribed a PRN bronchodilator delivered via inhaler with a spacer for relief of shortness of breath and a steroid inhaler with a spacer once a day. The nurse asked the patient how often he used the inhalers. He said he used the PRN bronchodilator 4 to 6 times a day but did not use the steroid inhaler very often because "it has a bad taste, it dries out my mouth, and it ruins the taste of good food." He said he would rather use the PRN inhaler. The nurse explained the value of the steroid medication in preventing asthma symptoms and why it should be taken regularly. He said, "*Yeah, I know.*"

The nurse then asked to see his PRN inhaler, which he had with him, and noticed that he was not using the spacer. He said he didn't use the spacer because with it the inhaler doesn't fit in his shirt pocket. She asked whether he used the spacer on his steroid inhaler—*No.* She suggested that he use the spacer with the steroid inhaler as it would get the medication deeper into his airway and not so much in his mouth. She also suggested gargling with warm water and brushing his teeth after using the steroid inhaler. He could continue using the PRN inhaler without a spacer and they would see how that went. He seemed agreeable to that so she showed him how to use the spacer and gave him a pamphlet about its use.

At his next visit a month later, he said he was using the steroid inhaler with the spacer every morning before he brushed his teeth and that the mouth problem was *okay.* He also thought that he was using the PRN inhaler less often. He had no wheezing at the time of this visit.

This is individualized care. The nurse recognized the importance of the steroid inhaler as part of the asthma management protocol, but at the same time was attuned to his complaint about its oral effects. She asked the right questions to get at how he was using his inhalers and together they came up with an approach that was both effective and acceptable to the patient.

At the point of care, clinician and patient together decide if an evidence-based protocol endorsed by the agency or health system is acceptable and effective. The patient brings to this discussion responses to treatments, preferences, experiences, life goals, family support, and resources. The clinician brings clinical knowledge, prior experience with similar cases, interpersonal sensitivity, information about the patient's clinical condition, and professional judgment. Through such an exchange, evidence-based protocols are tailored to the individual patient (Flynn & Sinclair, 2005; van der Weijden et al., 2010).

Standardized protocols only go so far in specifying how care should be given. There still will be situations for which there is not an applicable protocol or when the protocol does not address a specific issue relating to the protocol. As a nurse committed to evidence-based practice you should think: *I wonder if there is any research evidence about this to guide what I do.* However, clearly you only have a limited amount of time in which to get an answer to your question. The rest of this chapter is about websites or apps that can be accessed with handheld e-devices. Importantly, many of these resources provide short form summaries in everyday language. In some cases the evidence has even been appraised and an overall statement of its quality included in the summary or for each recommendation.

Point-of-Care Evidence-Based Practice Story

A home health nurse was caring for two older persons with chronic lower leg ulcers. One was a 92-year-old man whose wound was shallow, just lightly exuding, and periodically had a small amount of necrotic tissue. Compression stockings had been tried but were not tolerated by the patient, so just leg elevation and ACE elastic bandages were being used. The dressing was being changed daily and the wound cleansed with sterile water; a 21-day treatment with an enzymatic debriding agent had removed necrotic tissue.

The nurse went to the National Guideline Clearinghouse, the Registered Nurses' Association of Ontario, and the Cochrane Collaboration websites to search for clinical practice guidelines and systematic reviews. She had heard about several medications that might promote healing. She searched the databases using the terms *leg ulcer* or *venous leg ulcers*. Among the helpful documents were three guidelines and several systematic reviews about the management of open wounds in patients with lower extremity venous disease.

From these the nurse got several e-b ideas for promoting healing of this man's leg ulcer, including recommending walking in place and/or calf muscle pumping every 2 hours to increase circulation. She also learned that leg elevation is most effective when the feet are above the level of the heart (e.g., putting the foot of the bed on blocks or placing a wedge under the foot end of the mattress). The strong research support for the effectiveness of compression therapy convinced her that they should reconsider compression alternatives to see if they could find one that he would tolerate—there are many products. So, for not a lot of effort (a little over an hour) she learned about some interventions she hadn't tried that have research support and learned about the strong support for compression therapy as the mainstay of treatment.

From Mobile Devices

Okay, so maybe you don't have an hour and need some information quicker. First a caveat: there are hundreds of health care and nursing sites and resources available for various clinical specialties areas and purposes, but they are not all evidence based. Some are designed to provide reference information such as normal lab values, drug interactions, medical diagnosis signs and symptoms, or drug calculation. But if you are looking for e-b information to guide you in giving care, you should rely on the sites of recognized organizations and association that inform users about how they produce their care guidance or systematic research reviews.

Getting to e-b information doesn't have to involve an extensive search every time. Rather, put together a list of bookmarks that make available e-b guideline or systematic reviews in your area of practice. You may also mark a few sites of organizations that produce EbCPGs and SRs quite broadly that you can check out when you encounter clinical issues outside your usual area of practice. The time spent compiling such a list could save you a lot of time later on and help you avoid having to do online searches using a general browser that brings up all kinds of commercial sites.

The websites and apps listed below should help you in starting your list of online resources. All are sites providing evidence-based care information in formats suitable for access from mobile devices. Some cover many areas of practice, whereas others are specific to a particular area of practice. Some include summarized forms of full guidelines or systematic reviews; others just access them in full. Some are free, some charge. Most are available for iPad/iPhone and Android devices. The information provided in the following sections is taken from the websites listed.

PubMed

PubMed databases can be searched for citations using *PubMed Mobile*. The site uses keyword search but also uses filters for article type, which makes it easy to zero in on systematic reviews. Questions can be asked in the PICOTS format, and there are links to full-text articles. It is available through multiple interfaces and in multiple languages.

http://www.ncbi.nlm.nih.gov/m/pubmed/

National Guideline Clearinghouse

The National Guideline Clearinghouse guideline summaries are available in HTML format downloadable to mobile devices—just click the HTML link at the top of any summary page.

http://www.guideline.gov/resources/mobile-resources.aspx

U.S. Preventive Services Task Force

The Electronic Preventive Services Selector (ePSS) is designed to help primary care clinicians and healthcare teams make timely decisions regarding appropriate screening, counseling, and preventive services for their patients. The ePSS is available both as a Web application and a mobile application. The ePSS information is based on the current, evidence-based recommendations of the U.S. Preventive Services Task Force and can be searched by specific patient characteristics, such as age, sex, and selected behavioral risk factors.

http://epss.ahrq.gov/PDA/index.jsp

Canadian Task Force on Preventive Health Care

The Canadian Task Force on Preventive Health Care (CTFPHC) mobile app helps primary care practitioners rapidly access CTFPHC guidelines and resources at the point of care and while on the go. The app contains guideline and recommendation summaries, knowledge translation tools, and links to additional resources.

http://canadiantaskforce.ca/resources/ctfphc-mobile-app/

Professional Associations

Many professional associations offer apps that access e-b guidelines and other information related to their specialties. Here are the ones I know about, but I'm sure there are others and new ones becoming available.

Registered Nurses' Association of Ontario   Condensed versions of a wide range of nursing best practice guidelines are available via its PBG app or via a Web version. Their guidelines are available in English and French.

http://rnao.ca/bpg/pda
http://pda.rnao.ca

Wound Ostomy and Continence Nurses Society   The app provides access to guidelines for prevention and management of pressure ulcers, management of the patient with a fecal ostomy, management of wounds in patients with lower extremity arterial disease, management of wounds in patients with lower extremity neuropathic disease, and management of wounds in patients with lower extremity venous disease.

> http://www.wocn.org/?page=guidelinesapp

National Association of Nurse Practitioners in Women's Health Oncology   This association offers a free app intended to be a convenient quick reference during a well-woman visit. It consists of the most commonly used clinical guidelines, and the recommendations are age based.

> https://www.npwh.org/pages/mobile-app

Association of Operating Room Nurses   The Association of Operating Room Nurses offers an ebook mobile app featuring e-b guidelines for perioperative practice. It is available for purchase via computer, smartphones, and tablets.

> http://www.aorn.org/aorn-org/guidelines/purchase-guidelines/
> ebook-mobile-app

Infectious Diseases Society of America   The Guideline Central app offers mobile versions of summarized Infectious Diseases Society of America's guidelines. This interactive app features keyword search of pocket cards and quick reference tools even when Internet access and cellular service are not available.

> http://www.idsociety.org/guidelinesapp/

Hartford Institute for Geriatric Nursing   The ConsultGeriRN feature aims to help professionals make care decisions right from the bedside. The information is based on the most current evidence-based practice standards; topics include delirium, agitation, confusion, and fall prevention. The app is available through iTunes.

> https://itunes.apple.com/us/app/consultgerirn/id5783601

American College of Physicians
The American College of Physicians' high-quality guidelines are available via a mobile app. Guidelines are in an easy-to-read, interactive format.

https://itunes.apple.com/us/app/acp-clinical-guidelines/id61831
   8388?mt=8
https://play.google.com/store/apps/details?id=com.ACP.Clinical
   Guidelines

Companies

The companies that produce clinical reference sources for mobile devices often include evidence-based information in the form of care sheets, care plans, monographs, and hyperlinks to research evidence. Several are designed specifically for nurses and others are interdisciplinary.

The Information Intersection

In a very real sense, the point of care is an information intersection (Porter-O'Grady, 2010). It is the point at which scientific knowledge, patient-specific information, e-b clinical protocols, available clinical services, and professional expertise converge as the basis for care design (see **Figure 19-1**). At present, electronic patient records, clinical decision support systems, bibliographic databases, electronic scheduling systems, and cross-settings information sharing help clinicians access various sources of information. In the future, Porter-O'Grady (2010) sees healthcare information

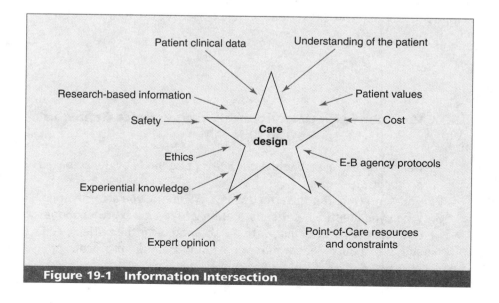

Figure 19-1   Information Intersection

systems as providing clinicians with a "seamless intersection of data" on which to decide and act (p. 22). Such an information system would make patient data, agency standards, research evidence, assessment guides, and decision support tools available at the point of care in easily searched and quick-to-read formats. Mobile devices will increase access to information and provide decision-making support. However, only the human decider can synthesize all the information to make a decision about what care should be given to a particular patient.

My Ending—Your Beginning

Evidence-based practice is not window dressing on *professional* nursing practice—rather it is an integral component of it. Some of the professional behaviors listed in **Box 19-1** will be part of your job expectations; others are activities you should do to contribute to quality care in your work setting and to give the most effective care to patients.

Reading research articles and e-b practice guidelines, appraising them, and deciding whether to change practice based on them compose a professional skill set. Like all new skills, there is a learning curve, but if you have paid attention, the steepest part of the curve is behind you. Like all skills, it requires some maintenance to keep the skill set sharp and current. Fortunately, a small amount of effort will benefit patients and make your professional dialogue and career more intellectually interesting.

Enough advice. Now I'll get out of here and leave the future to you.

BOX 19-1 Professional Evidence-Based Practice Behaviors of The BSN Nurse

1. Deliver care in accord with your unit's or agency's evidence-based protocols.
2. Constantly monitor the effectiveness of the care you are providing.
3. When you identify a patient situation where an e-b protocol does not seem to be effective, safe, or acceptable to the patient, consult with a nurse leader before deviating from the protocol.

4. Actively support implementation of evidence-based protocols in your unit, service, or agency.
5. Participate in the development of evidence-based protocols involving your clinical unit.
6. Be aware of quality improvement activities in your agency; actively participate.
7. Create an evidence-based practice folder in your e-device's bookmarks or favorites menu; add links to evidence-based practice resources that you find useful and to the evidence-based practice page of your specialty professional association.
8. Read research articles published in the clinical journals for your area of practice.
9. Bring credible e-b clinical methods to the attention of your peers and unit leaders.
10. Develop and maintain your knowledge and skills in evidence appraisal by appraising one research guideline/review/study report per month.

REFERENCES

Flynn, A. V., & Sinclair, M. (2005). Exploring the relationship between nursing protocols and nursing practice in an Irish intensive care unit. *International Journal of Nursing Practice, 11*(4), 142–149.

Porter-O'Grady, T. (2010). A new age for practice: Creating the framework for vidence. In K. Malloch & T. Porter-O'Grady (Eds.). *Introduction to evidence-based practice in nursing and health care* (2nd ed., pp.1–30. Sudbury, MA: Jones and Bartlett.

van der Weijden, T., Legare, F., Boivin, A., Burgers, J. S., van Veendaal, H., Stiggelbout, A. M., . . . Elwyn, G. (2010). How to integrate individual patient values and preferences in clinical practice guidelines? A research protocol. *Implementation Science 2010, 5*, 10. Retrieved from http://implementationscience.biomedcentral.com/articles/10.1186/1748-5908-5-10

Appraisal Guide:
Recommendations of a Clinical Practice Guideline

Citation:

_____

_____

_____

Synopsis

What group or groups produced the guideline?

What does the guideline address? Clinical questions, conditions, interventions?

What population of patients does the guideline address?

Did the panel use existing SRs or did it conduct its own?

What clinical outcomes was the guideline designed to achieve?

What are the main recommendations?

What system was used to grade the recommendations?

Credibility

Was the panel made up of people
with the necessary expertise?   ❑ Yes   ❑ No   ❑ Not clear

Are the goals for developing the
guideline explicit and clear?   ❑ Yes   ❑ No   ❑ Not clear

*Does the guideline production
process include all the widely
recognized steps?   ❑ Yes   ❑ No   ❑ Not clear

*Were the SRs used of high quality?   ❑ Yes   ❑ No   ❑ Not clear

Are differences in evidence for
subpopulations recognized?   ❑ Yes   ❑ No   ❑ Not clear

*Is the evidence supporting each
recommendation graded or stated
as adequate to strong?   ❑ Yes   ❑ No   ❑ Not clear

Is the guideline current? (based on
issue date and date of most recent
evidence included)   ❑ Yes   ❑ No   ❑ Not clear

ARE THE RECOMMENDATIONS
CREDIBLE?   ❑ Yes All   ❑ Yes Some   ❑ No

Clinical Significance

Are essential elements of any
recommended action or intervention
clearly stated?   ❑ Yes   ❑ No   ❑ Not clear

*Is the magnitude of benefit associated
with each recommendation clinically
important?   ❑ Yes   ❑ No   ❑ Not clear

*Is the panel's certainty or confidence
in each recommendation clear?   ❑ Yes   ❑ No   ❑ Not clear

Were patient concerns, values, and
risks addressed? ❑ Yes ❑ No ❑ Not clear

Were downsides or costs of each
recommendation addressed? ❑ Yes ❑ No ❑ Not clear

Was the guideline reviewed by
outside experts and a member of
the public *or* field tested? ❑ Yes ❑ No ❑ Not clear

**ARE THE RECOMMENDATIONS
CLINICALLY SIGNIFICANT?** ❑ Yes All ❑ Yes Some ❑ No

Applicability

Does the guideline address a problem,
weakness, or decision we are examining
in our setting? ❑ Yes ❑ No

Did the research evidence involve
patients similar to ours, and was the
setting similar to ours? ❑ Yes ❑ No ❑ Some

What changes, additions, training, or
purchases would be needed to
implement and sustain a clinical
protocol based on these conclusions? Specify.

---

*Is what we will have to do to implement
the new protocol realistically achievable
by us (resources, capability, commitment)? ❑ Yes ❑ No ❑ Not clear

Which departments and/or providers will
be affected by a change? Specify.

---

*How will we know if our patients are
benefiting from our new protocol?   Specify.

ARE THE RECOMMENDATIONS
APPLICABLE TO OUR SITUATION?   ❑ Yes All   ❑ Yes Some   ❑ No

SHOULD WE PROCEED
TO DESIGN A PROTOCOL
BASED ON THESE
RECOMMENDATIONS?   ❑ Implement All   ❑ Implement Some   ❑ No

* = Important criteria

Comments

Completed Appraisal:
Recommendations of
a Clinical Practice Guideline

Citation:

U.S. Preventive Services Task Force. (2014). *Final Recommendation Statement: Vitamin Supplementation to Prevent Cancer and CVD: Counseling.* Retrieved from http://www.uspreventiveservices taskforce.org/Page/Document/RecommendationStatementFinal/vitamin-supplementation-to-prevent-cancer-and-cvd-counseling

Synopsis

What group or groups produced the guideline?
U.S. Preventive Services Task Force develops recommendations about preventive services based on a review of high-quality scientific evidence and publishes its recommendations on its website and/or in a peer-reviewed journal.

What does the guideline address? Clinical questions, conditions, interventions?
Are multivitamin and single vitamin supplements effective in preventing cardiovascular disease (CVD) and cancer? Are any harms associated with taking these supplements?

What population of patients does the guideline address?
Healthy adults without special nutritional needs.

Did the panel use existing SRs or did it conduct its own?
The USPSTF commissions the Agency for Healthcare Research Quality to conduct systematic reviews for its recommendation task force. There is an agreed-upon and rigorous production process for conducting them (available on the USPSTF and AHRQ websites).

What clinical outcomes was the guideline designed to achieve?
Prevention of CVD and cancer and avoidance of harm. They also looked at all-cause mortality.

What are the main recommendations?
No recommendation regarding effectiveness of multivitamin and single vitamin supplements in preventing CVD and cancer is possible, except for vitamin E and β-carotene. There are recommendations against taking these two vitamins because the evidence indicated no benefits; in addition, β-carotene also has potential harm.

What system was used to grade the recommendations?
The USPSTF uses a five-level grading system focusing on certainty of net benefit, balance of benefit and harm, and insufficient evidence. The grading system is provided in the appendix of the article.

Credibility

Was the panel made up of people with the necessary expertise?   ☑ Yes   ☐ No   ☐ Not clear

Found on the USPSTF website: "The U.S. Preventive Services Task Force is made up of 16 volunteer members who are nationally recognized experts in prevention, evidence-based medicine, and primary care. Their fields of practice and expertise include behavioral health, family medicine, geriatrics, internal medicine, pediatrics, obstetrics and gynecology, and nursing." (http://www.uspreventiveservicestaskforce.org/Page/Name/our-members)

Are the goals for developing the guideline explicit and clear?   ☑ Yes   ☐ No   ☐ Not clear

The goals are not as explicit as they might be in this document but they are clear in the full report.

*Does the guideline production process ☑ Yes ☐ No ☐ Not clear
include all the widely recognized steps?
Definitely.

*Were the SRs used of high quality? ☑ Yes ☐ No ☐ Not clear
Definitely.

Are differences in evidence for ☑ Yes ☐ No ☐ Not clear
subpopulations recognized?

The special risk of current smokers taking β-carotene and the large study of multivitamins that found some cancer prevention benefit for men but not for women are noted. The dearth of research including women and minority groups was noted.

*Is the evidence supporting each ☑ Yes ☐ No ☐ Not clear
recommendation graded or stated
as adequate to strong?
Quite clear.

Is the guideline current? (based on ☑ Yes ☐ No ☐ Not clear
issue date and date of most recent
evidence included)

Issued 2014. The systematic review included original articles with up to 2013 dates of publication.

ARE THE RECOMMENDATIONS
CREDIBLE? ☑ Yes All ☐ Yes Some ☐ No

Clinical Significance

Are essential elements of any ☑ Yes ☐ No ☐ Not clear
recommended action or intervention
clearly stated?

As there are two non-recommendations and two recommendations against taking, this is not relevant. However, we note that the way in which dosages were addressed is not as clear as it might be, except the middle paragraph in the Potential Harms *section indicates they did not include studies with very high doses.*

*Is the magnitude of benefit associated with each recommendation clinically important?   ☑ Yes   ☐ No   ☐ Not clear

The section titled, Estimate of Magnitude of Net Benefit *addresses the issue of net benefit. Essentially for multivitamins and single vitamins except β-carotene and vitamin E, it was not possible to determine this. For β-carotene the net benefit was negative and for vitamin E it was zero. The size of benefit in the original studies was conveyed by relative risk with confidence intervals.*

*Is the panel's certainty or confidence in each recommendation clear?   ☑ Yes   ☐ No   ☐ Not clear

Quite clear on the table and in the text.

Were patient concerns, values, and risks addressed?   ☑ Yes   ☐ No   ☐ Not clear

Clearly patients want to avoid CVD and cancer as well as side effects of vitamin supplements.

Were downsides or costs of each recommendation addressed?   ☐ Yes   ☑ No   ☐ Not clear

The guideline document does not address cost other than to note the amount that Americans spent on dietary supplements in 2010.

Was the guideline reviewed by outside experts and a member of the public *or* field tested?   ☑ Yes   ☐ No   ☐ Not clear

A draft version of the guideline was posted for public review and several changes were made in response to that. In addition, the updated version addressed how the recommendations made align with the recommendations of other recognized organizations; essentially they are in agreement.

ARE THE RECOMMENDATIONS CLINICALLY SIGNIFICANT?   ☑ Yes All   ☐ Yes Some   ☐ No

Applicability

Does the guideline address a problem, weakness, or decision we are examining in our setting?   ☑ Yes   ☐ No

In our Healthy Aging workshops, several patients have asked about multi-vitamins and vitamin D as protective against cancer.

Did the research evidence involve ☑ Yes ☐ No ☐ Some
patients similar to ours, and was
the setting similar to ours?

We see mainly well adults age 55 to 75.

What changes, additions, training, or
purchases would be needed to implement
and sustain a clinical protocol based on
these conclusions? Specify.

We can add this content to our Healthy Aging session on diet and add it to the intake checklist to discuss with new patients who are taking vitamin supplements. We can also make a handout about it with a short summary and the website available in the waiting area.

*Is what we will have to do to implement ☑ Yes ☐ No ☐ Not clear
the new protocol realistically achievable
by us (resources, capability, commitment)?

Not a big deal, just a few minor changes.

Which departments and/or providers
will be affected by a change? Specify.

We will need to make all our primary care providers and RNs aware of this information so they can share it with patients when medications and supplements are discussed during intake interviews, when the medications of existing patients are reviewed, and when patients ask about it. We will emphasize that the information is about prevention of CVD and cancer in healthy persons and that persons with special nutritional needs such as those who are anemic or have gastrointestinal diseases should not be discouraged from taking vitamin supplements.

How will we know if our patients are
benefiting from our new protocol? Specify.

It is very difficult to know the impact of making information available to patients; this is particularly true of when it is provided to new patients. We could do some kind of chart review but that seems too demanding. But after 6 months or so we could talk about it in staff meetings and ask staff whether taking of vitamins is discussed very often and how this information about it is received by patients.

**ARE THE RECOMMENDATIONS
APPLICABLE TO OUR SITUATION?**   ☑ Yes All   ❑ Yes Some   ❑ No

**SHOULD WE PROCEED
TO DESIGN A PROTOCOL
BASED ON THESE
RECOMMENDATIONS?**   ☑ Implement All   ❑ Implement Some   ❑ No

This information should be offered at the time of intake of new patients either as a handout or in conversation.

* = Important criteria

Comments

_____

_____

Appraisal Guide:
Conclusions of a Systematic Review with Narrative Synthesis

Citation:

_____

_____

_____

Synopsis

What organization or persons produced the systematic review (SR)?

How many persons were involved in conducting the review?

What topic or question did the SR address?

How were potential research reports identified?

What determined if a study was included in the analysis?

How many studies were included in the review?

What research designs were used in the studies?

What were the consistent and important across-studies conclusions?

Credibility

Was the topic clearly defined?	❏ Yes	❏ No	❏ Not clear
Was the search for studies and other evidence comprehensive and unbiased?	❏ Yes	❏ No	❏ Not clear
Was the screening of citations for inclusion based on explicit criteria?	❏ Yes	❏ No	❏ Not clear
*Were the included studies assessed for quality?	❏ Yes	❏ No	❏ Not clear
Were the design characteristics and findings of the included studies displayed or discussed in sufficient detail?	❏ Yes	❏ No	❏ Not clear
*Was there a true integration (i.e., synthesis) of the findings—not merely reporting of findings from each study individually?	❏ Yes	❏ No	❏ Not clear
*Did the reviewers explore why differences in findings might have occurred?	❏ Yes	❏ No	❏ Not clear
Did the reviewers distinguish between conclusions based on consistent findings from several good studies and those based on inferior evidence (number or quality)?	❏ Yes	❏ No	❏ Not clear
Which conclusions were supported by consistent findings from two or more good or high-quality studies?	List		

ARE THE CONCLUSIONS
CREDIBLE?   ❏ Yes All   ❏ Yes Some   ❏ No

Clinical Significance

*Across studies, is the size of the
treatment or the strength of the
association found or the
meaningfulness of qualitative findings
strong enough to make a difference
in patient outcomes or experiences
of care?   ❏ Yes   ❏ No   ❏ Not clear

Are the conclusions relevant to the
care the nurse gives?   ❏ Yes   ❏ No   ❏ Not clear

ARE THE CONCLUSIONS
CLINICALLY SIGNIFICANT?   ❏ Yes All   ❏ Yes Some   ❏ No

Applicability

Does the SR address a problem,
situation, or decision we are addressing
in our setting?   ❏ Yes   ❏ No   ❏ Not clear

Are the patients in the studies or a
subgroup of patients in the studies
similar to those we see?   ❏ Yes   ❏ No   ❏ Not clear

What changes, additions, training, or
purchases would be needed to implement
and sustain a clinical protocol based
on these conclusions?   Specify and list

_____

_____

Is what we will have to do to implement
the new protocol realistically achievable
by us (resources, capability, commitment)?   ❏ Yes   ❏ No   ❏ Not clear

How will we know if our patients are
benefiting from our new protocol?   Specify

ARE THESE CONCLUSIONS
APPLICABLE TO OUR SETTING?   ❑ Yes All   ❑ Yes Some   ❑ No

SHOULD WE PROCEED TO DESIGN
A PROTOCOL INCORPORATING
THESE CONCLUSIONS?   ❑ Yes All   ❑ Yes Some   ❑ No

* = Important criteria

Comments

APPENDIX D

Completed Appraisal of a Systematic Review with Narrative Synthesis

Citation:

Graverholt, E., Forsetlund, L., & Jamtvedt, G. (2014). Reducing hospital admissions from nursing homes: A systematic review. *BMC Health Services Research, 14,* 36. Retrieved from http://www.biomedcentral.com/1472-6963/14/36; doi:10.1186/1472-6963-14-36

Synopsis

What organization or persons produced the systematic review (SR)?
Two authors are on the staff of the Centre of Evidence-Based Practice, Bergen University College, Norway; two are on the staff of the Norwegian Knowledge Centre for the Health Services.

How many persons were involved in conducting the review?
Three plus a research librarian.

What topic or question did the SR address?
To summarize the effects of interventions to reduce acute hospitalizations from nursing homes.

How were potential research reports identified?
Database searches were conducted using keywords. The search strategy is detailed in an accompanying file.

What determined if a study was included in the analysis?
This process is well described and detailed in a flow chart. Eligible studies were systematic reviews, randomized controlled trials, and quasicontrolled studies that examined the primary outcome of acute hospital admissions. Only studies of high methodological quality were included in the review. Forty-six studies were excluded, with the most frequent reason being they had no control group or were retrospective studies. (Table provided.)

How many studies were included in the review?
Nine with studies from a variety of countries.

What research designs were used in the studies?
Four systematic reviews and five primary studies.

What were the consistent and important across-studies conclusions?
Eleven different interventions to reduce hospital admissions were identified, but none was tested more than once; the overall quality of the studies was low. Interventions with positive effect on reducing hospital admissions in one study included advance planning intervention, use of palliative services, use of a care pathway for lower respiratory tract infections, and geriatric specialist services.

Credibility

Was the topic clearly defined?   ☑ Yes   ❏ No   ❏ Not clear
Most definitely.

Was the search for studies and other   ☑ Yes   ❏ No   ❏ Not clear
evidence comprehensive and unbiased?
As described previously.

Was the screening of citations for   ☑ Yes   ❏ No   ❏ Not clear
inclusion based on explicit criteria?
As described previously.

*Were the included studies assessed   ☑ Yes   ❏ No   ❏ Not clear
for quality?
The authors used Cochrane criteria for rating risk of bias of individual studies and GRADE to assess overall quality of the evidence.

Were the design characteristics and findings of the included studies displayed or discussed in sufficient detail?   ☑ Yes   ☐ No   ☐ Not clear

Per Tables 1 and 2, the Intervention column of Table 1 struck us in terms of the wide variation in approaches tried.

*Was there a true integration (i.e., synthesis) of the findings—not merely reporting of findings from each study individually?   ☐ Yes   ☐ No   ☑ Not clear

Limited because no intervention was tested more than once, but the division of interventions into three categories maximized the integration possible.

*Did the reviewers explore why differences in findings might have occurred?   ☐ Yes   ☐ No   ☑ Not clear

Again, not really possible because no intervention tested more than once.

Did the reviewers distinguish between conclusions based on consistent findings from several good studies and those based on inferior evidence (number or quality)?   ☐ Yes   ☐ No   ☐ Not clear

Not applicable, although they did consider the quality of the evidence as low or very low.

Which conclusions were supported by consistent findings from two or more good or high-quality studies?   List

None really. The reviewers said that several of the interventions to structure and standardize clinical practice and to use geriatric specialist services may have an impact of hospital admission—although their "confidence in the findings is weak."

ARE THE CONCLUSIONS CREDIBLE?   ☑ Yes All   ☐ Yes Some   ☐ No

This is a very well-conducted SR, and the authors' conclusion that all their findings are based on weak evidence is credible. So, not much for us to build on.

Clinical Significance

| *Across studies, is the size of the treatment or the strength of the association found or the meaningfulness of qualitative findings strong enough to make a difference in patient outcomes or experiences of care? | ❑ Yes ❑ No ☑ Not clear |

Overall size of treatments not possible to determine because of no intervention being studied more than once, but several individual studies found statistically significant reductions in admissions (e.g., the two geriatric specialists services studies) and reduced risk (RR) of hospitalizations (e.g., study in which the intervention was a half-day course for social workers in guiding residents and families about advance directives; the RR was 0.60 but the wide confidence interval makes no RR a possibility in the larger population). Overall, not impressive.

| Are the conclusions relevant to the care the nurse gives? | ❑ Yes ❑ No ☑ Not clear |

Some included multidisciplinary interventions that involved nurses, e.g., implementation of a national guideline for management of nursing home–acquired pneumonia. Evidence about the benefit of vaccinating staff was unclear, whereas vaccinating residents had a positive effect.

| ARE THE CONCLUSIONS CLINICALLY SIGNIFICANT? | ❑ Yes All ❑ Yes Some ☑ No |

Sadly, not convincing, so we will not proceed to consider the application of any of the interventions reviewed.

Applicability

| Does the SR address a problem, situation, or decision we are addressing in our setting? | ☑ Yes ❑ No ❑ Not clear |

Our numbers of admissions in comparison to other similar nursing homes look okay, but we have the sense that we could improve them. We were disappointed to see no studies about preventing pneumonia and urinary tract infections, or about managing flu season.

Are the patients in the studies or a subgroup of patients in the studies similar to those we see?	☑ Yes ☐ No ☐ Not clear

Generally yes.

What changes, additions, training, or purchases would be needed to implement and sustain a clinical protocol based on these conclusions? Specify.

Advanced care planning, palliative care geriatric specialists, and care pathways hold some promise, but not a lot of assurance that they will work.

Is what we will have to do to implement a new protocol realistically achievable by us (resources, capability, commitment)?	☐ Yes ☐ No ☐ Not clear

Not applicable due to lack of solid conclusions.

How will we know if our patients are benefiting from our new protocol?	Specify.

ARE THE CONCLUSIONS APPLICABLE TO OUR SETTING?	☐ Yes All ☑ Yes Some ☐ No

Some could be tried.

SHOULD WE PROCEED TO DESIGN A PROTOCOL INCORPORATING THESE CONCLUSIONS?	☐ Yes All ☐ Yes Some ☑ No

Although the SR is of good quality, the evidence itself provides no reason to think any of the interventions studied would reduce our hospital admissions.

* = Important criteria

Comments

Appraisal Guide:
Findings of a Qualitative Study

Citation:

_____

_____

_____

Synopsis

What experience, situation, or subculture does the researcher seek to understand?

Does the researcher want to produce a description of an experience, a social process, or an event, or is the goal to generate a theory?

How was data collected?

How did the researcher control his or her biases and preconceptions?

Are specific pieces of data (e.g., direct quotes) and more generalized statements (themes, theories) included in the report?

What are the main findings of the study?

Credibility

Is the study published in a source
that required peer review?   ❑ Yes   ❑ No   ❑ Not clear

Were the methods used appropriate
to the study purpose?   ❑ Yes   ❑ No   ❑ Not clear

Was the sampling of observations or
interviews appropriate and varied
enough to serve the purpose of the
study?   ❑ Yes   ❑ No   ❑ Not clear

*Were data collection methods
effective in obtaining in-depth data?   ❑ Yes   ❑ No   ❑ Not clear

Did the data collection methods
avoid the possibility of oversight,
underrepresentation, or
overrepresentation from certain
types of sources?   ❑ Yes   ❑ No   ❑ Not clear

Were data collection and analysis
intermingled in a dynamic way?   ❑ Yes   ❑ No   ❑ Not clear

*Is the data presented in ways that
provide a vivid portrayal of what was
experienced or happened and its
context?   ❑ Yes   ❑ No   ❑ Not clear

*Does the data provided justify
generalized statements, themes,
or theory?   ❑ Yes   ❑ No   ❑ Not clear

ARE THE FINDINGS CREDIBLE?   ❑ Yes All   ❑ Yes Some   ❑ No

Clinical Significance

*Are the findings rich and informative?   ❑ Yes   ❑ No   ❑ Not clear

*Is the perspective provided potentially useful in providing insight, support, or guidance for assessing patient status or progress?   ❑ Yes ❑ Some ❑ No ❑ Not clear

ARE THE FINDINGS CLINICALLY SIGNIFICANT?   ❑ Yes All ❑ Yes Some ❑ No

* = Important criteria

Comments

_____

_____

Appraisal Guide:
Findings of a Quantitative Study

Citation:

_____

_____

_____

Synopsis

What was the purpose of the study (research questions, purposes, and hypotheses)?

How was the sample obtained?

What inclusion or exclusion criteria were used?

Who from the sample actually participated or contributed data (demographic or clinical profile and dropout rate)?

What methods were used to collect data (e.g., sequence, timing, types of data, and measures)?

Was an intervention tested?   ❑ Yes   ❑ No

  1. How was the sample size determined?

  2. Were patients randomly assigned to treatment groups?

What are the main findings?

Credibility

Is the study published in a source
that required peer review?   ❑ Yes   ❑ No   ❑ Not clear

*Did the data obtained and the
analysis conducted answer the
research question?   ❑ Yes   ❑ No   ❑ Not clear

Were the measuring instruments
reliable and valid?   ❑ Yes   ❑ No   ❑ Not clear

*Were important extraneous
variables and bias controlled?   ❑ Yes   ❑ No   ❑ Not clear

*If an intervention was tested,
answer the following five questions: ❑ Yes   ❑ No   ❑ Not clear

1. Were participants randomly
   assigned to groups and were
   the two groups similar at the
   start (before the intervention)?   ❑ Yes   ❑ No   ❑ Not clear

2. Were the interventions well
   defined and consistently
   delivered?   ❑ Yes   ❑ No   ❑ Not clear

3. Were the groups treated
   equally other than the
   difference in interventions?   ❑ Yes   ❑ No   ❑ Not clear

4. If no difference was found, was
   the sample size large enough
   to detect a difference if one
   existed?   ❑ Yes   ❑ No   ❑ Not clear

5. If a difference was found, are
   you confident it was due to the
   intervention?   ❑ Yes   ❑ No   ❑ Not clear

Are the findings consistent with
findings from other studies?   ❑ Yes   ❑ Some   ❑ No   ❑ Not clear

ARE THE FINDINGS CREDIBLE?   ❑ Yes All   ❑ Yes Some   ❑ No

Clinical Significance

Note any difference in means, r^2s, or measures of clinical effects (ABI, NNT, RR, OR)

*Is the target population clearly
described?   ❏ Yes   ❏ No   ❏ Not clear

*Is the frequency, association, or
treatment effect impressive enough
for you to be confident that the finding
would make a clinical difference if used
as the basis for care?   ❏ Yes   ❏ No   ❏ Not clear

**ARE THE FINDINGS
CLINICALLY SIGNIFICANT?**   ❏ Yes All   ❏ Yes Some   ❏ No

* = Important criteria

Comments

_____

_____

_____

APPENDIX G

Completed Appraisal of the Findings of a Quantitative Study

Citation:

Canbulat, N., Ayhan, F., & Inal, S. (2015). Effectiveness of external cold and vibration for procedural pain relief during peripheral intravenous cannulation in pediatric patients. *Pain Management Nursing, 16*(1), 33–39.

Synopsis

What was the purpose of the study (research questions, purposes, and hypotheses)?
Hypothesis 1: Buzzy reduces procedural pain felt during peripheral IV cannulation; Hypothesis 2: Buzzy reduces procedural anxiety felt during IV cannulation.

How was the sample obtained?
Children ages 7–12 whose care required insertion of IV line and their parent(s) were asked to participate. They were in the surgical department of the medical center but it was not clear if they were inpatients or same-day outpatients. Importantly, none of the children had prior experience of peripheral IV cannulation.

What inclusion or exclusion criteria were used?
A list of 9 exclusions were applied; they were factors that would make insertion of the IV cannula difficult, exaggerate the child's response to the

procedure, or limit the child's ability to answer the required questions. These exclusions were used to control confounding variables.

Who from the sample actually participated or contributed data (demographic or clinical profile and dropout rate)?
All who agreed to participate completed data collection; no dropout.

What methods were used to collect data (e.g., sequence, timing, types of data, and measures)?
Questionnaire before, short questions before and after to child and parent. Data were all interval level data from widely used internal level scales.

Was an intervention tested?   ☑ Yes   ☐ No

    1. How was the sample size determined?
       Not known; no indication of power analysis having been done.

    2. Were patients randomly assigned to treatment groups?
       Yes

What are the main findings?
Children in the Buzzy group had significantly less pain than the control group. The Buzzy group also had significantly less anxiety during the procedure by parent and observer scoring.

Credibility

Is the study published in a source that
required peer review?   ☑ Yes   ☐ No   ☐ Not clear
Per website.

*Did the data obtained and the analysis
conducted answer the research question?   ☑ Yes   ☐ No   ☐ Not clear

Were the measuring instruments reliable
and valid?   ☑ Yes   ☐ No   ☐ Not clear
(per commentary in Chapter 10)

*Were important extraneous variables
and bias controlled?   ☑ Yes   ☐ No   ☐ Not clear

We like the fact that they checked for pre-op anxiety and body mass index equivalency between the groups. The only potential confounding variable we would have liked to have seen addressed was an indication of how many children in each group required more than two sticks to get the cannula in.

*If an intervention was tested, answer the following five questions:

1. Were participants randomly assigned to groups and were the two groups similar at the start (before the intervention)? ☑ Yes ☐ No ☐ Not clear

   As shown in Table 1 of the report.

2. Were the interventions well defined and consistently delivered? ☑ Yes ☐ No ☐ Not clear

   Delivered by one person, not several.

3. Were the groups treated equally other than the difference in interventions? ☑ Yes ☐ No ☐ Not clear

   Same nurse started all IVs.

4. If no difference was found, was the sample size large enough to detect a difference if one existed? ☑ Yes ☐ No ☐ Not clear

   Even though no power analysis was done, statistical results indicate the study was not underpowered.

5. If a difference was found, are you confident it was due to the intervention? ☑ Yes ☐ No ☐ Not clear

Are the findings consistent with findings from other studies? ☑ Yes ☐ Some ☐ No ☐ Not clear

Consistent with findings in the two cited studies where the Buzzy was tested with venipuncture in children.

ARE THE FINDINGS CREDIBLE? ☑ Yes All ☐ Yes Some ☐ No

Clinical Significance

Note any difference in means, r^2s, or measures of clinical effects (ABI, NNT, RR, OR)

*Is the target population clearly described? ☑ Yes ☐ No ☐ Not clear

Children 7 to 12 years old with no prior experience of IV cannulation.

*Is the frequency, association, or treatment effect impressive enough for you to be confident that the finding would make a clinical difference if used as the basis for care? ☑ Yes ☐ No ☐ Not clear

The difference in the means between groups is substantial, e.g., almost 3 points for child's rating of pain using the facial pictures pain scale. The procedural anxiety as rated by parents and observer is also considerable.

Using an online calculator, we determined that the 95% confidence interval for the difference in means using the WBFS scale is −3.84 to −2.06, so clearly in the target population children on whom Buzzy was used would have a pain score 2 and ~4 points lower than if Buzzy were not used.

ARE THE FINDINGS
CLINICALLY SIGNIFICANT? ☑ Yes All ☐ Yes Some ☐ No

* = Important criteria

Comments

_____

_____

_____

APPENDIX H

Completed Findings Table

Topic: Fatigue in Patients with Congestive Heart Failure				Date: July 2010
Author(s) and date	Questions, variables, objectives, hypotheses	Design, sample, setting	Findings	Notes
Evangelista et al., 2008	Fatigue-inertia, psychosocial and cardiac variables, QOL, depression, emotional health, physical health	Correlational 150 persons with HF awaiting transplant at tertiary center; mean age = 55; men = 73%; mean ef = 27% USA	1. 51% had high level of F 2. Maximal workload, physical health, emotional health, and depression explain 51% of F 3. Depression in > 28%	POMS-F; Minnesota Living with HF QOL overall; MN QOL physical; MN QOL emotional; Beck
Hägglund et al., 2008	Living with HF Experience of F	Qualitative Interviews and content analysis 10 women from outpatient clinic; mean age = 83 Sweden	1. Loss of physical energy 2. Experience of feebleness and unfamiliar body sensations 3. Experience unpredictable variations in physical ability 4. Need help from others 5. Strive for independence 6. Acknowledge remaining abilities 7. Being forced to adjust	

Topic: Fatigue in Patients with Congestive Heart Failure *(continued)*				Date: July 2010
Author(s) and date	Questions, variables, objectives, hypotheses	Design, sample, setting	Findings	Notes
Stephen, 2008	F intensity, global fatigue, symptom severity, trait negativity, functional status, exercise routine, QOL, satisfaction with life	Correlational 53 elders with stable HF, average age = 77; mean = 68%; average ef = 31% USA	1. F prevalence = 96% 2. F associated with QOL, perceived health, satisfaction with life 3. No relationship between F intensity and functional status 4. Being married predicted F 5. Regular exercisers reported less F	POMS-F; Visual analogue F; HF functional status inventory; MN overall; MN Satisfaction with Life Scale
Falk et al., 2009	General F, physical F, mental F, activity, motivation, anxiety, depression, symptom distress	Correlational 112 community-dwelling persons with worsening HF who sought care; average age = 77; men = 60% Sweden	1. F associated with emotional distress 2. Most intense symptoms: F, difficulty breathing, insomnia 3. Depression associated with activity	Multidimensional Fatigue Inventory; Symptom Distress Scale; Hospital Anxiety and Distress Scale

(continues)

Topic: Fatigue in Patients with Congestive Heart Failure *(continued)*

Date: July 2010

QOL = quality of life

HF = heart failure

F = fatigue

POMS-F = Profile of Mood States Scale, fatigue subscale

MN = Minnesota Living with Heart Failure Questionnaire

ef = ejection fraction

References

Evangelista, L. S., Moser, D. K., Westlake, C., Pike, N., Ter-Galstanyan, A., & Dracup, K. (2008). Correlates of fatigue in patients with heart failure. *Progress in Cardiovascular Nursing, 23*(1), 12–17.

Falk, K., Patel, H., Swedberg, K., & Ekman, I. (2009). Fatigue in patients with chronic heart failure—A burden associated with emotional and symptom distress. *European Journal of Cardiovascular Nursing, 8,* 91–96.

Hägglund, L., Boman, K., & Lundman, B. (2008). The experience of fatigue among elderly women with chronic heart failure. *European Journal of Cardiovascular Nursing, 7,* 290–295.

Stephen, S. A. (2008). Fatigue in older adults with stable heart failure. *Heart & Lung, 37,* 122–131.

Glossary

Absolute benefit increase (ABI) The difference between the percentage of persons in one treatment group who attained a clinical milestone and the percentage of persons in another treatment group who attained it.

Across-studies analysis Comparison, contrast, and pattern searching in findings from two or more studies; the analysis examines the studies as a body of evidence.

Algorithm A step-by-step instruction for solving a clinical problem; often consists of a series of yes/no questions leading to one of several possible decisions or actions.

Applicability The relevance of research evidence to a particular setting considering the similarity of the setting's patients to those in the studies, as well as the safety, feasibility, and expected benefit of implementing the findings.

Appraisal Making objective, systematic judgments regarding the credibility, clinical significance, and applicability of research evidence to determine if changes in practice should be made based on the evidence.

Bias A study influence or action (such as preconceptions or research methods) that produces distorted results, i.e., results that deviate from actuality. The most common sources of research methods bias are design bias, selection bias, measurement bias, and procedural bias.

Blinding Steps taken in experimental studies to keep study staff and participants from knowing which treatment group a person is in; the function of blinding is to prevent personal predilections from influencing responses to the treatment or rating of responses.

Bonferroni correction A lowering of the level at which a p-value is considered significant; it is used to prevent a type 1 conclusion error resulting from multiple tests on the same data.

Care bundle A group of e-b interventions related to a health condition that, when executed together, result in better outcomes than when implemented individually.

Care design The process of using knowledge, information, and data to develop a plan of care for a patient population or for an individual patient.

Case-control study A study in which patients who have an outcome of interest and similar patients who do not have the outcome are identified; then, the researcher looks back to determine exposures and experiences that could have contributed to the outcome occurring or not occurring.

Chance difference A difference in outcomes of a study that occurred in the sample of the study but would probably not be found in the target population. It is inferred from a nonsignificant statistical result (that is, a data-based p-value greater than the specified decision point p-level).

Chance variation The variability in sample averages that is expected whenever one measures a trait, behavior, physiological state, or outcome in two or more samples from the same population.

Clinical decision support The function of a computerized clinical information system that uses inputted patient data to provide agency protocols, information, and more general knowledge relevant to the care of the patient.

Clinical practice guideline A generic set of recommendations regarding the management of a clinical condition, problem, or situation. Ideally, the guideline is produced by a panel of experts and is based on rigorous analysis of research evidence.

Clinical protocol An agency standard of care that sets forth care that should be given to patients with a specified health condition, treatment, or circumstances. Protocols take a variety of forms including care maps, decision algorithms, standard order sets, clinical procedures, care bundles, and standardized plans of care; they guide care in combination with clinical judgment and patient preference.

Clinical significance In quantitative studies, an appraiser's judgment that a research finding indicates a large enough intervention effect or association between variables to have clinical meaning in terms of patients' health or well-being. In qualitative studies, an appraiser's judgment that the findings are informative and useful. The term can be applied in a more general sense to recommendations of clinical practice guidelines and conclusions of systematic reviews.

Coefficient of determination (r^2) The proportion (or percentage) of a variable that is associated with, or explained by, another variable.

Cohort study A study in which two groups of people are identified, one with an exposure of interest and another without the exposure. The two groups are followed forward to determine if the outcome of interest occurs.

Comparison group In an experimental study, the group that was not given the experimental treatment.

Conclusion error A wrong statistical conclusion reached because of a chance statistical result, a sample size that is too small, large variations in scores, or extraneous variables.

Confidence interval (CI) An extraneous interval that estimates the result that would be found if the whole target population were included in the study; it is an interval around the sample result.

Confounding variable A variable whose presence affects the variables being studied so that the results do not reflect the actual relationship between the variables being studied. It is an uncontrolled or unrecognized extraneous variable that exerted influence on the variables studied.

Consecutive series A method of obtaining a sample in which starting at a certain point, every person who meets the inclusion criteria is asked to participate in the study, and enrollment continues until the predetermined sample size is reached. It is essentially a convenience sample, although it is less prone to bias than the researcher inviting persons to participate based on his own schedule and inclinations.

Control Study methods that (1) decrease, isolate, or eliminate the influence of extraneous variables; (2) prevent bias from influencing the results; and (3) limit the amount of chance variation.

Control group See *Comparison group*.

Convenience sample A sample that is drawn from an accessible group of people who the researcher thinks are part of a larger target population.

Correlation A relationship between two interval or rank-order variables in which their values move in accordance with one another to a lesser, moderate, or greater degree.

Correlational research Research in which the relationship between two or more variables is studied without active intervention by the researcher.

Credibility A characteristic conferred on a finding. The judgment that a finding is trustworthy and not determined by bias, error, extraneous variables, or inaccurate interpretation of the data.

Database A structured, updated collection of informational records about articles, books, and other resources; access to the records is managed with computer software. Some examples are CINAHL, MEDLINE, and PsycINFO.

Delivery system The context in which direct clinical care is given; it is made up of a network of logistics including patient flow, scheduling, communications, supplies and equipment availability, role responsibilities, work patterns, accountability structures, and other work dynamics that support direct patient care.

Dependent variable Also called the outcome variable. In experimental research, the response or outcome that is expected to depend on or be caused by the independent variable. It occurs later in time than the independent variable.

Descriptive study A quantitative study that aims to portray a naturally occurring situation, event, or response to illness; data consists of counts of how often something occurs and breakdowns of various aspects of the situation into categories or levels.

Dichotomous variable A variable that has only two possible values, for example, readmitted/not readmitted.

Effect size A statistical representation of the strength of a relationship between two variables; commonly, the size of an intervention's impact on an outcome variable relative to the impact of the comparison intervention.

Error Distortion of data or results caused by mistakes in sampling or measuring or failure to follow study procedures.

Ethnographic research A qualitative research tradition that examines cultures and subcultures to understand how they work and the meaning of members' behaviors.

Evidence Objective knowledge or information used as the basis for a clinical protocol, clinical decision, or clinical action. Evidence sources include research, agency data regarding system performance and patient outcomes, large healthcare databases, and expert opinion.

Evidence-based clinical practice guideline A set of recommended clinical actions for a clinical problem or population that are based to some degree on research evidence.

Evidence-based practice (EBP) The use of care methods that have been endorsed by an agency because available evidence indicates they are effective.

Experimental group In an experimental study, the group that received the treatment of interest, which may be new or not yet definitively tested.

Experimental study A study aimed at comparing the effects of two or more interventions on clinical outcomes. It is characterized by random assignment of participants to treatment groups, careful measurement of outcomes, and control of as many extraneous variables as is feasible to achieve maximum confidence in causal conclusions.

Extraneous variable A variable that is outside the interests of the study but that may influence the data being collected and lead to wrong conclusions. Researchers try to identify them in advance so as to eliminate or control their influence.

Findings The interpretation of study results into statements that are slightly more general than the statistical results.

Generalizability A judgment about the extent to which the findings of a study will be similar outside the sample in which they were found, i.e., in other practice populations.

Grounded theory methodology A qualitative tradition of inquiry that is conducted to capture social processes that play out in situations of interest; the goal is to incrementally generate a theory that accounts for behavior or decisions.

Guideline See *Clinical practice guideline*.

Hawthorne effect A change in participants' responses or behaviors because they are aware they are in a study.

Hypothesis A formal statement of the expected results of a study. Hypotheses are tested by data collection and analysis.

Impact As used with the evidence-based practice impact model, it is the effect evidence-based practice has on patients' outcomes and experiences of health, illness, and health care.

Independent variable Also called the intervention/treatment variable. In an experimental study, the variable that is manipulated or varied by the researcher to create an effect on the dependent variable. It occurs first in time relative to the dependent variable.

Institutional review board (IRB) An agency or university committee that reviews the design and procedures of studies prior to their being conducted in the care setting. The purpose of the review is to ensure that the research is ethical and that the rights of study participants will not be violated. IRBs are federally regulated.

Instrument Also referred to as a measurement tool. A way of measuring something. The instrument can be a laboratory test, a questionnaire, a rating guide for observations, or a scored assessment form, to name a few.

Integrative research review A type of systematic review in which the findings from various studies are integrated using logical reasoning augmented by findings tables and lists. The goal of an IRR is to summarize the research knowledge regarding a topic.

Internal consistency An evaluation of the extent to which the items/questions that compose a measurement instrument capture the underlying concept. A commonly used measure of internal consistency is Cronbach's α.

Interrater reliability The degree to which two or more raters who independently assign a code or score to something assign the same or very similar codes/scores.

Intervention See *Treatment*.

Level of significance See *p-level*.

Measurement error The difference in a value obtained by a measurement activity and the actual/true value.

Meta-analysis A systematic research review involving a statistical pooling of the results from several (or many) quantitative studies examining an issue to produce a statistical result with the larger sample size.

Meta-synthesis A systematic research review in which findings from several (or many) qualitative studies examining an issue are merged to produce generalizations and theories.

Number needed to treat (NNT) A representation of treatment effect indicating the number of persons who would need to be treated with the more effective treatment to achieve one additional good outcome (over what would be achieved by using the less effective treatment).

Outcome measurement The instrument or tool used to quantify a dependent variable.

Outlier Data contributed by a single study participant that is extreme and considerably outside the range of the other scores in the data set.

Phenomenological research A qualitative research tradition used to examine human experiences. The methods seek to understand how the context of the persons' lives affect the meaning they assign to their experiences; the methods rely on inductively building understanding of the experience across several, a few, or a small number of persons.

PICOTS An acronym standing for the elements that should be considered when conducting an evidence-based project and when searching a database for studies. P = population; I = intervention or issue; C = comparison intervention; O = outcome(s); T = timing; S = setting.

p-level The prespecified decision point for the level of significance; data-based *p*-values above this level are considered statistically not significant.

Point-of-care design Care planning for a particular patient that takes place at the bedside or in the patient–nurse encounter; it includes either modification of a protocol or new courses of action not specified by an existing protocol.

Population A group of persons or entities with an important characteristic or characteristics in common.

Power analysis A way of determining sample size that factors in the size of the difference or association expected, the p-value cut point, and the probability of finding a difference or relationship that exists.

Projected population Based on the profile of a sample, the population to which the results of a study are believed to apply.

Protocol See *Clinical protocol*.

p-value The data-based probability that the obtained result is attributable to chance variation. This probability is compared to a previously chosen level of significance p-level to reach a conclusion about whether the relationship or difference found is statistically significant, i.e., likely to exist in the target population.

Qualitative content analysis A group of data analysis techniques used by qualitative researchers to derive meaning from the content of textual data. It typically involves developing a series of codes from the data.

Qualitative description A qualitative research method that produces straightforward descriptions of participants' experiences in language as similar to the participants' native language as possible.

Qualitative research Inquiry regarding human phenomena that refrains from imposing assumptions on study participants and situations. Its purposes include exploration, description, and theory generation.

Quality filter An assessment of the methodological quality of studies using explicit criteria; it is used in conducting systematic reviews to separate studies of different methodological soundness or to eliminate poorly conducted studies.

Quality improvement An agency's programs aimed at improving the safety, timeliness, patient-centeredness, and efficiency of care delivery systems.

Quantitative research Inquiry that (1) examines preidentified issues; (2) uses designs that control extraneous variables; (3) uses numeric measures to determine levels of various variables; and (4) analyzes data using statistical or graphing methods.

Quasi-experimental A type of intervention research in which either random assignment to control groups or control over the intervention and setting is not possible.

Random assignment A chance-based procedure used to assign study participants to a treatment or comparison group. Each participant has an equal chance of being assigned to either treatment group. It serves to distribute participant characteristics evenly in both groups.

Randomized clinical trial (RCT) An experimental study that involves advanced testing of an intervention using defined study protocols typically with a large, diverse sample.

Random sample A sample created by one of several methods by which every person in the population has a greater than zero chance of being included in the sample.

Relationship In research, a connection between two variables in which one influences the other, both influence each other, or both are influenced by a third variable.

Reliability The degree to which a measuring instrument consistently obtains the same or similar measurement values.

Research design A framework or general guide regarding how to structure studies conducted to answer a certain type of research question.

Research evidence Findings of individual studies, conclusions of systematic reviews of research, and research-based recommendations of soundly produced clinical practice guidelines.

Results The outcomes of the numerical and statistical analysis of raw data.

Rigor A quality of a research study that reflects its adherence to recognized standards for its type of study.

Sample Persons chosen from a target population to participate in a study. The ideal sample is representative of the target population.

Scope The range or breadth of a question, project, review, or guideline, including a description of what is included.

Search In the context of evidence-based practice, a pursuit to identify all research conducted relevant to a topic. More particularly, the use of a computer search engine to comb through bibliographic databases and other indexes to identify relevant research articles.

Simple random sample A sample that is randomly selected from a list of population members.

Statistical significance A statistical conclusion that a difference or association would likely be found in the population. It is based on a low probability of the result being just due to chance variation.

Study plan A term used in quantitative research to describe how the study will be conducted, including how the sample will be obtained; how the data will be measured, collected, and analyzed; and any control that will be used.

Systematic review (SR) A comprehensive and systematic identification, analysis, and summary of research evidence related to a specified issue. An SR can use statistics, tabulation, compare-and-contrast methods, or pattern identification to reach conclusions based on the body of studies in the review.

Target population The entire group of individuals or organizations to which the sample results are considered applicable. It may be the entire population from which the sample was randomly drawn or a projected population based on a convenience sample's profile.

Test-retest reliability A way of evaluating the consistency with which persons score themselves similarly on the questionnaire at two completions of the questionnaire separated by an appropriate period of time.

Theory Assumptions, concepts, definitions, and/or propositions that provide a cohesive (although tentative) explanation of how a phenomenon is thought to work.

Translational research Also called implementation research. The field of study that investigates how research evidence can effectively be integrated into agency and individual practice.

Treatment   In the research context, clinical interventions, therapies, action, or courses of action that are evaluated in the study. The treatment is the independent variable, and its effect on the dependent variables (outcomes) is what is being tested by the study.

True difference   A difference found in the study that is large enough that a difference would likely be found in the population; it is inferred from a significant statistical result (that is a data-based p-value less than the specified decision point p-level).

Type 1 conclusion error   The conclusion that there is a significant relationship between variables or a significant difference in groups' outcomes when in fact there is not a significant relationship or difference.

Type 2 conclusion error   The conclusion that there is not a significant relationship between variables or a significant difference in groups' outcomes when in fact there is a significant relationship or difference.

Validity   The degree to which a measuring instrument captures the concept it is intended to measure instead of another similar concept.

Variable   An attribute of a person, social group, thing, or situation that when measured has two or more categories or possible values.

Index

Page numbers followed by *f, t,* and *b* refer to figures, tables, and boxes, respectively.